AF344721

Substance Abuse Treatment: generalities and specificities

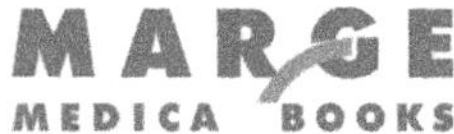

MARGE MEDICA BOOKS

Substance Abuse Treatment: generalities and specificities

Editors:
Ana Adan
Conrad Vilanou

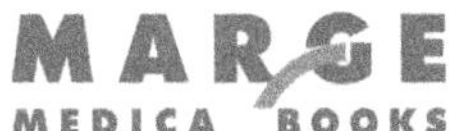

Substance Abuse Treatment: generalities and specificities
Editors: Ana Adan, Conrad Vilanou

First edition 2011

© Ana Adan, Conrad Vilanou (editors)
© of this edition, ICG Marge, SL

Publisher: Marge Médica Books - València, 558, ático 2.ª - 08026 Barcelona (España)
www.marge.es - Tel. +34-932 449 130 - Fax +34-932 310 865

Publishing director: Hèctor Soler
Managing editors: Ana Soto, Anna Palacios
Editing: Rosa Serra, David Soler
Editorial contributor: Tradusling
Make-up editor: Mercedes Lara
Printed by: Més Gran Serveis Gràfics i Digitals, SL, Santa Coloma de Cervelló (Barcelona)

ISBN: 978-84-15340-34-8
DL: B-42.293-2011

Index

Prologue
M. Teresa Anguera 11

BASIC ASPECTS AND RESEARCH

1. Is addiction a chronic relapsing disease?
Martien Kooyman 19

**2. In it for the long haul: recovery capital, addiction theory
and the inter-generational transmission of addictive behaviour**
Rowdy Yates 35

3. Self-Medication and addictions
Miquel Casas 51

**4. Promoting Best Practice in the drug addiction field:
the EMCDDA experience**
Marica Ferri 59

**5. Chronobiology and addiction: implications for treatment
and prevention**
Ana Adan 81

SEX DIFFERENCES

6. Biological bases of sex differences in drug addiction
Marta Torrens 101

**7. Female polydrug abuse and psychopathology – Gender differences:
an overview**
Edle Ravndal 115

**8. The impact of motherhood on recovery – Lessons we can learn
from the treatment journeys of mothers with problematic
substance misuse issues**
Karen Biggs 133

Therapeutic communities

9. **Quality of life in therapeutic communities for substance abuse**
Eric Broekaert 149

10. **The essential elements of treatment: a European therapeutic communities perspective**
Ilse Goethals 159

11. **MECETT, the journeymen model transferred to staff training in TC's**
George van der Straten 171

12. **The reasons for the rise and fall of the Bremberg empire**
Vera Segraeus 189

Social and politic factors

13. **The United Nations and drug demand reduction policies**
Xavier Fernández-Pons 203

14. **Factors for effective long-term recovery: risk and challenges during the economic crisis in Greece**
Charalampos Poulopoulos 219

15. **Getting regular, early and brief alcohol interventions into primary care in rural New South Wales: the origins of the Murdi Paaki Drug and Alcohol Network**
Rod MacQueen 239

16. **Social exclusion and immigration: new patterns of drug use among young marginal migrants**
Núria Empez 257

17. **Politics and ethics for a journal editor**
Richard Pates 277

Conclusions
Conrad Vilanou 289

Authors

Ana Adan
Department of Psychiatry
and Clinical Psychobiology
University of Barcelona.
Institute for Brain, Cognition
and Behaviour (IR3C)
Spain

Karen Biggs
Phoenix Futures
London, England

Eric Broekaert
Department of Orthopedagogy
Ghent University
Belgium

Miquel Casas Brugué
Department of Psychiatry
Hospital Universitari Vall d'Hebron
CIBERSAM.
Autonomous University of Barcelona
Spain

Núria Empez
Department of Theory and History
of Education
University of Barcelona
Spain

Xavier Fernández-Pons
Department of International
Law and Economics
Faculty of Law
University of Barcelona
Spain

Marica Ferri
European Monitoring Centre
for Drugs and Drug Addiction
Portugal

Ilse Goethals
Department of Special Education
Faculty of Psychology and Educational
Sciences
Ghent University
Belgium

Martien Kooyman
Psychiatrist and independent
treatment expert
The Netherlands

Rod MacQueen
Lyndon Withdrawal Unit
Bloomfield Hospital
Australia

Richard Pates
Cardiff School of Health Sciences
Llandaff Campus
University of Wales Institute Cardiff
United Kingdom

Charalampos Poulopoulos
KETHEA
Athens, Greece

Edle Ravndal
Norwegian Centre for Addiction
Research (SERAF)
University of Oslo
Norway

Vera Segraeus
National Board of Institutional Care
Uppsala University
Sweden

Marta Torrens
Addiction Programme,
Institute of Neuropsychiatry
& Addictions-Parc de Salut Mar.
Department of Psychiatry
Autonomous University of Barcelona
Spain

George van der Straten
Therapeutic Communitie Trempoline
Belgium

Conrad Vilanou Torrano
Department of Theory and History
of Education
University of Barcelona
Spain

Rowdy Yates
Scottish Addiction Studies
School of Applied Social Science
University of Stirling
Scotland

Prologue

Introducing a book is always a challenge, albeit a satisfying one. This is especially so in this case, where it is the University of Barcelona that is behind the initiative to publish the papers presented during the *13th International Symposium on Substance Abuse Treatment,* a scientific gathering that took place between the 23rd and 25th of March 2011, and that was held on the premises of our historic university, founded in 1550 by Alfonso V the Magnanimous. Congratulations are due to the fact that an international scientific event of this significance is now reflected here in black and white, in a book containing most of the papers that were presented over the three days.

We live in an age in which abundant material is published regarding almost all areas of knowledge, but the reader should have no problem discerning the relevance of the papers collected here to the section of the book in which they are presented, the overall effect being to provide a comprehensive approach to the treatment of substance abuse. Science often suffers as a result of the pressures facing many professionals, who are sometimes resistant to provide a conventional presentation of their work. In this regard, the book that I have the honour of introducing fulfils an important scientific purpose, that of offering a set of papers in a systematic and ordered way, which not only makes them easier to read and consult but also contributes to the exchange of ideas and the transfer of knowledge.

Nowadays no-one can doubt the significance of substance abuse in our postmodern society, one which is increasingly frenetic but often lacks a clear course.

Neither should we forget that the spirit of our age is characterised by a sense of widespread crisis, not only in economic terms but also a much deeper crisis that affects all spheres and levels of society. Ultimately we are facing an axiological crisis, for as the values of modernism wane we are now witnessing, rather impassively, the emergence of a new set of more volatile and ephemeral values that reflect a rapidly changing world, one that may even be ushering in a new era or period of history. All this creates problems not only for young people but also for adults who reach a point of transition in their lives and who often find it difficult to adapt to the sudden and unpredictable changes (technological, economic, social, political, etc.) that seem to rain down on them. Hence there are many vulnerable people who cannot match the pace of change, while numerous others become marginalised in relation to society, even from its most basic aspects. In the face of what is, at times, a bleak Outlook, it is no surprise that substance abuse, far from retreating, has actually increased in recent years and this is genuinely alarming. Times of crisis produce fear and instability, and likewise, some people become marginalised by the very workings of society, which expels citizens from the labour market who will have little opportunity to retrain and return to work. When this occurs many people resort back to old habits (alcohol, drugs, etc.), while others turn to them for the first time. Either way, this is a world that is easy to enter but difficult, although not impossible, to leave, at least not without pharmacological help and the support of family and the community.

Given the above, it was clearly an opportune moment to hold this international meeting on substance abuse, a gathering that has given rise to this book. The University of Barcelona, ever sensitive to the problems of society, took to this initiative from the outset and was ably supported by two notable agencies within the field of substance abuse research and treatment. The first of these was the Catalan NGO *Projecte Home Catalunya,* one of the most prestigious organisations in Spain with regards to the treatment of substance abuse. Indeed, Judge Baltasar Garzón, who spoke publicly of his commitment to combating the drug trade, is one of those who has given firm and enthusiastic support to the campaigns and programmes run by this NGO, whose work merits widespread public recognition. As regards the Symposium, it is also essential to acknowledge the role played by EWODOR (the European Working Group on Drugs Oriented Research), a long-established scientific network that not only brings together professionals and researchers from Europe but also attracts the attention of those from other parts of the world. Its work is always of high quality and this means that the *13th International Symposium on Substance Abuse Treatment* was backed by a scientific network with a proven track record. Indeed, if the Symposium was a success, which indeed it was, then this was due to the collaboration between three partners: firstly, a university that was established six centuries ago and whose lecturers have included famous physicians such as the Nobel Laureate Santiago Ramón y Cajal and psychologists of the prestige of Emilio Mira y López, a man who was ahead of his time and whose work is widely recognised; secondly, an organisation, *Projecte Home Catalunya,* which for over fifteen years has dedicated itself to the rehabilitation of people with substance abuse problems; and finally, the scientific network EWODOR.

In line with the initial proposal, the authors of the various papers offer a detailed analysis of all the key aspects to be considered and the editors have been skilled in organising this material. Their ideas should act as a seed that will take root, above all, in the receptive soil provided by those (researchers, specialist professionals, etc.) with the greatest interest in the field. For there is no better guarantee of the book's relevance than the solid and fertile ground produced by years of dedication to research on substance abuse. Yet every line of research is fertile and dynamic and constantly reveals new aspects and facets, the fruit of progress regarding the question at hand, whether this be in the form of the conceptual framework or in terms of substantive or procedural advances. This is particularly so when dealing with complex questions such as substance abuse, where we should always be aware of new aspects that need to be considered and optimised.

I would like to thank, on behalf of myself and the Rector of the University of Barcelona, Dr Dídac Ramírez, all those individuals who, in one way or another, helped to make the event a success. The benefits of scientific work sometimes need a long time to become apparent. I am sure, however, that the publication of this rigorous yet engaging book, which contains most of the papers that were presented in Barcelona back in March 2011, will make a decisive contribution not only in terms of raising awareness about the problem but also in relation to potential treatments. It may be just a small offering, but it more than fulfils its purpose. We all know, of course, that there are no easy solutions or magic bullets, but books such as this promote dialogue and the exchange of ideas, thereby fostering the transfer of knowledge, which is the basis for scientific progress and the creation of a better society. In this regard I would like to thank Ana Adan, a lecturer in the Faculty of Psychology of the University of Barcelona, for the enormous efforts and concern shown by her and her team in making this *13th International Symposium* a significant scientific event. I also offer my heartfelt congratulations to the editors of the book, Ana Adan and Conrad Vilanou, as well as to all the authors who have contributed to it, for a job well done, for their willingness to tackle a complex task with such rigour, and for their final achievements. I wish each of them success and good fortune within the line of work that has led to them collaborating with this project.

Finally, thanks are also due to all those whose presence, or assistance and support from afar, helped to ensure that the Symposium, which is so ably reflected in this book, constitutes a landmark in our understanding and treatment of substance abuse. The University of Barcelona, which I have the honour of representing, hopes and expects that this will indeed prove to be the case.

M. Teresa Anguera
Vice-Rector for Teaching and Science Policy,
University of Barcelona

Barcelona, 6 December 2011

Substance Abuse Treatment: generalities and specificities

Basic aspects and research

1 Is addiction a chronic relapsing disease?

Martien Kooyman

Psychiatrist and independent treatment expert
The Netherlands

martienkooyman@planet.nl

Abstract

Professionals are increasingly calling addiction a chronic relapsing disease. The term fits the medical model. However, efforts made by pharmaceutical industries have not been able to find a medical cure. Medical doctors ignore that addiction can be caused by a variety of factors. They mention that addiction to drugs or alcohol is a brain disease due to a genetic predisposition. Psychological and social factors are ignored. Hereditary factors may make a person more vulnerable to be addicted to the effects of drugs. Psychological factors, being victim of traumas, war and other violence and factors in the family may be the main factor leading to addiction.

It is questionable to call addiction a disease. Addiction is rather a symptom of something else in the same way as fever, high blood pressure or blindness is seen as a symptom. The definition of addiction as a chronic relapsing disease is not supported by research. Long-term follow up studies show that recovery is possible. Large samples of ex-clients of a variety of treatment programmes show that 40% of them are no longer addicted 20 years later. Also if relapses occur, they tend to happen with greater time intervals.

To call addiction a chronic relapsing disease has to be avoided as it causes unnecessary pessimism and a lack of motivation for treatment of addicted persons and primary care physicians. This definition can become a negative self-fulfilling prophecy. Addiction could rather be better called a dependency disorder from which recovery is possible.

Key words

Addiction definition; dependency disorder / disease; recovery; psychological factors; social factors.

Introduction

In recent years an increasing number of medical doctors became involved in the treatment of addiction resulting in a medicalization of the addiction problem. They define addiction as a chronic relapsing disease. Although addiction has medical consequences this definition of the problem is questionable. In this paper the different views on addiction will be discussed.

Often there is no clear distinction made between use and addiction. It is important to make a distinction between (non-problematic) use and addiction. Not every person using alcohol becomes addicted. Not everyone using drugs becomes a drug addict. There must be something else within the person or in his environment that leads to addiction.

The EMDDA (European Monitoring Centre) estimated in 2009 the lifetime use of cocaine in Europe at 13 million. The use last year was estimated at 4 million, last month at 1.5 million. The numbers of persons over 12 years old in the Netherlands who had at some time used cocaine in 2001 were 2.9%, recent use 1.2%. The numbers in the same year for the city of Amsterdam were: at some point used 10%, recent use 1.2% (Centre for Drug Research, University of Amsterdam).

When drugs are not available or when they are available and you do not use drugs you cannot become addicted to drugs. However when you use drugs this does not mean that you become addicted.

Not every person who uses alcohol becomes an alcoholic. Not every person who uses drugs becomes a drug addict.

Some people are apparently more vulnerable than others. Some people may have a genetic constitution that makes them more vulnerable. Some people live in circumstances whereby there is a high risk of becoming addicted.

Drug addiction is often correlated with other deviant or criminal behaviour and psychological disorders. In research on heroin addicts in the Netherlands, it was found that half of the addicts had already been in contact with the police for offences before they used their first drug (Jansen & Swierstra, 1983).

Addiction can be perceived in different ways.

In the moral view it is seen as a justice problem. The addict has to be punished. In the bio-medical view addiction is seen as a health problem, as a disease. The disease should be treated.

As a patient cannot be held responsible for a disease there is a dilemma: should a person who is not responsible for his condition be punished?

If addiction is seen as a disease is there a medical cure?

Medication to diminish craving has so far not shown any considerable results.

The medical profession in fact has created more addiction problems than finding a cure by overprescribing drugs, such as sleeping medication and tranquilisers.

Recently it was found that patients with Parkinson's disease treated with dopamine agonists can develop a loss of impulse control and an addiction to gambling, alcohol, drugs and sex.

In the past, addiction to opiates was treated with the prescription of heroin. Addiction to heroin was treated with the prescription of methadone. Lifelong substitution with methadone was recommended. In the Netherlands for some years, methadone together with heroin is distributed to people addicted to methadone and heroin without providing any further treatment. In all cases they appeared to continue to use cocaine together with these prescribed drugs.

It is only recently that there has been a growing consensus among researchers that by prescribing addictive drugs such as methadone for life without any incentives to stop, we may be creating chronic patients.

In 1964, the World Health Organization introduced the term: dependence.

In the International Classification of Disorders (ICD-10) the dependency syndrome was described as follows: "The dependency syndrome is a cluster of physiological, behaviour and cognitive phenomena in which the use of a substance or class of substances takes a much higher priority for a given individual than other behaviours that once had greater value".

The terminology dependence has been used later in the D.S.M. III and IV.

This Diagnostic and Statistic Manual for Mental Disorders is a classification system. It is not based on etiological theories and does not give therapists guidelines for treatment. The DSM IV describes substance dependence as a maladaptive pattern of substance use that leads to clinically significant impairment and distress and includes three or more of the following criteria: tolerance, withdrawal syndrome, more and longer use than intended, loss of control, most time spent in obtaining the substance, reduced activities (social, occupational, recreational) and continuation despite physical or psychological problems.

Explanation models for addiction

There are many explanation models for addiction:

- *The moral model:* Addictive behaviour is amoral and should be punished.
- *The pharmacological model:* Drug use leads to withdrawal symptoms when regular use is stopped causing physical and psychological dependence.
- *The psychodynamic model:* As a result of a disturbed childhood the child develops low self-esteem making the person, especially in late adolescence, vulnerable to developing a dependence on drugs.
- *The symptomatic model:* Addiction is a symptom of an underlying problem.
- *The self-medication model:* Drugs are used to cope with the symptoms of a disease such as schizophrenia or depression.
- *The disease model:* An inborn or acquired physiological condition makes the person vulnerable to addiction. It is part of the A.A. philosophy, advocating life-long abstinence to its members. Prescribing methadone to heroin addicts has been based on a biological theory, the metabolic deficiency theory of Dole and Nyswander (1976).
- *The consumer model:* Taking drugs is a matter of choice. The positive effects for the person make the person continue even if the consequences of addiction are known. The addict chooses to be addicted and is able to decide to stop. Addiction is self-correcting. Spontaneous recovery is possible.
- *The adaptive model:* Addiction is a way of coping with difficulties, with the problems of life. Addiction provides some kind of identity for people who have failed to achieve sufficient levels of self-confidence and social acceptance.

- *The behaviour-conditioning (learning) model:* Even if the euphoric effect of the drug has disappeared the addict wants to continue. There are other non-drug related sources of reinforcement. This model explains the onset of craving and withdrawal symptoms after detoxification when the person returns to environments where he used to take drugs.
- *The social model:* Drug abuse is seen as a result of a deficient society due to the pressure of the environment. This view is supported by the fact that most of the American veterans who had been addicted to heroin during the war in Vietnam could stop their use as soon as they had returned home.
- *The multi-dimensional model:* Addiction is a complex system of reinforcements due to a disturbed balance between outside pressure, support from the environment and the autonomy of the individual.
- *The bio-psycho-social model:* Biological, psychological and social factors together can explain how a person becomes addicted and also why they keep the person addicted.
- *The system-oriented model:* Addiction is the result of a pathological disturbance of the equilibrium in a relationship or in the family system. In a relationship the addict creates a possibility for the partner to be the strongest one of the two, while they also make the partner powerless. In a family system the addict has a role by distracting the attention from the problems in the family, keeping the family together by being the common focus of attention. Adolescent drug addicts have problems to separate from the family.
- *The existential disorder model:* Addiction is the result of not being able to find a meaning in life. It is an existential problem of a person who does not have the feeling of belonging to something greater than them self.

It is interesting that all of these views are partly true. However, they usually explain only one aspect of addiction. Recently the disease model is popular. Regarding addiction as a disease is only one of many views.

In the medical field, much interest is now also paid to research on hereditary and neurobiological factors. There are findings indicating that hereditary factors can make some individuals more vulnerable to developing an addiction than others. However, this knowledge has not yet resulted in improving the treatment of addiction. Describing addiction as a chronic relapsing disease fits the medical model.

In the medical model the doctor is responsible and in charge of the treatment. The patient is passive and not responsible for his condition. The disease can be treated with prescribed medication.

Some authors describe addiction as a brain disease. However, an "addiction gene" has not been discovered.

Is addiction a disease?

Regarding addiction as a disease is only one of many views and the only one, which in my opinion is not based on evidence. Medical consequences do not make a disease. To describe addiction as a disease leads to a number of questions.

Parson (1951) described that the individual cannot be held responsible for his illness.

How is that with addiction?

Are dysfunctions of the brain the result of chronic use or the cause?

Are the aetiology and the course of addiction controllable by the addicted person?

Can the addict be held responsible for the damage, harm and nuisance caused to others?

Does an addict seek help for the addiction problem? Usually a person who has a disease seeks help to stop the diseases. Addicts in general seek help to be able to continue their addiction.

Only one in ten of the alcoholics who visit their family doctors for various complaints are known by their doctors to be addicted to alcohol.

Although addiction is often regarded as a disease, addiction is in my opinion as much a disease as fever or high blood pressure or blindness, although persons suffering from these conditions, which may have various causes, can be regarded as being ill.

Addiction is a condition caused by something else, usually a combination of different factors.

Is addiction chronic?

Gerard Schippers concluded in a study of 5 reviews based on 56 original studies with data from more than 30,000 drug abusers (the DARP and TOPS follow-up data were included) that, where after 20 years 20% are seen with problem use and

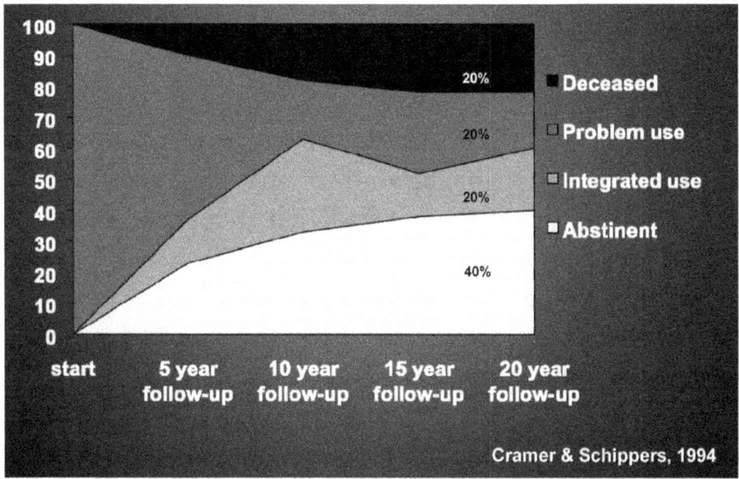

Figure 1. Long-term drug use (excl. unknown).

another 20% with integrated use, there is a slow increase in the number of deaths (around 20% after 20 years) and a steadily growing number of abstainers (40% after 10 to 20 years). See Figure 1.

In contrast with the maturing-out theory, the percentages of abstainers, abusers and non-problematic users tend to stabilise in the 10-20 year follow-up figures (Schippers, 2006). These studies were carried out on ex-clients of drug treatment programmes.

For alcohol, there are also studies in the general population showing that after 18 years, around 40% of alcoholics were abstinent 18 years later.

Schippers concluded that of the people with alcohol dependency entering treatment for their alcohol problems, 60% are no longer in that condition several years later (Schippers, 2006).

These findings show that chronic addiction is less common than often assumed.

So to call addiction a chronic relapsing disease has to be avoided as it causes unnecessary pessimism and a lack of motivation for treatment among primary care physicians (De Bruijn, c.s., 2005).

Is addiction a relapsing condition?

In the review of alcohol studies, it was found that the hazard of relapse was higher in the first 4 years than after that period (Schippers, 2006). The longer the person abstains the less likely there will be a relapse.

Harriet Barr found in a seven-year follow up of ex-residents, including all drop-outs of the Eagleville TC in Philadelphia, that over time more people remained clean without relapses (Barr, c.s., 1980).

Relapse into addiction after treatment is most frequent in the first year after finishing the treatment. In a follow-up study of first admissions in the Emiliehoeve Therapeutic Community, two years after they had left the programme, 32% of the sample had no relapse after leaving treatment. In the six months before the interview, 49.4% had no relapse (Kooyman, 1993).

Thousands of graduates from therapeutic communities were abstinent for more than ten years without a relapse, and are the living proof that abstinence is possible.

Therefore, we can say that a relapse does not always have to occur when a person is abstinent after having been addicted and that the longer a person is addicted the less likely he or she is going to have a relapse.

"What is in a name?" one could say.

Well, the name: chronic relapsing disease is not only incorrect; it ignores the facts that contradict this, such as the long-lasting positive successes of drug-free treatment. When you add, "chronic relapsing" it offers an excuse when treatment fails.

To call addiction a chronic relapsing disease has to be avoided as it causes unnecessary pessimism and a lack of motivation for treatment among primary care physicians (De Bruijn, c.s., 2005).

What is addiction?

If addiction is not a chronic relapsing disease, what is it?

Addiction is a self-inflicted disorder with multiple causes.

There are hereditary factors, biological factors, psychological factors, traumas, family factors, peer pressure, other environmental factors and factors in society.

Usually it is a combination of different actors that causes a person to become addicted. There is evidence that hereditary factors can be present that make a person more vulnerable to developing an addiction. It appears that hereditary factors do apply in alcohol as well in drug dependence (De Jong, 2006). Twin studies indicate a cross inheritance for anti-social personality and alcoholism (Enoch, 2003).

There are biological factors. The drug itself may cause changes in the body. To reach the same effect, higher dosages may be needed. Withdrawal symptoms may cause a need to use again. If addiction was only caused by biological factors, compulsory detoxification could be the answer. The truth is that treatment really starts after detoxification.

Understanding how to prevent a relapse is more important in the treatment of addiction than how to detoxify the addict.

Ten years after Dole and Nyswander had introduced the prescription of methadone as a substitute drug to heroin addicts they wrote:

> Perhaps the limitations of medical treatment for complex medical-social problems were not sufficiently stressed. No medicine can rehabilitate persons. But to succeed in bringing disadvantaged addicts to a productive way of life, a treatment program must enable its patients to feel pride and hope in accepting responsibility (Dole & Nyswander, 1976).

Addiction can start as self-medication with drugs and alcohol and medicine can reduce the symptoms caused by an existing disorder. However, a developing dependence can become a problem in itself.

Traumatic experiences are often present in the history of addicted persons. Traumas in youth such as physical and sexual abuse, incest and separation from the parents apparently make young people more vulnerable to drug addiction. There is evidence that this vulnerability can partly develop through changes in the brain caused by exposure to traumatic events.

The effect of traumas on the development of addiction has been studied in animals. Traumatised animals are more vulnerable to becoming addicted to alcohol and drugs as is shown in experiments. Rats in boxes can easily become addicted when offered morphine. There is some evidence in animal experiments that early deprivation by separation from the mother does not only produce psychological effects but also biological and physiological traumas, making the young animal more vulnerable to addiction. This may well also be the case in young children. Van der Kolk (1987) stated, that early traumatisation by parents leads to a "negative bonding". Although insufficient research has been carried out to support the hypothesis that traumatic experiences in early childhood make someone especially vulnerable to becoming addicted at a later age, there are many indications to support this. It seems probable that a lack of affection and tenderness in early childhood causes the person to be more vulnerable to the pain of a rejection by others. In addicts, we often see a tendency to repeat the trauma. More than half of the female residents in therapeutic communities were victims of incest or sexual abuse in their childhood. Addiction to drugs and alcohol is frequently seen among war veterans, civilian war refugees and other migrants.

In general, it can be said that traumatic experiences in childhood as well as traumas occurring at a later age can lead to an addiction to drugs or alcohol (Kooyman, 2000).

Stressful circumstances in society such as poverty, unemployment and war can also lead to addiction.

There are common psychological characteristics of the addicted person. Drug addicts have a failure identity and are unable to sustain long lasting relationships (Bassin, 1980). The addict who comes to treatment has low self-esteem, a failure identity and an inability to sustain intimate relationships.

Although insufficient research has been carried out to support the hypothesis that unsafe attachment and traumatic experiences in early childhood make someone especially vulnerable to becoming addicted at a later age, there are many indications to support this. It seems that a lack of affection and tenderness in early childhood makes an individual more vulnerable to rejection.

Rejection in early childhood leads to the development of a negative self-image. If the child does not feel love and affection from the parents, the child feels rejected and then starts thinking: "I am bad". But not knowing the reason why is unbearable for the child so they start be naughty, start to steal or later to abuse drugs. Out of fear of rejection, they are unable to ask for help. When they become addicted they deny addiction. Manipulative behaviour, which develops in early childhood, serves in particular to avoid possible rejection (Kooyman, 1986).

Intimacy is avoided in order to avoid the pain caused by a possible rejection (Kooyman, 1992). Amongst most addicts there is a fear of closeness related to a fear of rejection. Leaving the family of origin and leaving home becomes problematic. This may well be an explanation why addiction often develops in adolescence. We know from research that drug addicts have more frequent contact with their parents than persons of the same age who are not addicted. Not being able to deal with the painful emotions of being rejected and feelings of guilt and lack of self-esteem can lead to substance abuse and addiction. Factors in the family such as physical or sexual abuse of the child, or problems between the parents can lead to problematic drug use and addiction. The addict's drug problem can draw the attention away from other problems in the family. Stanton (1982) described the tendency of the addict who has stopped using drugs and has successfully started to live his own life, to relapse into his old habits of drug abuse and to return home when a crisis in the family has occurred.

Negative influences from peers can lead to abuse of drugs and addiction especially if it fills the need to belong to a group.

Factors in society such as poverty, unemployment and war can lead to addiction. Drugs or alcohol use offers an escape from the pressure and painful emotions.

In view of the above risk factors in developing addiction it can be said that addiction is usually a symptom of an underlying problem and is not a disease in itself. It is a self-induced condition to make the user feel better and in which control has been lost.

The vicious circles of addiction

When a person has become addicted he is caught up in a vicious circle: "I drink because my wife is angry at me because I drink".

Van Dijk pointed out that the addicted person is trapped in several vicious circles (Van Dijk, 1971).

The addict is caught up in:

- a pharmacological vicious circle (stopping use produces effects that force him to use again),
- a psychological vicious circle (stopping no longer hides negative thoughts or feelings such as guilt that make a person use again),
- a vicious circle of the primary group (using peers reject a person who stops, the addict helps the parents to stay together, these problems make it difficult to stop) and
- a vicious circle of society (the ex-addict is not trusted: "once an addict, always an addict").

For some drugs causing damage to the brain a cerebro-ego weakening vicious circle can play a role in keeping the person addicted.

See Figure 2.

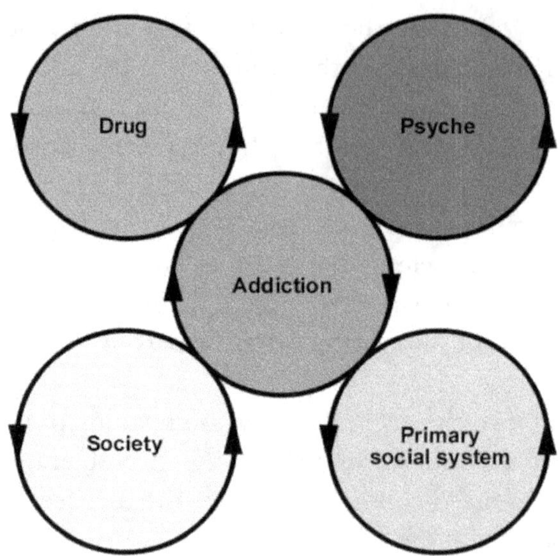

Figure 2. The vicious circles of addiction.

The definition of addiction

Addiction is a self-inflicted disorder with multiple causes.

Addiction is a condition caused by something else. It can be seen as an adjustment to exceptional circumstances by means of adaptive behaviour that has become uncontrollable. Addiction can arise when control over this behaviour is lost.

Addiction is a self-inflicted disorder with multiple causes.

The definition of addiction that follows from this is:

- Addiction is a self-continuing harmful process resulting from the loss of control over adaptive behaviour which then itself becomes a problem (Kooyman, 1992, p. 223).
- or in line with the description in the DSM IV: Addiction is a dependency disorder from which recovery is possible.

Consequences for treatment

In the discussion on drug policies here are two conflicting views. Harm reduction or recovery-oriented.

The harm reduction view is that a person has the right to use. Only the risks to the users and society should be minimal. The goal of the policies should be a reduction of harm.

In Europe most supporters of harm reduction regard addiction to drugs as normal behaviour. So there is no pressure in the harm reduction programmes to stop using the drugs. In America harm reductionists seem to look upon drug addiction as a disease. Those who had no success in abstaining should be helped to improve their condition. Harm reduction strategies have that goal. They are usually only meant for addicted users, while in Europe also non-addicted users are helped, for instance with leaflets on how to shoot dope properly and with volunteer organisations testing the quality of the users' drugs. The recovery-oriented view is that a person has the right to treatment. All addicts should be treated with abstinence as the ultimate goal.

The advocates of harm reduction are often in favour of legalising all drugs and ignoring the serious effects of an addiction. The recovery-oriented people often ignore the fact that many users will never become addicted. Harm reduction is not treatment. Harm reduction is a medically supervised continuation of a potentially self-destructive lifestyle. Treatment is harm reduction. The goal of the treatment is recovery from the addiction. Readiness and motivation for treatment are important factors for reaching a successful outcome. The goal is to change learned helplessness by stimulating self-help and activities, changing passivity into active participation and changing negative attitudes towards oneself and others into positive ones.

The best way to treat addiction is to first try to help stop the addictive behaviour, the use of drugs that became a problem in itself, and then to treat the cause. Treatment of addiction has to be directed at breaking down all four vicious circles and has to be directed not only at the symptom but also at the underlying cause. In treatment in drug-free therapeutic communities, the negative influences of the drug, the family and fellow users and society are first excluded. Methods directed at overcoming the psychological problems are applied. In the community a resident learns to help himself with the help of others.

The tools of the classic therapeutic community such as the work structure and encounter groups are useful to increase awareness and self-esteem. Medication for psychiatric or somatic illnesses should be used; even in drug free programmes, if needed. Parents and other relatives should be involved in the programme. And lastly, society should be made aware that successful treatment is possible.

In the Therapeutic Community the resident learns to ask for help to solve problems, learns how to make mistakes and not feel a failure as a person, learns to sustain long-lasting friendships and not be afraid of success. He can also learn how to respond to stress and also how to have pleasure without the use of drugs or alcohol. We know from research that longer periods of time spent in a programme is linked to successful outcomes and that parent involvement in the treatment is linked to longer periods of time in a programme. Drug-free treatment is relatively inexpensive and successful (De Leon, 2000; Pitts, 2002).

Conclusions

There are many views on addiction. The various models are all partly true. If only one model is getting attention other views are ignored. A reductionist approach will work only partly.

The model of addiction that is used has great consequences for drug policies. For instance, in the consumers' model the addict has a choice and is responsible for the consequences of his use. All drugs can be legalised.

In the disease model the addict is a patient, a victim, and is not responsible for the problem. Medication, substitute drugs and harm reduction programmes should be available. The concept of chronic relapsing disease fits the medical model.

This concept of a chronic relapsing disease is not supported by research and should be avoided as it creates unnecessary pessimism and a negative self-fulfilling prophesy.

Calling addiction a chronic relapsing disease is incorrect. It gives therapists an excuse for failing treatments and creates a lack of motivation among addicts and primary care physicians.

The term dependency disorder, from which recovery is possible, should be used instead.

References

Barr H & Antes D (1980). Seven years after treatment: A follow-up study of drug addicts and alcohol addicts treated in Eagleville Hospital's Inpatient Program. Final Report to N.I.D.A. Eagleville Hosp. Research Report, Eagleville, Penn.

Bassin A (1980). Reality Therapy in the Therapeutic community. In: readings of the 5th World Conference of Therapeutic Communities, Noordwijkerhout, 109-110. Samsom/ Sijthoff, Alphen a/d Rijn.

De Bruijn C, van den Brink W de Graaf R & Vollebergh W (2005). Alcohol abuse and dependence criteria as predictors of a chronic course of alcohol use disorders in the general population. Alcohol, 40, 441-446.

De Leon G (2000). The Therapeutic Community. Theory, Model, Springer Publ. Comp., New York, NY.

Dijk WK van (1971). Complexity of the Dependence Problem: Interaction of Biological Psychogenic and Sociogenic Factors in Drug Dependence in: H.M. van Praag (ed), Biochemical and Pharmacological Aspects of Dependence and Reports on Marijuana Research, 26-32, Boon, Haarlem.

Dole VP & ME Nyswander (1976). Methadone maintenance treatment. A ten-year perspective. J.A.M.A., 235 (19), 2117-2119.

Enoch MA (2003). Pharmacogenomics of alcohol response and addiction. Am J. Pharmacogenomics, 3 (4), 217-233.

Janssen O & K Swierstra (On defining "hard core Addict", Instituut voor Criminologie, Gronningen.

Jong de CAJ, Schellekens AFA, Ellenbroek B, Franke B & Verkes R-J (2006). Results: Human genetics. In: Verslaving, 2, 14-26, ZonMW, Den Haag.

Kolk BV van der (1987). The separation cry and the trauma response. Chapter in: Psychological Trauma, 31-62, Washington.

Kooyman M (1986). The psychodynamics of therapeutic communities for treatment of heroin addicts. In: De Leon & Ziegenfuss (Eds.) Therapeutic Communities for addictions. Readings in Theory, Research and Practice, 29- 41. Charles C. Thomas, Springfield, Ill.

Kooyman M (1992). The Therapeutic Community for Addicts, Intimacy, Parent Involvement and Treatment outcome. Universiteitsdrukkerij Erasmus Universiteit Rotterdam

Kooyman M (1996). La comunidad terapeutica para drogodependientes. Intimidad, implicacion de los padres y exito del tratamiemto. Ediciones Mensajero., S.A. Sancho de Azpeitia,2, 48014 Bilbao.

Kooyman M (2000). Trauma and addiction. In: Greenberg, B. (ed.). Proceedings of the 20th World Conference of Therapeutic Communities 26-29. Walden House San Francisco

Kooyman M (2009). The multiple causes of addiction and the response of Therapeutic communities. Paper presented at the South African Therapeutic Communities Conference, Cape Town, December 2009.

Kooyman M (2009). What is therapeutic in the therapeutic community? Paper presented at the 24th World Conference of Therapeutic Communities Lima. Peru, February.

Parsons T (1951). The social system. Glencoe, The Free Press, New York, N.Y.

Pitts JA (2002). Cost Benefits of Therapeutic Community Programming, Results of a National Survey. Paper presented at the 21st World Conference of Therapeutic Communities, 17-21 February 2002, Melbourne.

Schippers GM & Broekman, TG (2006). The course of drug dependence. In: Verslaving, deel 3, 34- 44, ZonMW Den Haag,

Schippers GM & Broekman, TG (2006). The course of alcohol dependence. In: Verslaving, deel 3, 6- 26, ZonMW Den Haag.

Stanton MD & TC Todd (1982). The family therapy of drug abuse and addiction, Guildford Press, New York.

2 In it for the long haul: recovery capital, addiction theory and the inter-generational transmission of addictive behaviour

Rowdy Yates

Scottish Addiction Studies
School of Applied Social Science
University of Stirling, Scotland

p.r.yates@stir.ac.uk

Abstract

An understanding of addiction as a complex disorder involving biological/physiological; psychological; socio-cultural; and socio-economic elements is well established as a foundation for good practice in treatment interventions. More recently, we have begun to view recovery from this disorder as being reliant upon a realignment of all these elements within the context of a sustained structure of encouragement and support rather than as an illness which will respond to a short, time-limited intervention such as treatment. Drug treatment-seeking populations have been rigorously researched and we know much about their journey towards and through treatment and even into post treatment. However non treatment-seeking populations are far less well known and we know almost nothing about their experiences of long-term recovery. What is known is that "natural" recovery, from even the most serious episodes of addiction is widespread; perhaps even commonplace. In Europe, the majority of these natural recovery episodes appear to take place outside formal treatment and even in defiance of the injunctions and advice of treatment providers. Understanding this process of natural remission and the structures or elements that both make remission possible and sustain it over the long-term will help to identify the most critical aspects of treatment interventions in general and after-care processes in particular. This chapter reviews the literature on recovery and addiction theory in order to examine commonalities in the maintenance of drug-free recovery and propose ways in which treatment interventions might better prepare their clients for the post-treatment journey.

Key words

Treatment interventions; natural remission; recovery; long-term recovery.

Introduction

In recent years, there appears to have been a growing interest both in a wider view of addiction and its treatment in general and of the issue of recovery in particular (Betty Ford Consensus Panel, 2007; Scottish Govt., 2008; HM Govt., 2008). In part this rebirth of interest in recovery appears to have been driven by a media-led dissatisfaction with the perceived failures of the substitute prescribing policy of the previous two decades (Ashton, 2007). In part also, though, it appears to owe much to a largely grassroots led movement to redefine the nature and direction of the treatment process (Day *et al.*, 2005).

This chapter briefly charts the early history of the recovery movement and outlines its beliefs. Most of these groups were self-help mutual-aid groups with little or no input from the mainstream treatment providers who were largely content to leave the state response to excessive alcohol use to the relevant criminal justice systems (Peele, 1995; Berridge, 1999; Yates & McIvor, 2003; Yates & Malloch, 2010).

It was not until the middle of the Twentieth Century that the scientific and academic community began to seriously explore the theoretical frameworks of addictive behaviour. Prior to that time, there was a general acceptance of the broad position within the various temperance movements that the addictive element was firmly located within the substance: the Devil was in the bottle (Peele, 1995; Berridge, 1999; Roizen, 2004). With the development of competing theoretical models of addiction came the associated treatment and, though more gradually, changes in public perception and attitude (Roizen, 1987; Room, 2003). The history of addiction theory and its implications for treatment are outlined here and in the latter part of this chapter, the relevance of these two associated histories for the modern recovery movement is set out.

The Early Recovery Movement

Some of the earliest examples of self-help mutual-aid fellowships appeared amongst the Native American population (White, 2000). Both Kenekuk, the so-called Kickapoo prophet and Handsome Lake, a Seneca chief,[1] founded popular movements in the Eighteenth Century (White, 2000), built around the concept of recovery and sobriety but extending across much of the cultural life of their tribe (Herring, 1877; White & Whiters, 2005; Parker, 2008). Both Kenekuk and Handsome Lake were reformed drinkers. Both saw sobriety as a first step in restoring cultural integrity and "upright living" to a people humiliated and disenfranchised by decades of white aggression and deceit.

Handsome Lake did much to restore the broken Iroquois Nation and rebuild the confederation as a respected force in Native American politics. His Gaiwiio (Good Message) runs to many pages and was (and still is) learnt by heart by many of his followers (Sturtevant & Trigger, 1978).

Both of these early movements, coming over 150 years before the establishment of Alcoholics Anonymous, recognised that simply stopping drinking was only a small part of the solution. What was required was a significant change in belief and behaviour. Kenekuk railed against the high prevalence of domestic violence amongst the Kickapoo and Handsome Lake argued that the work of a sober Indian was to organise and restore the dignity and cultural self-belief of the red man (Smith, 1985; White, 2000; Parker, 2008).

Similarly, the Washingtonian movement that flourished across America in the mid-Nineteenth Century argued that a reformed drunkard had a crucial duty to become the family's main breadwinner. The Washingtonians (more formally entitled the Washington Temperance Society), a recovery movement founded in 1840 by a group of former drinkers, eschewed religious doctrine and allowed only "reformed drunkards" to speak at their meetings (Maxwell, 1950; Peele, 1995). The Washingtonian meetings followed a format remarkably similar to that adopted by the Alcoholics Anonymous fellowship almost a hundred years later.

---

[1] The Seneca people were one of the six tribes that constituted the Iroquois Nation.

T. S. Arthur (1848), in a temperance tract published some eight years after their formation, paints a vivid picture of his attendance at Washingtonian meetings in Philadelphia and offers a series of somewhat romanticised vignettes of the lives and tribulations of some of its members. Even within this short space of time, the Washingtonians were holding regular meetings in most East-coast cities in America and had already established a number of lodging houses for the respite of their fallen members. On the anniversary of the 110th anniversary of the birth of George Washington, Abraham Lincoln chose the meeting of the Springfield Washingtonians to deliver his memorial address (Basler, 1953). At its peak, the Washingtonians numbered between 300,000 and 600,000 (reports vary wildly) and could boast at least 150,000 members in long-term recovery (Maxwell, 1950; Peele, 1995; White, 2001).

Although the organisation allowed only those in recovery to speak at their meetings, both membership and attendance was open to all. As a result, membership appears to have been swelled by an influx of temperance campaigners and religious proselytisers. This resulted in a series of damaging and, ultimately fatal, internal schisms with some members insisting that the organisation should be more active in the prohibition campaign, more meaningfully connected to the established church and even, more active in the anti-slavery movement. For some twenty years, the Washingtonians flourished, founding new branches across America but by the 1860s, the internal feuds caused the organisation to implode. Some of its sober houses continued, often under the management of other temperance organisations, the sober house in Chicago became the Washington Hospital and continued to offer alcohol treatment up until the 1980s. But mostly, the organisation simply crumbled. Members left to join other related organisations and, by the 1940s, the dissolution was so complete that the founders of Alcoholics Anonymous claimed never to have heard of it (Peele, 1995).

In the early years of the Twentieth Century, the Emmanuel Movement, based in the Emmanuel Baptist Church in Boston, began to achieve significant attention for their blend of spirituality, medicine and a kind of basic psychotherapy. The movement attracted serious criticism from Freud, during his brief visit to the United States in 1909. Freud was, perhaps understandably, particularly scathing about the limited medical qualifications of the movement's main protagonists (Dubiel, 2004). Despite Freud's scepticism and that of many other medical professionals the movement grew and in 1909, Ernest Jacoby began to organise weekly meetings at Emmanuel Church. More meetings began to be established as Jacoby Clubs, ("A Club for Men to Help Themselves by Helping Others") and Jacoby Clubs and their weekly meetings flourished (McCarthy, 1984). In Boston, the Jacoby Club provided meeting space for one of the earliest Alcoholics Anonymous (AA) groups but the two organisations remained separate and the Jacoby Clubs gradually lost out to their newer, more vigorous fellow traveller (White, 2000; Dubiel, 2004).

What seems striking about these early recovery groups is the similarity of their insistence that stopping drinking alone was not enough to sustain recovery. What was required was a much more radical alteration in the former addict's thinking about themselves and how they behaved towards others and the company they kept. In this, they foreshadowed the central tenets of the Black Power movement – similarly led by a reformed criminal and multi-drug user, Malcolm X – in the 1960s (White & Whiters, 2005). Malcolm X argued that stopping using drugs and drinking and stopping offending was not enough. Members of the movement were exhorted to be "black and proud" (Johnson, 1986).

The Alcoholics Anonymous fellowship has been one of the most successful mutual-aid groups and has spawned a number of parallel organisations including Narcotics Anonymous, Gamblers Anonymous and Cocaine Anonymous. They too have, from their earliest writings, discussed the concept of the "dry drunk": the former drinker who continues to behave in ways that are unacceptable and that were the hallmark of their former drinking career (Mäkelä, 1996).

Largely informed by the work of therapeutic community (TC) pioneer, Charles Dederich at the experimental commune, Synanon and bolstered by the 'second generation of therapeutic communities on the East coast of America (Rawlings & Yates, 2001; Broekaert *et al.*, 2006), the residential self-help community, modelled on AA practices, rapidly gained a foothold in Europe in the early 1970s. In Europe, this development was melded with the existing therapeutic community practice in psychiatry pioneered by Jones, Laing, Clark and others and grafted onto a century long tradition of caring for (and addressing the needs of) "maladjusted" children (Rawlings & Yates, 2001). Even with this rich history however, the notion that a community of addicts could manage and control the elements of their own recovery was initially greeted with scepticism within mainstream addiction treatment (Yates, 2003; Broekaert *et al.*, 2006).

Perhaps one of the most telling clues to the origins of the TC movement lay in its insistence on the AA concept of the "dry drunk". Early in the history of Synanon, Dederich argued that Synanon was emphatically not a treatment service, rather, he said, it was a school where people learned to "live right". Subsequently, De Leon, one of the foremost evaluators of the TC and undoubtedly its foremost chronicler, argued that the notion of "right living" lay at the heart of the TC approach (De Leon, 2000). The TC, he suggested was more school than hospital and could better be viewed as a learning environment where individuals learned (or relearned) correct behaviour. Abstinence was not a goal, necessarily, rather a serendipitous outcome of overall behaviour change.

Addiction Theory

Peele (1995) has noted that the vigorous promotion of alcoholism as a chronic, relapsing disease by the scientific medical community in the 1950s and 1960s (Jellinek, 1952, 1960; Glatt, 1952; Keller, 1962) has effectively embedded the notion of addiction, in both the public consciousness and (to a lesser, though significant extent) within the academic discourse, as an incurable condition that can, at best, be managed and contained. Room (1983) has charted the opposition to this position by sociological researchers and proponents of the behaviourist schools, but, although these arguments gained significant ground during the 1970s and early 1980s, the increasing focus, during the past two decades, upon infection control and crime reduction has resulted in a general return to a medical model of addiction treatment predicated upon the management of the problem and containment of its physiological and criminological sequalae.

The notion of a disease, which robs those afflicted with it, of their individual will, is embedded in a cultural context where individuality and liberty is a paramount aspiration and where appropriate behaviour is an individual personal responsibility. This, of course, is precisely the cultural matrix that developed with the industrialization of previously rural communities, where controls had tended to be vested more explicitly within the family or "tribe" than in the individual.

These concepts have proved to be of an enduring nature. The current definition of addiction or dependence, as set out in the *International Classification of Diseases* (ICD-10) (World Health Organisation, 1992), neatly sets out this diagnostic requirement as, "Impaired capacity to control substance-taking behaviour in terms of onset, termination or level of use". ICD-10 lists a number of other manifestations of addiction,[2] including a preoccupation with the substance of choice, which disregards other important concerns or alternatives. Room (2003) argues that this definition again, is culturally specific, relating to a social structure in which time

---

[2] The WHO uses the term "dependence" – currently, the preferred terminology.

has become a commodity in itself, "a cultural frame in which time is... used or spent rather than simply experienced" (Room, 2003, p. 226).

Thus, the discovery of addiction (and, consequently, of "recovery") came during a period of extraordinary social upheaval and change. In America, in particular, the period was also associated with additional changes in established communities as existing residents moved out to explore and settle new territories and were replaced by significant numbers of immigrants from Europe. In the period between 1785 and 1835, the population of the United States almost doubled (Peele, 1995). In the newly-settled territories, drinking houses were largely rudimentary, frequented by prostitutes and gamblers, and generally structured to encourage drunkenness and heavy, drink-related spending; a far cry from the community-oriented taverns in the close-knit communities most settlers had left behind. In the cities and established communities, the new immigrants brought with them European drinking practices, which were often frowned upon and largely misunderstood.

The publication of Jellinek's (1952) work on phases of alcoholism and its subsequent incorporation into World Health Organisation guidelines (Room, 1983), significantly influenced discussions on the nature of addiction and recovery for most of the 1950s and 1960s. This disease model of addiction was not without its critics. Trice and Wahl (1958) tested Jellinek's hypothesis and concluded, "if the concept of a disease process in alcoholism is valid, only the earliest or the most advanced stages are reliably indicated." Similarly, the presentation of alcoholism as an *irreversible* disease, has been subjected to much debate and criticism.

Davies (1962) provided an early challenge to this notion with a paper in the *Quarterly Journal of Studies on Alcohol,* which noted the capacity of many of his patients to return to normal drinking patterns. Commentaries in subsequent issues –on both his findings and his diagnostic methodology– was heated but largely scholarly. This was not the case with the response to the Rand Report, *Alcoholism and Treatment* (Armor *et al.,* 1976). The controversy that surrounded the publication of this report, with its finding that not only was a reversion to controlled drinking possible but that it was the most likely successful outcome, sparked a public argument that refused to die down. Room (1983) has noted that some studies of controlled drinking had their funding withdrawn at this time and that the debate became at times, extremely emotive. The authors were accused of providing struggling abstainers with a "scientific excuse for drinking" (Room, 1983) and numerous commentators predicted dire consequences as a result of its publication (Roizen, 1987). However, as Roizen points out, subsequent studies

(Hingson *et al.,* 1977) indicated that this apprehension had been misplaced and the publication of the report – and its interpretation in the media – had had little or no impact on drinking behaviour.

By this time also, the notion of addiction as a disease was being increasingly challenged; particularly by sociological and psychological theorists. As social concern switched from being largely dominated by alcohol misuse and began to respond to increasing use of illicit drugs, particularly heroin and cocaine, the emergence of theories based upon psychodynamic, socio-cultural and behaviourist traditions multiplied inexorably.

Khantzian (1974a,b), Wurmser (1974) and others suggested that the origins of addiction might lie in deep-rooted childhood trauma. Psychoanalytic and psychodynamic theorists have been prominent in developing theories of drug dependence based on personality factors. Early psychoanalytic theories suggested that alcohol abuse reflected an individual who was experiencing severe conflict concerning dependence that was expressed by oral fixation. Over the years, these theories have ranged from suggestions that drug dependence reflects low self-esteem to sex-role conflicts, or feelings of powerlessness that are masking a need for control (Blane & Leonard, 1987). According to Wurmser, addiction is the result of a "narcissistic crisis" that creates "neurotic conflict" (Wurmser, 1974, 1987). In this model, a harsh superego creates intense feelings of rage, fear, guilt, and anxiety. The use of drugs is a way of escaping these feelings.

Others (Ellis & Harper, 1975) proposed a behavioural origin to the addiction phenomenon based largely upon the work of Skinner and Pavlov. Addiction was, they argued, a learned behaviour that could in turn be unlearned or, perhaps more accurately, be replaced with less self-destructive behaviours. These theories, in their turn, spawned a raft of cognitively based interventions still in use today, including motivational interviewing (Miller & Rollnick, 1991) and relapse prevention (Marlatt & Gordon, 1985).

Perhaps the greatest leap forward in understanding addiction, came with the work of theorists such as Engel (1980), Robbins (Robbins *et al.,* 1970) and Zinberg (1984) through the development of models of addiction –most often described as biopsychosocial– that are multi-dimensional.

Bio-psychosocial theories of addiction argue that the addiction experience is impacted upon by three distinct factors. These factors –Zinberg's "drug, set and setting"– are the chemical interaction and any biological or genetic predisposition to intoxication; the individual's psychological and spiritual state; and the environment in which he or she exists. This three-part model has been hugely influential in the drug treatment field in the past thirty years. Some practitioners have argued that the model provides an essential framework for assessment and treatment planning (Yates, 1985) and most validated instruments, such as the Maudsley Addiction Profile, the Addiction Severity Index and the Client Treatment Matching Protocol would appear to owe their genesis to this layered and individualistic approach to the problem.

Subsequently, a number of practitioner authors argued that the model was not only a tool for understanding addiction but could also be used to assess problems and plan treatment interventions. Yates (1979, 1984) developed an assessment model that set out the various questions that would need to be asked to ascertain the balance of difficulties experienced by the individual in each of the three domains. Thus, if the level of drug-taking was relatively low and of short duration, whilst self esteem and the availability of non-using friends and relatives was correspondingly high, then a fairly low intensity intervention would be required. Madden (1977) similarly argued that the three domains outlined by Zinberg could be used in an understanding of the "treatment strengths" with which the addict came to their first appointment.

Addiction Theory and Long-Term Recovery

Addiction theory matters not simply because it underpins the approaches used in drug treatment interventions[3] but because it also has implications for recovery and for the long-term sustainment of recovery.

If indeed, addiction is a result of a fluid interaction between the biological propensity, the environmental setting and the self-esteem and self-belief of the individual, then clearly, an intervention must address all three elements if it is to be successful. Treatment interventions that are limited to a concentration on the addict's consumption of substances will at best, deliver a level of stability. At the worst, they will attempt abstinent recovery for which the individual will – without radical

---

[3] At least, this should be the case. Paradoxically, it can be argued that many substitute prescribing agencies, whilst espousing a bio-psychosocial approach, actually operate as if their central principle was the disease model. Equally, 12-step fellowships, despite arguing for the disease model, in practice place as much, or more emphasis on securing changes in personal self-perception and the socio-cultural environment.

changes to his/her environment and their own self-esteem – be both ill-prepared and ill-equipped.

The term "social capital" is generally used by sociologists to describe the connections within and between social networks. The term was probably first used by the American schools inspector, Lyda Hanifan. Introducing the term in a 1916 report on rural schools in Virginia, Hanifan explained:

> I do not refer to real estate, or to personal property or to cold cash, but rather to that in life which tends to make these tangible substances count for most in the daily lives of people, namely, goodwill, fellowship, mutual sympathy and social intercourse among a group of individuals and families who make up a social unit… (Hanifan, 1916, p. 130).

Sheldon & MacDonald (2009) note that Hanifan's notion of "social capital" was rooted in a belief in self-help and peer support. Hanifan himself was content to conclude that: "It was not what they [professionals] did for the people that counts in what was achieved; it was what they led the people to do for themselves that was really important" (Hanifan, 1916, p. 138). Whatever its origins, it is clear that the term has become a shorthand for all that is good about community spirit in the related fields of sociology, social policy and social work. Significantly, Hanifan maintained that social capital, unlike other forms of capital was not depleted with use. On the contrary, it's use resulted in an increase, a phenomenon that Hanifan described with the pithy slogan, "use it or lose it" (Hanifan, 1916, p. 139): a concept not a million miles from the therapeutic community principle, "you can't keep it unless you give it away", a slogan designed to describe the personal benefit that those in recovery receive by helping others with their own recovery.

More recently, writers on recovery, such as White & Cloud (2008) and Best & Laudet (2010), have taken this idea and coined the term "recovery capital" to describe changes they have observed in the resilience and robustness of people's social and emotional circumstances in long-term, abstinent recovery. There are, they argue, dramatic improvements in self-esteem, civic and social engagement, physical and psychological health and overall well-being. These changes, they argue, are fundamental to the successful outcome of any abstinence-based recovery journey (Best *et al.*, 2010):

> The best predictor of the likelihood of sustained recovery is the extent of "recovery capital" or the personal and psychological resources a person has, the social

supports that are available to them and the basic foundations of life quality, i.e. a safe place to live, meaningful activities and a role in their community (however this is defined) (Best *et al.*, 2010, p. 8).

Cloud & Granfield (2009) have recently suggested that this concept can be further refined as four individual, though overlapping, categories: social, physical, human and cultural. Best & Laudet (2010) endorse this view but note that of these, the social, human and cultural capital "reserves" are probably of the most significance, particularly in group or community settings:

Although the focus here is primarily on individual factors, it is the meshing of three of these components – social, human and cultural capital – that may be particularly important in assessing recovery capital at a group or social level (Best & Laudet, 2010, p. 4)

But significantly, these categories bear a striking resemblance to Zinberg's "drug, set and setting" (and to Madden's "the seed, the soil and the atmosphere", op cit.; and Yates' effect, expectation and situation', op cit.). In all of these analyses, it is argued that changes in these three central areas are vital for both a comprehensive assessment and the development of a person-appropriate treatment plan. What was not examined in any systematic way in these earlier writings was the use of this model to measure long-term improvements in individual resilience and social reintegration. What is argued here is that the use of the bio-psychosocial model in all phases of the recovery journey would provide a coherence to the role of various interventions throughout the process and enable drug treatment practitioners –even those who remain sceptical of the so-called "recovery agenda"– to view their role in the process from within an accepted scientific framework.

Conclusions

Numerous authors (Best *et al.*, 2000a; White and Whiters, 2005; White, 2009; Yates & Malloch, 2010) have commented upon the apparent antipathy, even occasionally outright hostility, of mainstream treatment practitioners to the "unscientific" nature and ungrounded optimism of the self-help recovery movement (Best *et al.*, 2000a; Yates & Malloch, 2010). In order for this scepticism to be modified, the recovery movement in all its forms (spiritual healing communities, 12-step groups, therapeutic communities etc.) will need to demonstrate an openness to research and innovation and a willingness to debate their role and responsibility within the wider sphere.

Why this seems important is not only because of issues of individual well-being but about the wider issue of intergenerational transmission of addiction and its associated problems: low educational achievement, unemployment, offending behaviour, teenage pregnancy, physical and mental ill-health. Numerous authors have noted this phenomenon (Peele & Brodsky, 1975; Peele, 1985; Best *et al.*, 2010; Gilman & Yates, 2011) and argued that improvement in this area is the ultimate prize for treatment intervention. Whilst some have argued that this apparent inheritance of problematic behaviour may have its roots in genetics (Goodwin, 1990), the argument for a mixture of the biological, social and psychological (echoing the bio-psychosocial model) seems particularly compelling. Since long-term, abstinence-oriented recovery appears to require significant improvements in all three domains it seems appropriate to explore whether such recovery journeys have an impact upon parenting and subsequent behaviour in drug-affected families.

Andreas & O'Farrell (2009) have noted improvements in behaviour and attitude amongst the children of parents in long-term engagement with mutual-aid fellowships. Similarly, in a large Australian study, Callan & Jackson (1985) reported significantly better behaviour and well-being of children in families where one or both parents had achieved long-term recovery than amongst children where parental drug use was continuing.

Conversely, numerous studies have shown that long-term substitute prescribing, concentrating as it does on the biological elements of the addiction experience, whilst having a significant impact upon illicit drug use and its consequent criminality and joblessness, seems largely unable to completely eradicate these behaviours in the majority of individuals (Best *et al.*, 1998, 1999; Best & Ridge, 2000b, 2003). Illicit drug use and criminality appears to continue at a reduced level in most thus prescribed (Eley-Morris *et al.*, 2002; Eley *et al.*, 2002; Yates *et al.*, 2005; McIvor *et al.*, 2006).

Thus, whilst long-term substitute prescribing might seem to offer the greatest gains –in terms of treatment expenditure– over the short-term, it would appear that long-term abstinence-oriented recovery is likely to deliver the most significant gains when examine over a more significant period.

References

Andreas, J & O'Farrell, T (2009). Alcoholics anonymous attendance following 12-step treatment participation as a link between alcohol-dependent fathers' treatment involvement and their children's externalising problems. *Addiction, 36,* 87-100.

Armor, D, Polich, J & Stambul, H (1976). *Alcoholism and Treatment.* Santa Monica CA: Rand Corp. Publications (R 1739).

Arthur, P (1992). Temperance Tales or Six Nights with the Washingtonians. Philadelphia: W A Leary & Co.

Ashton, M (2007). *The New Abstentionists. Druglink,* (Special Insert).

Basler, R P (Ed.) (1953). *The Collected Works of Abraham Lincoln,* New Brunswick: Rutgers University Press.

Berridge, V (1999). Opium and the People: Opiate use and drug control policy in nineteenth and early twentieth century England, London: Free Association Books.

Best, D, Lehmann, P, Gossop, M, Harris, J, Noble, A. & Strang, J (1998). Eating too little, smoking and drinking too much: wider lifestyle problems among methadone maintenance patients. *Addiction Research, 6,* 489-498.

Best, D, Gossop, M, Stewart, D, Marsden, J, Lehmann, P & Strang, J (1999). Continued heroin use during methadone treatment: relationships between frequency of use and reasons reported for heroin use. *Drug and Alcohol Dependence, 53,* 191-195.

Best, D & Ridge, G (2003). Using on top and the problems it brings: additional drug use by methadone treatment patients. In: G Tober & J Strang (Eds.) *Methadone matters: evolving community methadone treatment of opiate addiction.* 141-154. London: Martin Dunitz.

Best, D, Harris, J & Strang, J (2000a). The NHS AA/NA: NHS attitudes to 12 step help. *Addiction Today, 11,* 17-19.

Best, D, Harris, J, Gossop, M, Farrell, M, Finch, E, Noble, A & Strang, J (2000b). Use of non-prescribed methadone and other illicit drugs during methadone maintenance treatment. *Drug and Alcohol Review, 19,* 9-16.

Best, D & Laudet, A B (2010). *The Potential of Recovery Capital.* London: Royal Society for the Arts.

Best, D, Rome, A, Hanning, K A, White, W, Gossop, M, Taylor, A & Perkins, A (2010). *Research for Recovery: A Review of the Drugs Evidence Base.* Edinburgh: Scottish Government.

Betty Ford Institute Consensus Panel (2007). What is recovery? A working definition from the Betty Ford Institute, *Journal of Substance Abuse Treatment, 33,* 221-228.

Blane, H T & Leonard, K E (Eds.) (1987). *Psychological theories of drinking and alcoholism.* Guilford: New York.

Broekaert, E, Vandervelde, S, Soyez, V, Yates, R & Slater, A (2006). The third generation of therapeutic communities: the early development of the TC for addiction in Europe. *European Addiction Research, 12,* 2-11.

Callan, V & Jackson, D (1985). Children of alcohol fathers and recovered alcoholic fathers: personal and family functioning. *Journal of Studies on Alcohol, 47,* 180-182.

Cloud, W & Granfield, W (2009). Conceptualising recovery capital: expansion of a theoretical construct. *Substance Use and Misuse, 43,* 1971-1986.

Day, E, Gaston, R, Furlong, E, Murali, V & Coppello, A (2005). United Kingdom substance misuse treatment workers' attitudes toward 12-step self-help groups, *Journal of Substance Abuse Treatment, 29,* 321-327.

De Leon, G (2000). *The Therapeutic Community: Theory, Model and Method.* New York: Springer Publishing Company.

Dubiel, R (2004). The road to fellowship: The role of the Emmanuel Movement and the Jacoby Club in the development of Alcoholics Anonymous. New York: Universe, Inc.

Eley, S, Malloch, M, McIvor, G, Yates, R & Brown, A (2002). *Glasgow's Pilot Drug Court in Action: The First Six Months,* Edinburgh: Scottish Executive Social Research.

Eley-Morris, S, Gallop, K, McIvor, G, Morgan, K & Yates, R (2002). *Drug Treatment and Testing Orders: Evaluation of the Scottish Pilots,* Edinburgh: Scottish Executive Social Research.

Ellis, A & Harper, RA (1975). *A New Guide to Rational Living*. Oxford: Prentice-Hall.

Engel, GL (1980). The clinical application of the biopsychosocial model. *American Journal of Psychiatry, 137*, 535-544.

Goode, E (2007). Theories of drug use. In Goode, E. (Ed.) *Drugs in American Society. 7th Edition*. 58-88. Columbus OH: McGraw-Hill.

Goodwin, D (1990). Evidence for a genetic factor in alcoholism. In: R Engs (Ed.) *Controversies in the Addiction Field*. 10-16. Dubuque, Kendall Hunt.

Gilman, M & Yates, R (2011) North-West Recovery Forum: recovery and harm reduction, the odd couple of drug treatment, *Journal of Groups in Addiction and Recovery, 6*, 49-59.

Glatt, M (1952). Drinking habits of English middle-class alcoholics. *Acta Psychiatrica Scandinavica, 37*, 88-113.

Hanifan, LJ (1916) "The rural school community centre" *Annals of the American Academy of Political and Social Science, 67*, 130-138.

Herring, JB (1877). *Kenekuk, the Kickapoo Prophet*. Lawrence KS: University of Kansas Press.

Hingson, R, Scotch, N & Goldman, E (1977). Impact of the Rand Report on alcoholics, treatment personnel and Boston residents. Journal of Studies on Alcohol, 38, 2065-2076.

HM Government (2008). Drugs: Protecting families and communities: The 2008 drug strategy. London: HMSO.

Jellinek, E (1952). Phases of alcohol addiction. *Quarterly Journal of Studies on Alcohol, 13*, 673.

Jellinek, E (1960). *The Disease Concept of Alcoholism*, New Haven: Hillhouse Press.

Johnson, TV (1986). *Malcolm X: A Comprehensive Annotated Bibliography*. New York: Garland Publishers.

Keller, M (1962). The definition of alcoholism and the estimation of its prevalence. In: D Pittman & C Snyder (Eds.) *Society, Culture and Drinking Patterns*. 310-329. New York & London: Wiley.

Khantzian, EJ (1974). Opiate addiction: A critique of theory and some implications for treatment. *American Journal of Psychotherapy, 28*, 59-70.

Khantzian, EJ, Mack, JE & Schatzberg, JF (1974). Heroin use as an attempt to cope: clinical observations. *American Journal of Psychiatry, 131*, 160-164.

Madden, JS (1977). A psychiatric view of substance abuse. In: JS Madden, R Walker & WH Kenyon (Eds.) *Alcoholism and Drug Dependence: A Multidisciplinary Problem*. 115-121. New York: Plenum.

Mäkelä, K (Ed.) (1996). Alcoholics Anonymous as a mutual-help movement: a study in eight societies. Geneva: World Health Organisation.

Marlatt, A & Gordon, J (1985). Relapse Prevention: Maintenance strategies in the treatment of addictive behaviour. London: Guilford Press.

Maxwell, M (1950). The Washingtonian movement, *Quarterly Journal of Studies on Alcohol, 11*, 410-451.

McCarthy, K (1984). Early Alcoholism Treatment: The Emmanuel Movement and Richard Peabody. Journal of Studies on Alcohol, 59-74.

McIvor, G, Barnsdale, L, Eley, S, Malloch, M, Yates, R & Brown, A (2006). *The Operation and Effectiveness of the Scottish Drug Court pilots*. Edinburgh: Scottish Executive Social Research.

Miller, W & Rollnick, S (1991). Motivational Interviewing: Preparing people to change addictive behaviours, New York: Guilford Press.

Parker, AC (2008). *The Code of Handsome Lake, the Seneca Prophet*. Charleston SC: Forgotten Books.

Peele, S and Brodsky, A (1975). *Love and Addiction*. New York: Taplinger Publishing.

Peele, S (1985). The Meaning of Addiction: Compulsive experience and its interpretation. Lexington: Lexington Books.

Peele, S (1995). *The Diseasing of America*. New York: Lexington Books.

Roizen, R (1987). The Great Controlled-Drinking Controversy. In: M Galanter (Ed.) *Recent Developments in Alcoholism* (vol. 5). 245-279. New York: Plenum Press.

Roizen, R (2004). "How does the nation's 'alcohol problem' change from era to era?", in: S Tracy & C Acker (Eds.) *Altering American consciousness: The history of alcohol and drug use in the United States 1800–2000*. 61-89. Amherst, MA: University of Massachusetts Press.

Room, R (1983). Sociological aspects of the disease concept of alcoholism. In R. Smart, F Glaser &

Y Israel (Eds.) *Alcohol and Drug Problems. Vol. 7*. New York and London: Plenum.

Room, R (2003). The cultural framing of addiction. *Janus Head, 6*, 221-234.

Scottish Government (2008). The Road to recovery: A new approach to tackling Scotland's drug problem. Edinburgh: Scottish Government.

Sheldon, B & MacDonald, G (2009). *A Textbook of Social Work*. London: Routledge.

Smith, DG (1985). Handsome Lake Religion. In: *Canadian Encyclopaedia*, vol. ii, Toronto: Historica Foundation.

Sturtevant, W & Trigger, B (1978). *Handbook of North American Indians: Northeast. Vol.15*. Washington DC: Smithsonian Institute.

Trice, H & Wahl, J (1958). A rank order analysis of the symptoms of alcoholism. *Quarterly Journal of Studies on Alcohol, 19*, 636.

White, W (2000). The history of recovered people as wounded healers: from Native America to the rise of the modern alcoholism movement. *Alcoholism Treatment Quarterly, 18*, 1-23.

White, W & Whiters, D (2005) "Faith-based recovery: its historical roots", *Counselor, 6*, 58-62.

White, W & Cloud, W (2008) "Recovery capital: a primer for addictions professionals", *Counselor, 9*, 22-27.

White, W (2009). *Peer based addiction recovery support: History, theory, practice and scientific evaluation*. North East Addiction Technology Transfer Centre/Great Lakes Addiction Technology Transfer Centre/Philadelphia Department of Behavioural Health & Mental Retardation Services.

Wurmser, L (1974). Psychoanalytic considerations of the etiology of compulsive drug use. *Journal of the American Psychoanalytic Association, 22*, 820-843.

Wurmser, L (1987). Flight from conscience: Experiences with the psychoanalytic treatment of compulsive drug abusers. *Journal of the Substance Abuse Treatment, 4*, 169-179.

Yates, R (1979). *Recreation or Desperation*. Manchester: Lifeline Project.

Yates, R (1984). Addiction: An everyday disease. In: J. Lishman & G. Horobin (Eds.). *Research Highlights*. 63-75. London: University of Aberdeen/Kogan Page.

Yates, R (2003). A brief moment of glory: the impact of the therapeutic community movement on drug treatment systems in the UK. *International Journal of Social Welfare, 12*, 239-243.

Yates, R & McIvor, G (2003). Alcohol and the criminal justice system in Scotland. In: S Kilcommins & I O'Donnell (Eds.) *Alcohol, Society and Law*. Chichester: Barry Rose Law Publishers.

Yates, R, McIvor, G Eley, S, Malloch, M & Barnsdale, L (2005). Coercion in drug treatment: the impact on motivation, aspiration and outcome. In: Pedersen, M, Segraeus, V and Hellman, M eds. *Evidence Based Practice - Challenges in Substance Abuse Treatment: Proceedings of the 7th International Symposium on Substance Treatment, November, 25-27, 2004, Aarhus*. 159-170. Helsinki, Nordic Council for Alcohol and Drug Research/University of Aarhus/EWODOR/EFTC.

Yates, R & Malloch, M (2010). A road less travelled: a short history of addiction recovery. In: R Yates & M Malloch (eds.) *Tackling Addiction: Pathways to Recovery*, London: Jessica Kingsley Publishers.

Yates, R, McIvor, G, Eley, S, Malloch, M & Barnsdale, L (2005). Coercion in drug treatment: the impact on motivation, aspiration and outcome. In: M Pedersen, V Segraeus & M Hellman (Eds.) *Evidence Based Practice - Challenges in Substance Abuse Treatment: Proceedings of the 7ᵗʰ International Symposium on Substance Treatment, November, 25-27, 2004, Aarhus*. 159-170. Helsinki: Nordic Council for Alcohol and Drug Research/University of Aarhus/EWODOR/EFTC.

Yates, R & Malloch, M (2010). The road less traveled? A short history of addiction recovery. In: R Yates & M Malloch (eds.) *Tackling Addiction: Pathways to Recovery*. London: Jessica Kingsley.

Zinberg, N (1984). Drug, Set and Setting: The basis for controlled intoxicant use. New Haven: Yale University Press.

3 Self-Medication and addictions

Miquel Casas

Department of Psychiatry
Hospital Universitari Vall d'Hebron
CIBERSAM.
Autonomous University of Barcelona, Spain

mcasas@vhebron.net

Abstract

Within the neuropsychobiological purview concerning addictive behaviours, or "addictions," as they will be termed in the new psychiatric classifications of the DSM-V and the ICD-11, there are different research lines, including that of the "Self-Medication Hypothesis", formulated by Edward Khantzian in the 1970s and 1980s. It is a working hypothesis that makes it possible to combat the very erroneous and deeply entrenched notion that addictions are a "vice", indicative of moral turpitude. Rather, the Self-Medication Hypothesis proposes new etiopathogenic explanations, which, admittedly, await empirical confirmation, and let the patient, the family, and, in part, society as a whole, off the hook as being directly responsible for that group of disorders known as addictions. Support for the Self-Medication Hypothesis continues to increase, despite the determination of its detractors who assert that it is a hypothesis past its expiry date.

Key words

Addictions; neuroadaptation; self-medication hypothesis; vulnerability.

Introduction

Over the past few decades there has been a considerable increase in the consumption of psychoactive substances that work on the Central Nervous System (CNS), substances that have a high potential for abuse and dependence, and are commonly known as "drugs". A number of different explanations have been proffered, including the ready availability of these psychotropic substances, the presence of a predisposed or "addictive" personality, the decline of "family values", the failure in both teaching and prevention in schools, the voluntary desire of youth to alter their state of consciousness be it for curiosity or pure hedonism, the quest for instant gratification without concern for the relevant psychic or organic risks, the stress generated by the lack of work in a classist and repressive society, etc.

When these sorts of theoretical presuppositions are deployed to explain drug use, it becomes customary to conclude that the solution to the problem should come from a new "moral rearmament" at the socio-familial level, from improvement in drug use prevention programmes, from an increase in the war against drug trafficking, from a search for new psychological and psychiatric therapies for when the patient is ready to abandon drug use, etc. Although all of these proposals are good and desirable, the results from implementing preventive and therapeutic strategies based on these theoretical principles have not led to the expected outcomes, and in the majority of cases have simply failed.

Of all users who share the same problematic drug use patterns and, family, ethnic, socio-cultural, and environmental contexts, only a select few end up in a process of abuse and dependence. All the evidence would appear to suggest that in addition to factors related to the intrinsic effect of drugs and the influence of the socio-familial context, a large number of personal factors mediate the addictive effect of these substances.

Perhaps because of all of this, many professionals, associations of users and their families, and public and private institutions, are increasingly looking to etiopathogenic explanations deriving from the neurosciences. These explanations propose the existence of a series of neurobiological factors operating at the level of the CNS; vulnerable individuals who were once in contact with these substances initiate a process of dependence. All of which are a counterpoint to the "protective factors" presumed to benefit the majority of the population, and that allow people to consume the same substances without becoming addicted.

A clear example of this is that in Western societies, a majority of people have had repeated contact with alcohol and tobacco without developing problems of abuse or dependence. That is, drug dependence, from the perspective of the neurosciences, is not a vice but rather a neurobiological condition. Such a perspective affords a response to the question that is constantly being asked by those professionals who work in the addictions: Why is it that only some of the individuals who try drugs end up as addicts? And, quite simply, the answer is, it is neither desire nor circumstances that makes an addict, but rather, unfortunately, because they are predisposed to the addictive effects of drugs. This causal determinism has a neurobiological foundation that finds its expression in terms of individual vulnerability.

Within the neuropsychobiological purview concerning addictive behaviours, or "addictions", as they will be termed in the new psychiatric classifications of the DSM-V and the ICD-11, there are different research lines, including that of the "Self-Medication Hypothesis", formulated by Edward Khantzian in the 1970s and 1980s. Khantzian proposed that drug dependence could be explained as a functional alteration at a biological level, a predisposition, a vulnerability, a dysfunction or indeed the result of a mental disorder, which, together or independently, in effect force the addict to take drugs as a sort of self-treatment. As they attempt to relieve their distress with drugs, vulnerable individuals develop neuroadaptation phenomena that in turn generate addictive processes.

The Self-Medication Hypothesis, as its name indicates, is a working hypothesis that makes it possible to combat the very erroneous and deeply entrenched notion that the addictions are a "vice", indicative of moral turpitude. Rather, the Self-Medication Hypothesis proposes new etiopathogenic explanations, which, admittedly, await empirical confirmation, and let the patient, the family, and, in part, society as a whole, off the hook as directly responsible for that group of disorders known as addictions. Nevertheless, proponents of the Self-Medication Hypothesis by no means claim that it explains the totality of addictive phenomena, or that it can be applied systematically to all who have substance abuse problems.

Lines of work and research of the Self-Medication Hypothesis

The Self-Medication Hypothesis is characterised by four major complementary lines of work and research:

1. The first line proposes the existence of an acquired or genetic dysfunction in the neuromodulation-neurotransmission systems at the level of the

CNS. This dysfunction gives rise to severe alterations in the regulation of analgesic, homeostatic, sexual response, affective, and higher order cognitive processes. The individual affected by this dysfunction experiences a combination of psycho-organic disorders that provoke significant distress and a marked reduction in quality of life. If this individual, who should be considered to be ill, comes into contact with psychoactive substances with high levels of abuse potential, he or she could rapidly enter a process of dependence if these substances function as highly effective medications for the disorders from which he or she suffers. In such cases, should the organic dysfunction not normalise spontaneously or with psychopharmacological help, detoxification and relapse prevention treatments are doomed to failure, given that the affected patient will, sooner or later, seek a rapid solution to her or his problems. This solution, all too often, though toxic, takes the form of drugs, which, of course, furthers the addictive process.

2. The second line is a variation of the first and proposes the hypothesis that neuromodulation-neurotransmission system dysfunction does not have a genetic origin, nor are they a product of individual development, but rather are a result of the existence of a special vulnerability of these central systems to the effects of drugs. In view of this vulnerability, drug use generates functional alterations that severely and possibly permanently deregulate the homeostatic systems, basic psychic functions, and higher order cognitive processes. In the event that neither psychology nor psychiatric resolve these problems, the individual is sentenced to further drug use in a somewhat futile effort to re-establish her or his quality of life.

3. The third line proposes the existence of mental disorders prior to the initiation of drug use as predisposing factors for substance dependence. Predicated on the recognised antipsychotic, antidepressive, and anxiolytic effects of many of the substances categorised as "drugs", the Self-Medication Hypothesis suggests that these addicted patients are in fact psychiatric patients (Dual Disorder patients) who self-medicate with relative success. This "secondary" drug use, then, makes it very difficult to achieve and maintain abstinence after detoxification given the incomplete therapeutic action and the bothersome undesired side-effects of the psychiatric medication, (e.g. neuroleptics, antidepressants, anxiolytics, etc.) prescribed to treat the psychiatric disorders that sustain the addictive process.

4. The fourth line is a variation of the third and proposes that the psychiatric disorders that predispose an individual to addictions are not prior but subsequent to psychoactive substance use. That is, there are some individuals, who, with no history of mental illness, but with a special vulnerability to the psychotropic effect of the so-called "drugs", develop serious long-term, low remission psychiatric disorders as a consequence of drug use. Once the drug-induced psychopathology is established, the patient may well resort to compulsive substance use in an effort to contain the resulting symptomatology.

As is the case with all scientific working hypotheses in medicine and psychology, the Self-Medication Hypothesis is an instrument, a tool, a reflexive process based on data published in accredited journals, clinical experience, and common sense. It opens the possibility of elaborating new lines of research for complex pathologies such as addictions, and thus to propose more efficacious, effective, and efficient therapeutic approaches that could improve the course and evolution of these disorders, with a special emphasis on the quality of life of both the patients and their families.

The designation of "HYPOTHESIS" means, of course, a case that has yet to be proven. Were this to be so, or indeed shown to be erroneous, it would cease being a "hypothesis". It is a scientific reflection of which the proponents aspire towards and hope for scientific corroboration, and yet accept, of course, the difficulties, delays, and misunderstandings that are inevitably involved in the study of a highly stigmatised brain disorder. A highly stigmatised brain disorder that has its origins in brain regions that regulate pleasure, reinforcement, basic psychic functions, emotion, and so on, and which is characterised by disruptive and antisocial behaviour, which, appears to be under the voluntary control of the afflicted individuals.

Conclusions

The Self-Medication Hypothesis does not seek to blame anyone, or to pontificate with arguments that are admittedly difficult to accept at first. Proponents of the hypothesis simply present logical and common sense arguments, hoping that scientific support will follow. There is no ambition of proposing absolutist or universal reasons, nor is there any aspiration to provide the definite causal explanation for all of the addictions. Rather, what is hoped for is a symbiotic co-existence with other etiopathogenic hypotheses which accept (and this is not negotiable) scientific methods as an instrument of knowledge and progress. In addition, proponents of the Self-Medication Hypothesis dedicate a large part of their efforts to liberate patients and their families from being viewed as accomplices who are guilty of the development of these addictive disorders. Finally, proponents of the hypothesis propose and defend theoretical arguments to support the new harm-reduction strategies and substitution maintenance programmes as long as psychopharmacological and psychotherapeutic treatment approaches are not more effective.

Support for the Self-Medication Hypothesis continues to increase, despite the determination of its detractors who assert that it is a hypothesis past its expiry date. One sure-fire indication of this is that 20 years ago, noone with the exception of Khantzian and his disciples discussed the hypothesis. 10 years later, the hypothesis began to be defended or challenged in scientific articles, and, currently, it is almost impossible to find an article that addresses etiopathogenic aspects of the addictions without the authors making some sort of reference to the hypothesis, be they defenders or detractors, as a possible causal explanation of the origin of addictive disorders.

References

Arendt, M, Rosenberg, R, Fjordback, L, Brandholdt, J, Fodlager, L, Sher, L & Jorgensen, P (2007). Testing the self-medication hypothesis of depression and aggression in cannabis-dependent subjects. *Psychological Medicine, 37,* 935-945.

Bizarri JV, Rucci, P, Sbrana, A, Gonnelli, C, Massei, GJ, Ravani, L, Girelli, M, Dell'Osso, L & Cassano, GB (2007). Reasons for substance use and vulnerability factors in patients with substance use disorders and anxiety or mood disorders. *Addictive Behaviors, 32,* 384-391.

Casas, M (2000). Trastornos Duales. In: Vallejo, J & Gastó, C. *Trastornos Afectivos: Ansiedad y Depresión.* 2ª Edition. Barcelona: Masson.

Casas, M, Pérez de los Cobos, J, Salazar, I & Tejero, A (1992). Las conductas de automedicación en drogodependencias. In: Casas, M (coord.). *Trastornos Psíquicos en las Toxicomanías.* 291-304. Barcelona: Ediciones en Neurociencias.

Castaneda, R (1994). Empirical assessment of the self-medication hypothesis among dually diagnosed inpatients. *Comprehensive Psychiatry,* 35, 180-184.

Castaneda, R, Galanter, M & Franco, H (1989). Self-medication among addicts with primary psychiatric disorders. *Comprehensive Psychiatry,* 30, 80-83.

Dervaux, A, Baylé, FJ, Laqueille, X, Bourdel, M-C, Borgne, M-H, Olié, J-P & Krebs, M-O (2001). Is substance abuse in schizophrenia related to impulsivity, sensation seeking or anhedonia? *American Journal of Psychiatry,* 158, 492-494

Goswami, S, Mattoo, SK, Basu, D & Singh, G (2004). Substance-Abusing Schizophrenics: Do they Self-Medicate? *The American Journal on Addictions,* 13, 139-150.

Gregg, L, Barrowclough, C & Haddock, G (2007). Reasons for increased substance use in psychosis. *Clinical Psychology Review,* 27, 494-510.

Hall, DH & Queener, JE (2007). Self-medication hypothesis of substance use: testing Khantzian's updated theory. *Journal of Psychoactive Drugs,* 39, 151-158.

Henwood, B & Padgett, DK (2007). Reevaluating the self-medication hypothesis among the dually diagnosed. *American Journal on Addiction,* 16, 160-165.

Khantzian, EJ (1974). Opiate addiction: A critique of theory and some implications for treatment. *Journal of American Psychotherapy,* 28, 59-70.

Khantzian, EJ (1985). The self-medication hypothesis of addictive disorders: focus on heroin and cocaine dependence. *American Journal of Psychiatry,* 142, 1259-1264.

Khantzian, EJ (1997). The ego, the self, and opiate addiction: Theoretical and treatment considerations. *International Review of Psychoanalysis,* 5, 189-199.

Khantzian, EJ (1997). The self-medication hypothesis of addictive disorders: a reconsideration and recent applications. *Harvard Review of Psychiatry,* 4, 231-244.

Khantzian, EJ (1999). *Treating Addiction as a Human Process.* London: Aronson.

Sivapalan, H. (2009). Khantzian's 'self-medication hypothesis' of drug addiction and films by Martin Scorsese. *International Review of Psychiatry,* 21, 285-288.

Tomlinson, KL, Tate, SR, Anderson, KG, McCarthy, DM & Brown, SA (2006). An examination of self-medication and rebound effects: Psychiatric symptomatology before and after alcohol or drug relapse. *Addictive Behaviors,* 31, 461-474.

4 Promoting Best Practice in the drug addiction field: the EMCDDA experience

Marica Ferri

**European Monitoring Centre
for Drugs and Drug Addiction
Portugal**

marica.ferri@emcdda.europa.eu

Abstract

Best Practice is the best application of the available evidence to current activities in the drug field. Evidence-based knowledge and practice, i.e. the experience and lessons learned from the implementation of evidence-based intervention, are two key dimensions of the Best Practice concept.

The objective of creating the Best Practice Portal[1] on the EMCDDA website is to develop a knowledge database providing reliable information on the latest scientific evidence as well as on the practical aspects of implementation throughout Europe.

Search for systematic reviews is performed and results are summarised in plain language modules following the Patients-Interventions-Comparisons-Outcomes-Type of studies logic. Interventions are scored for the level of evidence based on the GRADE assessment system and results are grouped according to the level of impact on patients (the highest being "Beneficial"; the lowest "Evidence of ineffectiveness"). Currently the Portal contains modules on treatment, harm reduction and prevention. The modules are updated annually with new evidence.

---

[1] http://www.emcdda.europa.eu/best-practice

Experience gained from practice is presented in a separate section, including a collection of European standards and guidelines and a collection of real-life projects from 30 European countries (EDDRA database). The EMCDDA's network of national focal points regularly submits examples of interventions that are assessed according to the level of evidence and internal consistency.

Identifying evidence and implementation experiences has important implications in highlighting research gaps as well as defining research priorities. The BPP is the result of an initial effort to bridge together evidence and practice to disseminate and promote evidence-based interventions throughout Europe and foster a common approach.

Key words

Best practice; evidence; drug addiction; treatment; EMCDDA.

Best Practice: the meeting of two worlds

A definition of Best Practice

The term "best practice" is commonly used in many different fields from information technology to social sciences, but there are no universally accepted definitions.

Over the last decade an increasingly frequent use of the term has been observed in scientific literature. A search on *Pubmed*[2] for "best practice" in titles and abstracts, found 470 results before 2000, which increased to 4066 in 2011.

The frequent use of the term "best practice" in many documents that have a substantial impact on research, implementation and evaluation activities such as the latest EU Drug Strategy and Action Plans, requires a straightforward definition of "best practice" in the drug demand reduction field.

---

[2] The freely available platform to access the U.S. National Library of Medicine (www.ncbi.nlm.nih.gov/pubmed).

Best practice is composed of two main aspects: the evidence-based knowledge on specific interventions and the "practice", i.e. the experience of implementing an intervention.

The term "evidence" and evidence base, were first introduced in the medical field: "Evidence-based medicine is the conscientious, explicit, and judicious use of current best evidence in making decisions about the care of individual patients. The practice of evidence-based medicine means integrating individual clinical expertise with the best available external clinical evidence from systematic research (Sackett *et al.,* 2007)". It was then applied to the social sciences and policy-making science by, for instance, the Campbell Collaboration,[3] which aimed at helping people to make well-informed decisions by preparing, maintaining and disseminating systematic reviews on the existing scientific evidence of interventions in education, crime and justice, and social welfare.

This first area requires a clear methodology to identify, assess and synthesise the proof of the effectiveness of interventions. Effectiveness stands for proof of obtaining the expected effects under different circumstances.

The second area (the practice) needs a safe methodology to identify, collect and synthesise relevant experiences of implementation and lessons learned in the practical application of evidence-based interventions.

The whole process is a reiterative cycle where new evidence and new experiences can modify the results at any time.

The EMCDDA recently developed a definition of Best Practice in the drug field, taking into consideration the different aspects involved and establishing a consensus among national experts and authorities in the field:

Best Practice is the best application of the available evidence to current activities in the drug field.

- underlying evidence should be relevant to the problems and issues affecting those involved (professionals, policymakers, drug users, their families);
- methods should be transparent, reliable and transferable and all appropriate evidence should be considered in the classification process;
- experience in implementation, adaptation and training should be systematically collected and made available;

---

[3] http://www.campbellcollaboration.org

    – contextual factors should be studied by modeling different prevalence
levels so as to assess the impact of an intervention on the population; and
    – evidence of effectiveness and feasibility of implementation should both
be considered for the broader decision-making process.

This definition orients the activities undertaken at EMCDDA to develop best practice promotion.

Methods to develop the definition of Best Practice

A content analysis of the published articles about "best practices" was presented to a group of experts in the different fields (treatment and rehabilitation, harm reduction and prevention) of several European Countries. The different components identified were therefore discussed in order to create a definition that was both exhaustive and flexible.

To search the articles, we firstly identified a series of keywords that were then used to search the relevant databases. Only the abstracts of the eligible articles were considered for the analysis. References to "best practice" linked to drug demand reduction (prevention, treatment, harm reduction, rehabilitation) in EU policy and research funding documents were also included in the analysis.

We therefore identified the context in which the word: "best practice" was used -for the purpose of this exercise, context was considered to be the paragraph in which the reference to "best practice" was made. With a grounded theory approach, we identified two main "families" of keywords: one pertaining to "evidence" (for example RCT, systematic reviews, meta-analysis etc.); a second family pertaining to "practice" (consensus, programs, strategies, care etc). We then coded and mapped the documents to find associations between words pertaining to the two "families" and to recognise possible patterns. The resulting outcome was the identification of key dimensions related to both "evidence" and "practice".

A panel of European experts was convened to discuss the outcomes of the content analysis exercise and each expert was requested to present a suitable definition in their field of expertise. The aim was to reach a consensus on a definition of best practice in the drug field. A final proposal was drafted and approved by email consultation.

Promoting Best Practice: the production cycle

The EU drugs strategy (2009-2012) and the subsequent action plans have reinforced the principle that the exchange of best practice among Member States in the field of drugs is a prerequisite for effective drugs policy.

The EMCDDA committed to build on existing tools and projects (e.g., Best Practice Portal, EDDRA) to develop a comprehensive package of services for the promotion of Best Practices in Europe.

The production cycle of BP includes 5 key steps:

a) *Identification of relevant questions.* This means that the questions should come from daily activity in the field by enquiring practitioners, drug users and their families rather than being based on mere academic curiosity for knowledge. The efforts to create a Best Practice information service should focus on answering those questions.

b) *Search and retrieval of the available evidence.* Comprehensive and reproducible search for all the available evidence is essential to make sure that all the existing information is used to answer the questions and, more importantly, that the process is transparent and objective.

c) *Synthesis of the evidence.* The available information needs to be synthesised and made understandable in order to be directly applicable to the practice. Shared and standardised methods to synthesise the evidence are applied and they are those developed by the GRADE working Group (Guyatt *et al.*, 2011) and by the Cochrane Collaboaration (Amato *et al.*, 2011).

d) *Identification of implementation experiences (and possibly monitoring the impact).* It has been noted that the efforts spent during the last years on developing guidelines should now be redirected toward an increased implementation rate of these guidelines (Grol, 2009). Implementation encompasses all the activities aimed at studying the actual practice, identifying possible obstacles and barriers to changes, and promote the intended improvements. Many countries undertook such activities at different levels, both centrally and locally, and those experiences need to be identified and shared. A future objective should be also to monitor the impact of such implementation over the intervention outcomes.

e) *Identification of gaps and generation of further questions.* Imagining the whole process as a cycle (see below), the final output should become the starting point from which to draw further questions.

As mentioned above, the information process starts by collecting relevant questions from the field. Once those questions are translated into answerable queries, and the supporting evidence is researched, assessed and synthesised, it is inevitable that some gaps will be identified. This means that the results of the process are not only constituted of the answers but, more importantly, they create further questions. See Figure 1.

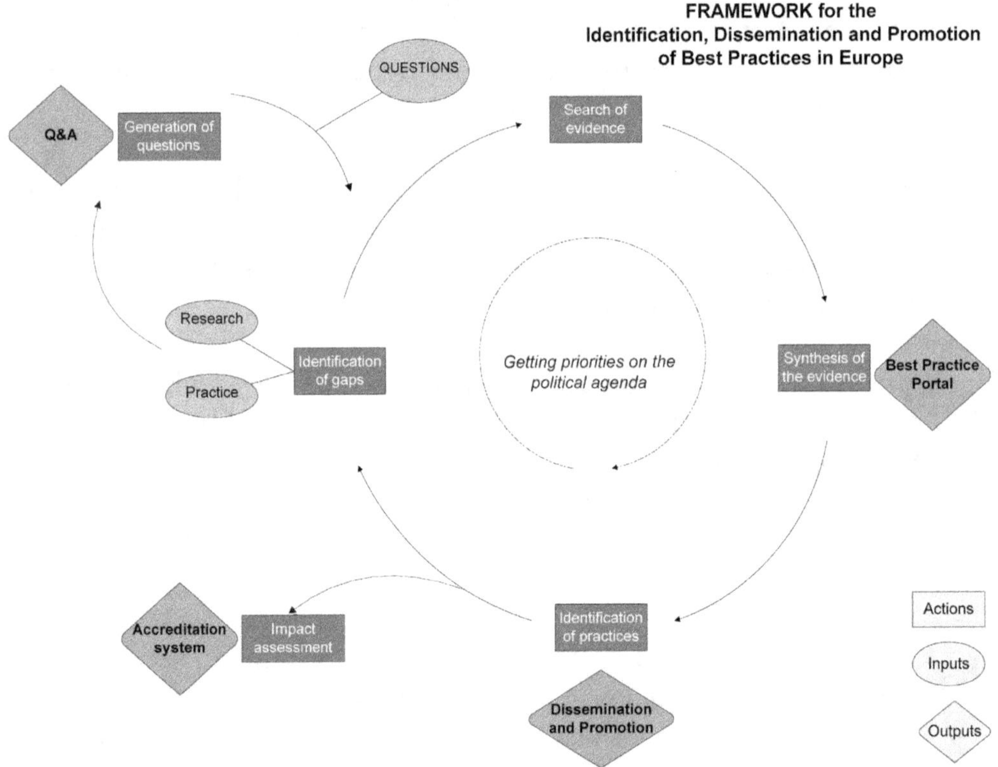

Figure 1. Illustrates the information cycle for promoting Best Practice. The starting point is the upper left corner in which the questions are generated with the contribution from the practitioners. In the top centre, the research for the evidence (in terms of published and unpublished studies) is shown, followed to the right by the publication of the synthesis of evidence in the Best Practice Portal. A key step is the identification and promotion of existing implementation examples. A logical future development would be to measure the impact of implementation (lower left) but this may require further planning.

Synthesising and grading evidence

Synthesis of the evidence

We consider "best practice" to be the answers resulting from the available and methodologically sound literature applied to interventions for drug users, as depicted by EMCDDA data.

The interventions presented in the Best Practice Portal are ranked according to their potential to achieve the intended results in different European contexts.

Each of the modules available in this portal – specifically prevention, treatment and harm reduction (social reintegration and supply reduction will be developed in the future) – includes results of the appraisal and synthesis of available and reliable literature. For the literature search we considered including the study designs that most appropriately answer the key question: "is the intervention likely to achieve the expected results in different contexts?".

After having searched the available information on the effect of specific interventions that are currently provided to drug users in Europe, we adopted the following ranks:

- *Beneficial.* Interventions for which precise measures of the effects in favour of the treatment were found in the systematic review of randomised controlled trials (RCTs), and that were recommended in guidelines with reliable methods for assessing evidence (such as GRADE)[4]. A treatment ranked as "beneficial" is suitable for most patients.

- *Likely to be beneficial.* Interventions that were shown to have limited measures of effect, which are likely to be effective but for which evidence is limited, and those that are recommended with some caution in guidelines with reliable methods for assessing evidence (such as GRADE). A treatment ranked as "likely to be beneficial" is suitable for most patients, with some discretion.

---

[4] *GRADE* is an approach to grading quality of evidence and strength of recommendations. The categories of effectiveness were created following those adopted by *BMJ Clinical Evidence* that were originally developed in the Cochrane Collaboration first editorial group for the publication "A guide to effective care in pregnancy and childbirth".

- *Trade-off between benefits and harms.* Interventions that obtained measures of effects in favour of treatment and are recommended in guidelines with reliable methods for assessing evidence (such as GRADE), but that showed some limitations or adverse effects that need to be assessed before providing them to patients.

- *Unknown effectiveness.* Interventions for which there are not enough studies or where available studies are of low quality (with few patients or with uncertain methodological rigour), making it difficult to assess whether they are effective or not. Interventions for which more research should be undertaken are also grouped in this category.

- *Evidence of ineffectiveness.* Interventions that gave negative results if compared with a placebo, for example.

Measures of effect reported in the Best Practice Portal

In order to grant transparency and synthesis of the information, we included the measures of effect obtained for each considered outcome in the Best Practice Portal. It is our aim to clarify and underline that the interventions are not effective in absolute, but, on the contrary, they are effective in reaching some outcomes that have been considered desirable.

In order to provide a synthetic quantification of the effectiveness of interventions, some measures have been commonly adopted and they are:

a) *Relative Risk (RR).* The Relative Risk (RR) is used to compare the risk in comparison groups of people (enrolled in the epidemiological studies), i.e. treated and control groups, to see whether belonging to one group or another increases or decreases the risk of developing certain outcomes. This measure of effect shows the number of times an outcome is more likely (RR > 1) or less likely (RR < 1) to happen in the treatment group compared with the control group.

   Practical interpretation:

   - If the RR (the relative risk) = 1, or the CI (the confidence interval) includes 1, then there is no significant difference between treatment and control groups

- If the RR > 1, and the CI does not include 1, events are significantly more likely in the treatment than the control group
- If the RR < 1, and the CI does not include 1, events are significantly less likely in the treatment than the control group

b) Confidence Interval (CI). The Confidence Interval (CI) is a measure of the precision (or uncertainty) of study results. It is the interval that most likely includes the true value of the parameter we are calculating, where "most likely" is taken by common usage to be a 95% probability thus the current expression of "95% CI". A wide CI indicates less precise estimates of effect and vice versa.

c) Standardised Mean Difference (SMD). The Standardised Mean Difference (SMD) is the difference in means divided by a standard deviation. Note that it is not the standard error of the difference in means (a common confusion). The standardised mean difference has the important property that its value does not depend on the measurement scale. It may be useful if there are several trials assessing the same outcome, but using different scales.

Identification of practices

As stated above, one crucial aspect of promoting best practice is the identification of the actual practice. For the time being, two strategies have been adopted and they consist of collecting national guidelines and standards on one hand, and local projects on the other.

Standard and guidelines

The European Monitoring Centre for Drugs and Drug Addiction created an inventory of National Guidelines for the Treatment of Drug Addiction by collecting information on 30 European Countries, thanks to the invaluable collaboration with the EMCDDA's National Focal Points. The Guidelines were in fact collected through a two-round survey and an international experts meeting. The guidelines identified in this way were described in general terms (target population, clinical conditions, treatment considered). In addition, the EMCDDA's network of national focal points performed a benchmark exercise comparing 15 recommendations from an evidence-based guideline (WHO, 2009) with similar recommendations in their National Treatment Guidelines, specifically regarding opioid substitution treatment.

The guidelines in national languages are available in portable format document on the Best Practice Portal (http://www.emcdda.europa.eu/best-practice/standards/treatment) and as of July 2011, 141 guidelines have been available.

A more comprehensive overview of those guidelines will be published by the end of 2011 in the EMCDDA collection, "Selected Issue".

Along with the guidelines, a managerial instrument has been adopted and it is being developed in Europe to ensure the quality of interventions. This is the development of quality standards that some countries developed further with the creation of an accreditation system for interventions that provide services.

Recently the European Commission, Directorate-General for Justice, commissioned a European Study aimed at creating a framework for minimum quality standards and benchmarks in drug-demand reduction (EQUS).[5] EMCDDA was actively involved in the steering committee of the Project and the development will be followed up with information made available in the Best Practice Portal.

Another Project that focused on the Standards for Prevention has been completed as part of the ongoing activities in the area for drug-prevention standards under the Programme of Community Action in the field of Public Health (2003-2008) and a handbook containing the results will be published by EMCDDA and made available in the Best Practice Portal.

Living Projects

Many years ago, well before the Best Practice Portal was created, a database of European projects was created and this was the Exchange on Drug Demand Reduction Action (EDDRA). It provides details on a wide range of evaluated prevention, treatment, harm reduction interventions as well as interventions within the criminal justice system and is primarily designed to help professionals and policy-makers. Currently EDDRA contains more than 400 entries. Some of these have been linked to the Best Practice Portal in order to highlight the projects that are putting evidence-based interventions into practice.

---

[5] http://www.equs-drugs-conference-registration.net/project.jsp

Sources

The information about guidelines, systematic reviews and studies was obtained through structured search strategies consulting the resources shown below.

- The National Health Library platform: Pubmed;
- the Cochrane Library (specifically the Cochrane Drugs and Alcohol Group);
- the primary international databases for guidelines (such as: the Scottish Intercollegiate Guidelines Network; published NICE clinical guidelines; New Zealand Guidelines Group; National Guideline ClearingHouse; Guidelines International Network; La Haute Autorité de Santé; National Institute for Health and Welfare and others)
- direct consultation with the Network of EMCDDA's National Focal Points;
- information retrieved from the registries of ongoing studies (Current Controlled Trials; ClinicalTrials.gov; http://www.who.int/ictrp/en; https://www.clinicaltrialsregister.eu/ctr-search);
- direct contact with leading researchers of the studies.

The EMCDDA Best Practice Portal: synthesis of the evidence

The module on Treatment provides some synthesis of the current evidence available for each type of illicit substance used. Even though in reality people may be using more than one substance, for clarity, the modules have been divided into: Opioid users, Cocaine users, Cannabis users, Amphetamine users.

For opioid users, some of the strongest existing evidence is found for the psychologically-assisted pharmacological treatment that helps people to remain in treatment, to reduce the use of illicit opioid and to reduce mortality. Remaining in treatment also helps people to avoid criminal activity and imprisonment. The intervention that has the greatest evidence of effectiveness is long-term methadone maintenance treatment, but buprenorphine has also proved to be effective. Psychosocial support improves outcomes either in pharmacological maintenance or in detoxification interventions. In terms of psychological interventions, better results among the studied interventions were found for case management that reduce drug use better than psycho-education and drug counselling. Methadone maintenance can also be helpful for heroin-addicted pregnant women in order to prevent further risks deriving from their use of illicit substances, even though the effects on the foetus and the neonatal abstinence syndrome need to be considered.

When it comes to comparing detoxification interventions for opioid addiction, methadone and buprenorphine gave similar results and buprenorphine appears to be better than alpha2 agonists. In order to maintain abstinence, naltrexone was found to be more effective than placebo but it did not affect retention in treatment.

A considerable investment in the research of the pharmacological treatment of cocaine dependence is not producing the desired results, at least for the time being. The only intervention that has evidence of effectiveness is disulfiram (a substance that interferes with alcohol metabolism), which proved to retain patients in treatment and reduce cocaine use better than placebo and than non-pharmacological interventions.

The remaining interventions for cocaine dependence that gave positive results are cognitive behavioural interventions and among them contingency management, which proved to help people reduce their use of cocaine.

The studies on the effectiveness of treatment for cannabis use are now increasing together with the treatment demands for cannabis users. Psychosocial interventions and in particular cognitive behavioural interventions and family therapy appear to be the most promising and new results are expected to corroborate this evidence.

The current reviews of evidence do not support a single treatment to approach that is able to tackle the multidimensional facets of amphetamine addiction patterns, some evidence shows that the antidepressive agent fluoxetine, as a short-term treatment, can decrease craving for amphetamine (if compared with an adrenergic uptake inhibitor, imipramine); while the adrenergic uptake inhibitor imipramine, in medium-term treatment, significantly increased the duration of adherence to treatment.

Some systematic reviews tried to analyse and synthesise the results from studies on therapeutic communities, concluding that there is little evidence that therapeutic communities offer significant benefits in comparison with other residential treatment, or that one type of TC is better than another. The methodological limitations of the available studies prevented firm conclusions on the basis of the existing evidence.

See table for a complete overview:

Summary table of evidence of treatment effectiveness

	Beneficial	Likely to be beneficial	Trade-off between benefits and harms	Unknown effectiveness	Evidence of ineffectiveness	N and type of Studies	Outcomes and measure of effect
Opioid dependence							
Methadone maintenance therapy	x					3 RCTs (N=505)	Increasing retention in treatment (RR 3.05, 95% CI 1.75 to 5.35); Reducing illicit opioid use (RR 0.32, 95% CI 0.23 to 0.44).
						1 RCT (N=253)	Reduce the risk of HIV infection by approximately 50% (RR 0.45, 95% CI 0.35 to 0.59)
						3 obs. studies* (N=43035) f.u. 2.5-21yrs *Observational follow up studies	Mortality (RR 0.37, 95% CI 0.29 to 0.48).
						2 obs. Studies (N=876) f.u. 5yrs	Reduction in seroconversion rates (RR 0.36, 95% CI 0.19 to 0.66) compared to withdrawal or no treatment.
Buprenorphine maintenance therapy (16mg vs 1mg)	x					1 RCT (N=366)	Improving retention in treatment (RR 1.52, 95% CI 1.23 to 1.88); reducing the number of morphine-positive urines (SMD –0.65, 95% CI –0.86 to –0.44) than a placebo.
Psychosocial interventions in maintenance treatment	x					3 RCTs (N=388)	Methadone treatment plus psychosocial intervention comparedwith methadone treatment only is more effective in reducing heroin use (RR 0.69, 95% CI 0.53 to 0.91)

Continues

Continuation

Psychosocial assistance in addition to pharmacological assistance for opioid withdrawal	x					5 RCts (N=184)	Combined psychosocial (contingency management, community reinforcement, psychotherapeutic counselling and family therapy) and pharmacological assistance were found to be effective in: increasing rates of completion of treatment (RR 1.68, 95% CI 1.11 to 2.55, moderate quality evidence); reducing rates of relapse at follow-up (RR 0.41, 95% CI 0.27 to 0.62, moderate-quality evidence).
Case management	x					1 RCT (N~500)	Case management proved to be more effective than psycho-education and drug counselling in reducing drug use (RR 0.24, 95% CI 0.06, 0.42).
Opioid assisted withdrawal with buprenorphine	x					8 RCTs (N=884)	Buprenorphine for opioid assisted withdrawal was found to be effective in: achieving higher completion rates than alpha-2 agonists (RR 1.67, 95% CI 1.24 to 2.25, moderate-quality evidence); lowering the peak of objective withdrawal scores (SMD –0.61, 95% CI –0.86 to –0.36, moderate-quality evidence); lowering overall self-reported levels of opioid withdrawal (SMD –0.59, 95% CI –0.79 to –0.39, high-quality evidence).
Naltrexone for preventing relapse		x				10 (N=696)	Naltrexone was found to be effective in preventing relapse inuse in detoxified patient: naltrexone was more effective than a placebo in reducing heroin use (RR 0.72, 95% CI 0.58 to 0.90, low-quality evidence); naltrexone did not affect retention in treatment (RR 1.08, 95% CI 0.74 to 1.57) or relapse at follow-up post-treatment (RR 0.94, 95% CI 0.67 to 1.34).

Continues

Continuation

Maintenance agonist treatments for opiate dependent pregnant women	x					3 RCTs (N=96)	Significant difference between methadone and buprenorphine treatment in: use of primary substance (RR 2.50, 95% CI 0.11 to 54.87) Oral slow morphine seemed superior to methadone in abstaining women from the use of heroin: use of primary substance (RR 2.40, 95% CI 1.00 to 5.77)
Psychosocial interventions	x					3 RCTs (N=500)	Psychosocial interventions in addition to Methadone maintenance treatment is more effective than methadone only in: retaining patients in treatment (RR 0.94, 95% CI 0.85 to 1.02).
Heroin maintenance treatment for chronic heroin users		x				8 RCTs (N=2007)	Supervised Injected Heroin helps people: To remain in treatment (RR 1.44 95% CI 1.19-1.75) heterogeneity P=0.03), and to reduce use of illicit drugs. Mortality (RR 0.65 (95% CI 0.25-1.69) heterogeneity P=0.89), But it exposes a greater risk of adverse events (Risk Ratio 13.50 (95% CI 2.55-71.53) heterogeneity P=0.52).
Naltrexone in place of methadone			x				No studies
Assisted opioid withdrawal with methadone or alpha-2 agonists			x			7 RCTs (N=577)	No significant difference between methadone and alpha-2 agonists in: treatment completion (RR 1.09, 95% CI 0.90 to 1.32); relapse at follow-up (intention-to-treat analysis) (RR 1.06, 95% CI 0.55 to 2.02, low-quality evidence).
Assisted opioid withdrawal with methadone or buprenorphine			x			2 RCTs (N=63)	There was no significant difference in: completion of treatment between methadone and buprenorphine (RR 0.88, 95% CI 0.67 to 1.15).

Continues

Continuation

Maintenance agonist treatments (methadone compared with buprenorphine) for opiate dependent pregnant women				x		3 RCTs (N=96)	Maintenance treatment for pregnant women: was no different from buprenorphine in: drop out rate (RR 1.00, 95% CI 0.41 to 2.44)
Pharmacological detoxification treatment for adolescent opioid users				x		2 RCTs (N= 190 participants between 13–18 years of age)	Detoxification treatment alone or in combination with psychosocial intervention compared to no intervention, other pharmacological interventions found no conclusive results in: completion of treatment; reducing the use of substances; and improving health and social status.
Cocaine dependence							
Cognitive behavioural interventions [+]	x					27 RCTs (N=3 663)	Cognitive behavioural interventions were found to be effective in: reducing dropouts from treatment and reduction in the use of cocaine, when compared with drug counselling.
Behavioural interventions	x					27 RCTs (N=3 663)	Behavioural interventions clearly performed better than clinical management in the number of psychotherapy sessions attended. Behavioural interventions clearly performed better than clinical management in reducing the number of patients using cocaine at one and three months
Disulfiram for the treatment of cocaine dependence	x					7 RCTs (N=492)	Disulfiram was found not to be statistically significantly better than a placebo in: retaining patients in treatment (RR 0.82, 95% CI 0.66 to 1.03); reducing cocaine use (WMD 4.50, 95% CI 2.93 to 6.07). Disulfiram was found to be not statistically better than naltrexone in: reducing dropouts (RR 0.67, 95% CI 0.45 to 1.01).

Continues

Continuation

							Disulfiram was found to be better than no pharmacological treatment in: reducing cocaine use (WMD 2.10 (95% CI 0.69 to 3.51); number of subjects achieving three or more weeks of consecutive abstinence (RR 1.88, 95% CI 1.09 to 3.23).
Psychostimulant drugs to reduce heroin use	x					16 RCTs (N=1345)	Psychostimulants were found to be effective in: reducing heroin use (SMD 0.29, 95% CI: –0.02 to 0.61, p= 0.07).
Psychostimulants for sustained abstinence			x			8 RCTs (N=800)	Psychostimulants (bupropion and dextroamphetamine, and modafinil) showed a statistical trend over improving sustained cocaine abstinence (RR 1.41, 95% CI 0.98 to 2.02, p=0.07)
Antipsychotic medications for cocaine dependence			x			7 RCTs (N=293)	The antipsychotic drugs studied were risperidone, olanzapine and haloperidol, and no significant differences were found for any of the efficacy measures comparing any antipsychotic with placebo. Risperidone was found to be superior to placebo in diminishing the number of dropouts (RR 0.77, 95% CI 0.77 to 0.98).
Psychostimulants to reduce use and dropouts, and to increase retention				x		16 RCTs (N=1345)	Psychostimulants were found in not effective in: reducing cocaine use (SMD 0.11, 95% CI –0.07 to 0.29); retention in treatment (RR 0.97, 95% CI 0.89 to 1.05); reducing the dropouts caused by adverse events (RD 0.01, 95% CI –0.02 to 0.03).
Anticonvulsants for cocaine dependence				x			There is no current evidence supporting the clinical use of anticonvulsant medication in the treatment of cocaine dependence.

Continues

Continuation

							Evidence	Description
Cannabis use								
Psychotherapies in individual or group sessions		x					5RCTs (N=1297)	Psychotherapies (cognitive behavioural (CBT), motivational enhancement) in individual or group sessions have been found to be effective in reducing cannabis use.
Cognitive behavioural therapy in individual sessions		x					1RCT (N=450)	Cognitive behavioural therapy (nine sessions or more) in individual sessions proved to be more effective than brief motivational therapy in reducing cannabis use and symptoms of dependence.
Voucher-based incentives			x				5 RCTs (N=125)	Voucher-based incentives associated with effective psychotherapeutic interventions were found to be likely to enhance treatment acceptability (defined as the number of participants who attended more than one therapy session). However, they were not effective in improving rates of treatment completion (defined as attending at least one session and giving one urine specimen).
Multidimensional family therapy				x				Results are expected in 2010 from the INCANT study, a multi-site trial on multidimensional family therapy (MDFT). The study was conducted in Belgium, France, Germany, the Netherlands and Switzerland. See Liddle (2008) and Rigter (2010).
Amphetamines use								
The antidepressive agent fluoxetine as a short-term treatment			x				5 RCTs (N=150)	The antidepressive agent fluoxetine (40 mg/day) as a short-term treatment* was found to be effective in significantly decreasing craving (if compared with an adrenergic uptake inhibitor, imipramine). * defined by the authors and not specified.
The adrenergic uptake inhibitor imipramine as a medium-term treatment			x					The adrenergic uptake inhibitor imipramine (150 mg/day), in medium-term treatment*, significantly increased the duration of adherence to treatment. * defined by the authors and not specified.

EMCDDA Best Practice Portal: collection of treatment guidelines

As of July 2011, 144 National Treatment Guidelines from 28 (out of 30) Countries were identified and for 141, the full text was obtained (available on our website: http://www.emcdda.europa.eu/best-practice). Almost half of them (68/144) are about opioid dependence and 55 guidelines from 13 countries state Methadone Maintenance as the main treatment. Overall, the recommendations included in the guidelines are similar, for instance, recommending an integrated package of long-term substitution treatment with psychological support, yet some guidelines are based on evidence and others rely more on consensus from experts. Differences exist with regard to the choice between Buprenorphine or Methadone for first-line treatment and about drug dosages. Psychosocial interventions often accompany these pharmacological treatments, in some cases there are more detailed recommendations and in others just a mention is made.

Opioid dependence is the most frequent problem dealt with in the guidelines but it is not the only one; a number of guidelines, for instance, do not specify a single substance but are aimed more generally at drug dependence, and others address cocaine, other stimulants, cannabis and alcohol.

Detoxification from opioid dependence is the second most frequent pharmacological subject for the guidelines on treatment across the European countries.

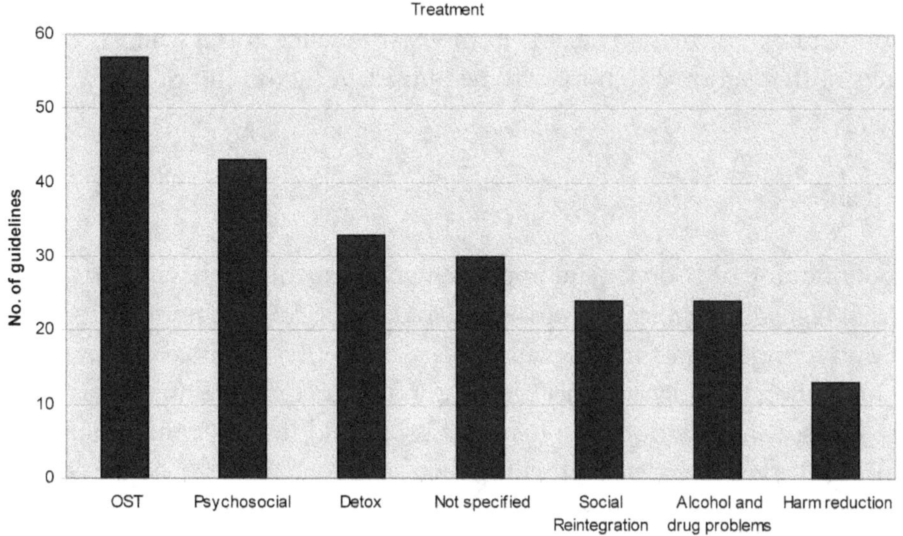

Graph 1. Number of guidelines by type of intervention.

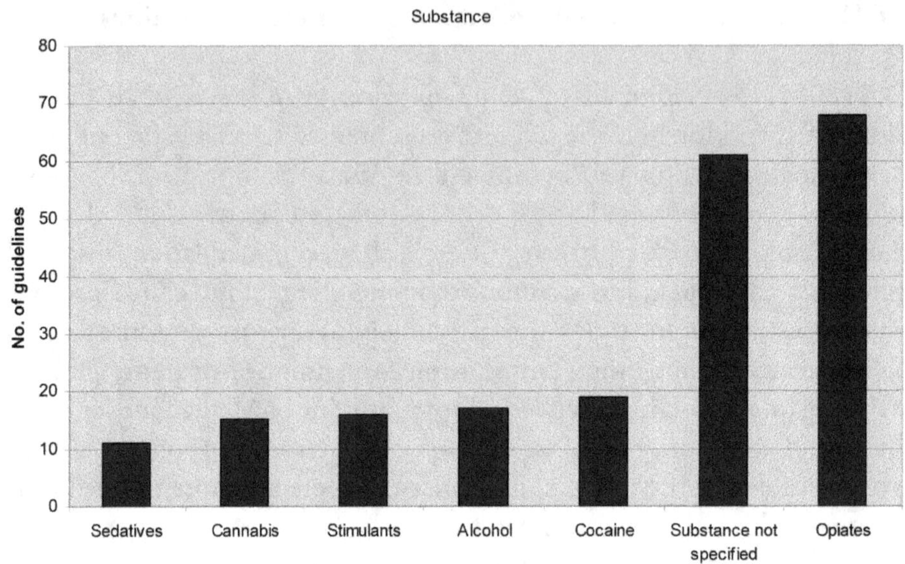

Graph 2. Number of guidelines by type of substance

The medications suggested for this purpose are methadone, buprenorphine, lofex-idine, clonidine, alpha2adrenergic agonists and benzodiazepine for the control of withdrawal symptoms.

A detailed description of the guidelines, their context and the future plan for development will be made available in the Best Practice Portal where the relevant chapters of the National Reports will be published by the end of 2011.

Conclusions

The identification of evidence and implementation experiences has important impli-cations in highlighting research gaps as well as defining research priorities. The Euro-pean Monitoring Centre for Drugs and Drug Abuse's Best Practice Portal is the result of an initial effort to bridge together evidence and practice to disseminate and promote evidence-based interventions throughout Europe and foster a common approach.

During the last decades, a growing body of evidence in the field of drug ad-diction has developed and continues to grow. For the time being, this is more prominent in the field of treatment and is slowly increasing in Prevention, Harm Reduction and Social Rehabilitation.

EMCDDA is in partnership with the most advanced methodological working groups (such us GRADE working group and the Cochrane Collaboration) and with its stakeholders, represented by the National Focal points and the European Scientific Community, created a unique system to search, synthesise and make available existing and upcoming evidence.

To make it practical and useful, the evidence is synthesised and linked to real world experiences from different European countries. It is a circular process that benefits from interaction with people working in the field.

For this reason we consider the opportunity to participate in the EWODOR initiative an important source of inspiration and improvement.

References

Amato, L, Minozzi, S, Pani, PP & Davoli, M (2007). "Antipsychotic medications for cocaine dependence", Cochrane Database of Systematic Reviews, Issue 3, Art. No. CD006306, DOI: 10.1002/14651858.CD006306.pub2.

Amato, L, Davoli, M, Vecchi, S, Ali, R, Farrell, M *et al.* (2011). "Cochrane systematic reviews in the field of addiction: What's there and what should be", *Drug Alcohol Depend.* 113(2-3), 96-103.

Castells, X, Casas, M, Pérez-Mañá, C, *et al.* (2010). "Efficacy of psychostimulant drugs for cocaine dependence", Cochrane Database of Systematic Reviews, Issue 2. Art. No.: CD007380. DOI: 10.1002/14651858. CD007380.pub3.

Denis, C, Lavie, E, Fatseas, M & Auriacombe, M (2006). "Psychotherapeutic interventions for cannabis abuse and/or dependence in outpatient settings", Cochrane Database of Systematic Reviews, Issue 3.

Ferri, MMF, Davoli, M & Perucci, CA (2005). "Heroin maintenance for chronic heroin dependents", Cochrane Database of Systematic Reviews, Issue 2, Art. No. CD003410, DOI: 10.1002/14651858.CD003410.pub2.

Grol, R (2009). "Implementation of changes in practice", in R. Grol, M.W.a.M.E.e. (editor), *Improving patient care: the implementation of change in clinical practice*, 6-14, Elsevier, Edinburgh.

Guyatt, GH, Oxman, AD, Schunemann, HJ, Tugwell, P & Knottnerus, A (2011). "GRADE guidelines: A new series of articles in the Journal of Clinical Epidemiology", *J Clin. Epidemiol.* 64(4), pp. 380-2 (available at:PM:21185693).

Knapp, WP, Soares, B, Farrell, M & Silva de Lima, M (2007). "Psychosocial interventions for cocaine and psychostimulant amphetamines related disorders", Cochrane Database of Systematic Reviews, Issue 3, Art. No. CD003023, DOI: 10.1002/14651858. CD003023.pub2.

Liddle, HA, Dakof, GA, Turner, RM, Henderson, CE & Greenbaum, PE (2008). "Treating adolescent drug abuse: a randomized trial comparing multidimensional family therapy and cognitive behavior therapy". Addiction 103, 1660–1670.

Minozzi, S, Amato, L, Vecchi, S *et al.* (2006). "Oral naltrexone maintenance treatment for opioid dependence", Cochrane Database of Systematic Reviews, Issue 1, Art. No.: CD001333, DOI: 10.1002/14651858. CD001333.pub2.

Minozzi, S, Amato, L, Vecchi, S & Davoli, M (2009). "Maintenance agonist treatments for opiate dependent pregnant women", Cochrane Database of Systematic Reviews 2008, Issue 2. Art. No.: CD006318. DOI: 10.1002/14651858.CD006318.pub2

Pani, PP, Trogu, E, Vacca, R, *et al.* (2010). "Disulfiram for the treatment of cocaine dependence", Cochrane Database of Systematic Reviews, Issue 1. Art. No.: CD007024. DOI: 10.1002/14651858.CD007024.pub2.

Rigter H, Pelc I, Tossmann A *et al.* (2010). "INCANT: a transnational randomized trial of Multidimensional Family Therapy versus treatment as usual for adolescents with cannabis use disorder", BMC Psychiatry 2010, 10:28 (doi:10.1186/1471-244X-10-28).

Sackett, DL, Rosenberg, WM, Gray, JA Haynes, RB & Richardson, WS (2007). "Evidence based medicine: what it is and what it isn't. 1996", *Clin. Orthop. Relat Res.* 455, 3-5 (available at:PM:17340682).

Smith, LA, Gates, S & Foxcroft, D (2006). "Therapeutic communities for substance related disorder", Cochrane Database of Systematic Reviews, Issue 1, Art. No. CD005338, DOI: 10.1002/14651858.CD005338.pub2.

Srisurapanont, M, Jarusuraisin, N & Kittirattanapaiboon, P (2001). "Treatment for amphetamine dependence and abuse", Cochrane Database of Systematic Reviews, Issue 4, Art. No.: CD003022. DOI: 10.1002/14651858. CD003022.

WHO (2009). "Guidelines for the Psychosocially Assisted Pharmacological Treatment of Opioid Dependence", World Health Organization Dept. of Mental Health and Substance Abuse.

5 Chronobiology and addiction: implications for treatment and prevention

ANA ADAN[1,2]

[1] Department of Psychiatry and Clinical Psychobiology
  University of Barcelona, Spain
[2] Institute for Brain, Cognition and Behaviour (IR3C), Spain

aadan@ub.edu

Abstract

This work reviews the findings of chronobiology in the field of addiction and its application possibilities both in preventive and therapeutic approaches. Different works have provided evidence that drug consumption, even in moderate doses, produces a reduction in the amplitude of circadian rhythms, the time lag of maximum values and even the disappearance of rhythmicity. Recently some circadian genes *(Clock, Period)* have been implied as biological risk factors for drug addiction, and the modification of their genetic expression has been found in patients with addiction disorders, regardless of the pharmacological effects of the drug taken. Moreover, the evening-circadian typology is currently being considered as an endophenotype for the onset and maintenance of drug consumption. Preventive and therapeutic approaches to addiction should take into account circadian rhythmic organisation, with special emphasis on redirecting the time patterns towards a better entrainment with the light-dark cycle. In many cases it may suffice to establish regular time patterns of wake-sleep, meals and daily activity with a tendency towards a morningness pattern of functioning. Light therapy or exposure to morning light may also be considered, as well as the administration of exogenous melatonin at the end of the day. These chronobiological strategies may be applied for long periods of time, even for life, since they have shown an excellent degree of security. This field of research is still in its infancy, but it shows great potential for the management of substance use disorders in the future.

Key words

Addiction; chronobiology; circadian rhythm; circadian typology; bright light therapy; melatonin.

Introduction

There are several biological rhythms, although the most studied ones, due to their clinical interest, are the circadian rhythms (24 hour duration). These are produced endogenously by the organism's biological clock, which is anatomically located in the suprachiasmatic nucleus (SCN) of the hypothalamus, located above the crossing of the optic nerves. In normal conditions, circadian rhythmic expression is entrained to the environmental light information and, especially, to the cycle of light-darkness (Herzog, 2007; Levi & Schibler, 2007). The information from the environmental light is transmitted to the SCN through the retinohypothalamic tract and, although this is the main *zeitgeber* (time-giver) of the biological clock, a number of other cues have been identified including food, locomotor activity and social cues (Kosobud *et al.,* 2007). The endogenous clock is extremely precise in its functioning, and also has the ability to adjust to environmental changes, such as a transmeridian journey or subject to shift work, in the fastest possible time. The SCN works closely with the pineal gland, which produces melatonin, the darkness signal in the organism (see Figure 1). To read further on the neuroanatomical and functional aspects of circadian rhythmic expression, Rosenwasser's (2009) excellent revision should be consulted.

Chronobiology is the science studying the rhythmic phenomena, and it has developed mostly since the second half of the 20th century. The correct rhythmic expression is an indicator of health and quality of life in all the phases of the vital cycle, and this is a universal feature both in Nordic countries with a very variable light-dark cycle depending on the season of the year, as well as in those countries with more benign conditions. Although the Nordic countries are very sensitive to the possible risks of having too little or too much light throughout the year, in the Mediterranean countries it is common to neglect this factor, and therefore the problems related to a bad adjustment of the endogenous clock according to the environmental signals reaches a similar prevalence. Thus, those people with individual biological vulnerability to the seasonal rhythmic changes do not take the necessary preventive precautions and, many times, despite the good environmental conditions, they live almost without taking light into account.

There are several outputs with circadian rhythmicity (biochemical, physiological, behavioural), and the most obvious one is the sleep-wake cycle. Among these, some have become measurements considered to be markers of the functionality of the circadian system, thanks to their robustness and implications both in health and in sickness, mainly body temperature (central/core and peripheral/skin) and the hormones cortisol and melatonin. Central temperature, with a sinusoidal function whose maximum appears between 17-20 h and its minimum between 3-5 h in the morning, is considered an estimator of brain activity and its disorganisation is well known in several mood disorders, especially endogenous depression. Peripheral temperature, with an inverse function to that of central temperature, has been recently proposed as an excellent record to perform outpatient assessments with the minimum disturbance for patients (Sarabia *et al.,* 2008). We should also notice the recent proposal of a new integrated measure based on thermometry, actimetry and body position to assess the circadian system status

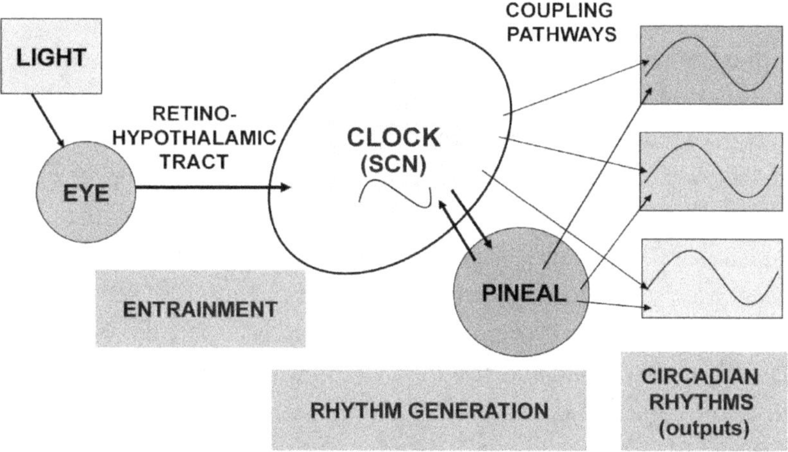

Figure 1. Circadian system organisation with the endogenous clock in the suprachiasmatic nucleus (SCN) of the hypothalamus.

of humans (Ortiz-Tudela *et al.*, 2010), an outpatient system that is easy to use and to interpret the data. Cortisol's circadian rhythm is characterised by a marked secretion peak near the time of awakening and minimum during the first half of the sleep (Kripke *et al.*, 2007). The production of cortisol is highly sensitive to inputs from the limbic system and the prefrontal cortex during times of stress and may be altered under different psychopathological circumstances (Lovallo, 2006). Finally, melatonin presents a secretion with a marked night peak dependent on the duration of the environmental photoperiod, and with minimum values during the wake period. The loss of the melatonin peak produces a clear impairment of sleep, and at the same time it decreases the organism's antioxidant and immuno-logical activity (Reiter, 2007; Tekbas *et al.*, 2008; Jung-Hynes *et al.*, 2009).

The interest in the study of the relations between rhythmic expression and the consumption of psychoactive substances is recent. With the exception of specific works, most of the research has been developed during the last decade, and the data currently available provides evidence of its importance both in basic and ap-plied levels of knowledge. All the existing data suggest that the biological clock affects our physical and psychological response to casual drug intake, as well as to the vulnerability to develop an abuse or dependence disorder. The current work reviews the available results and their practical implications both for prevention and for the treatment of drug addictions.

Drug consumption and circadian rhythms

Several studies have shown that the chronic consumption of psychoactive substances has a negative effect on the expression of circadian rhythmicity. Broadly speaking, drug addicts have reduced amplitude and a time lag in the maximum values of their circadian functions. There is also some desynchronisation of the circadian function between the CNS and peripheral organs (Wang *et al.*, 2006). Circadian rhythm may even disappear in extreme cases, which suggests a lesser quality of the wake and sleep periods. Moreover, a disrupted functioning of the circadian system results in a less favourable adaptation to environmental changes and is associated with a wide variety of diseases such as metabolic and reproductive abnormalities, cancer development, aging, and neurological and psychiatric problems in humans (Barnard & Nolan, 2008: Huang *et al.*, 2010). The studies with human drug addicts show circadian rhythm variations mostly ruled by factors associated to the type of drug, such as metabolism, tolerance and sensitivity to the drug reward (Kosobud *et al.*, 2007).

The lack of regularity in the circadian rhythms has been mostly studied with alcohol dependence, cocaine and tobacco. However, most of the evidence suggests that the data compiled may be generalised to most types of drugs, independently of their pharmacological effects on the organism (Perreau-Lenz & Spanagel, 2008; Perreau-Lenz *et al.*, 2009). The effects of drug addiction on the circadian rhythmic expression persists for a long time –weeks or even months- after drug use has ceased (Falcon & McClung, 2009), although more longitudinal studies are needed to obtain data on this subject and also to find predictive variables associated to the recovery time of the circadian system.

Chronic consumption of alcohol reduces the rhythmic amplitude both of the core body temperature and of melatonin, and there is a maximisation of this process during the withdrawal syndrome. Thus, there is hypothermia during the wake period and hyperthermia during the night hours, together with a considerable reduction of the secretion of night melatonin and higher values during the day (Danel & Touitou, 2004, for a revision). Patients dependent on alcohol or other drugs may show the loss of a normal diurnal secretion of cortisol, which may regain a relatively normal pattern at about one to four weeks from abstinence, although the hypothalamic-pituitary-adrenocortical axis may not be completely normal (Lovallo, 2006). The affectation in the melatonin circadian rhythm is also seen in young healthy individuals with a sporadic evening administration of alcohol at a moderate dose (Rupp *et al.*, 2007). This piece of data is especially relevant and alerts us on the need to do further research on heavy episodic drinking in teenagers and young adults (Scaife & Duka, 2009; Adan, 2010), in order to delimit both the possible impact on circadian rhythmicity and on its duration. Although it is unclear how melatonin regulates the behavioural responses to drugs, there is evidence that it has an inhibitory effect on dopamine release (McClung, 2007). A recent study by Reinberg *et al.* (2010) also provides evidence that the simple intake of a glass of red wine during dinner (20.5 g alcohol / 24 h) may desynchronise circadian time organisation, and reduce the subjects' night performance (reaction time).

The affectation of the circadian rhythmic expression has also been seen in young healthy smokers. These subjects have a lesser amplitude and a time lag of the maximum or acrophase in the day values of subjective activation and affect state in comparison to non-smokers (Adan & Sánchez-Turet, 2000), and this is especially relevant for those subjects with high dependency (Adan *et al.*, 2004). See Figure 2. Similarly, day variations of cardiovascular parameters show a phase delay and higher values in the second half of the day in smokers

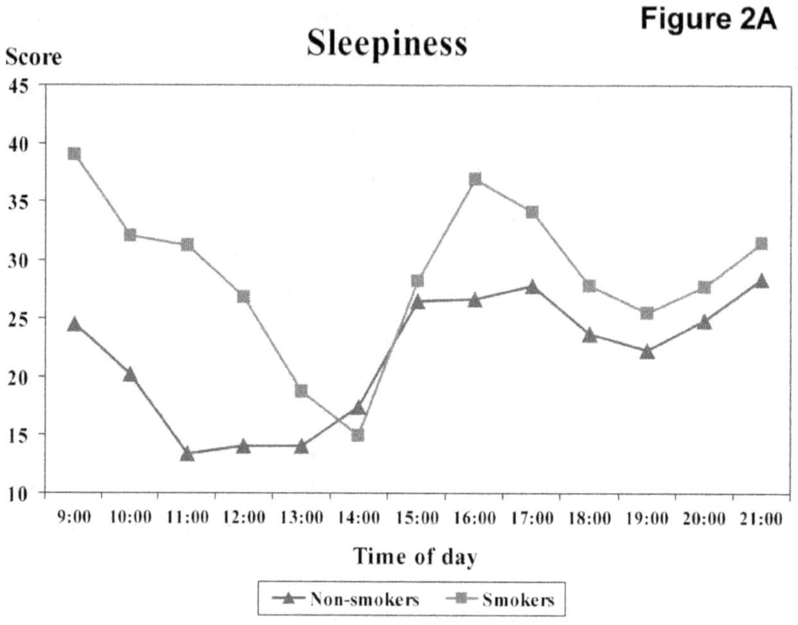

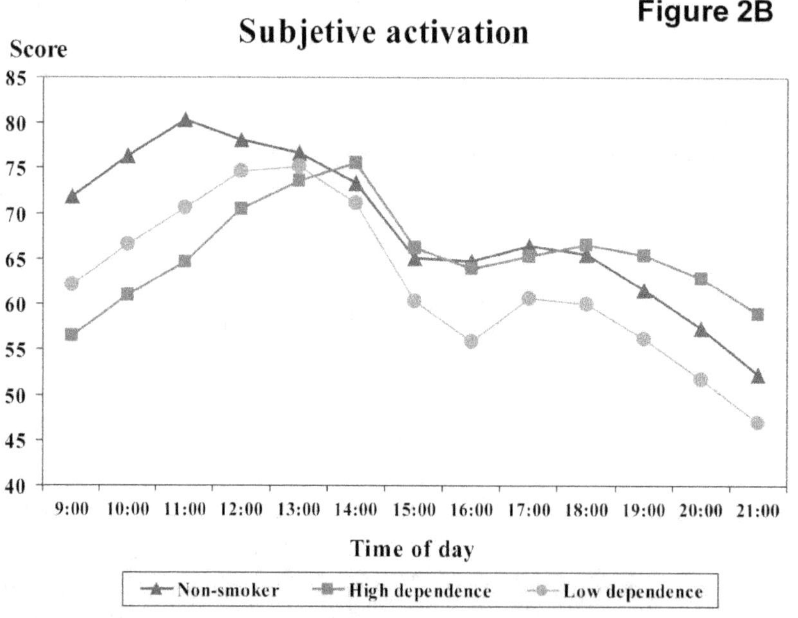

Figure 2. Diurnal functions of sleepiness in smokers and non-smokers (2A; modified from Adan & Sánchez-Turet, 2000) and of subjective activation, taking into account the level of dependency of the smokers (2B; modified from Adan et al., 2004). The scores in both cases range from 0 (totally awake / low activated) to 100 (very asleep / highly activated).

when compared to non-smokers (Adan & Sánchez-Turet, 1995). The rhythmic cardiovascular affectation in the initial phases of consumption may be a risk estimator for the development of acute and chronic pathologies associated to tobacco dependency.

In consumers of MDMA, the deterioration of the circadian rhythmic expression and, more specifically, the worse quality of sleep, have also been related to a greater risk of suffering serotoninergic neurotoxicity and mental pathologies associated to the use of this drug (McCann & Ricaurte, 2007; McCann *et al.*, 2007).

Drug addiction and circadian genes

Recent studies have implicated circadian genes in the neuroadaptive processes underlying drug reward and addiction (Manev & Uz, 2006; Falcon & McClung, 2009; Rosenwasser, 2010), as well as to a variety of other psychopathological (Herzog, 2007; McClung, 2007a) and neuroendocrinous disorders (Liu *et al.*, 2007). Individual differences in sleep quality and possible circadian organisation may predict initial susceptibility to drug abuse and dependence (Spanagel *et al.*, 2005) and there is more and more evidence of the association between circadian genes and drug-preference phenotypes. Thus, polymorphisms in the circadian genes may be a biological factor of vulnerability to addiction, and circadian rhythmicity must be considered in the multifactorial model of risk of developing and maintaining addictive behaviours. Most of these studies have been carried out using lab animals, cocaine and alcohol, but all the evidence points to this being transferable to humans and generalised to all abuse drugs (Perreau-Lenz & Spanagel, 2008; Falcon & McClung, 2009).

A relevant finding is that relating the activity of the reward system to circadian genes, specifically to the *Clock* gene, responsible for activating several circadian genes (McClung *et al.*, 2005). This study was done with mice carrying a mutated *Clock* gene. These mice were much more active both before and after cocaine administration in comparison to the control group. Moreover, the response of the reward system to the drug was much higher, and there was an increase in the levels of dopamine and their synthesising enzyme. The results point at the *Clock* gene as a direct regulator of the dopaminergic activity in the brain areas of reward (Lamont *et al.*, 2007). Mutations in the *Clock* gene produce a behavioural pattern not only at risk of developing an addiction but also very similar to manic states in humans (McClung, 2007b; Rosenwasser, 2010).

A recent study has evidenced that in human subjects the *Clock* variations may be a vulnerability factor to depression given the exposure to alcohol in individuals with alcohol abuse or dependence (Sjöholm *et al.*, 2010). Although the etiology of affective disorders is unlikely to be related to the *Clock* gene expression alone, the circadian genotype may be a contributing factor (Lamont *et al.*, 2007). This work opens a very interesting new line of research on the link between circadian genes and dual diagnosis.

The circadian genes *Period* (*Per1* and *Per2*) are also relevant in addiction. *Per1* has been related to the rewarding properties to the multiple substances in acute or specific administrations (Liu *et al.*, 2007; McClung, 2007b). The work by Wang *et al.* (2006) with morphine administration in mice has also revealed that morphine causes a desynchronisation of the circadian function between the Central Nervous System (CNS) and peripheral organs due to changes in the genetic expression of *Per1*. The mammalian *Per1* gene is a major participant in the molecular feedback loop that generates circadian rhythms and plays a role in the resetting of the SCN by light signals. *Per2* has been proven essential to modulate (inhibit) the sensitisation and reward of CNS to the effects of both cocaine (Abarca *et al.*, 2002) and alcohol (Spanagel *et al.*, 2005; Perreau-Lenz *et al.*, 2009). The animals with a mutant *Per2* gene, or with a lack or dysfunction of it, display enhanced cocaine consumption and alcohol drinking behaviour, as well as the loss of the well-known day variation of the sensitivity to the drug.

It has also recently been observed that in humans, variations in the *Per2* gene are associated to a higher consumption of alcohol (Spanagel, 2009) and, more specifically, a polymorphism in *Per2* has been associated to heavy drinking among alcoholics (McClung, 2007b). It is believed that the regulation of *Per2* in the dependence to alcohol and other depressive substances is mediated by its effects on the reuptake of glutamate and thereby may produce alterations in a variety of physiological and immune functions (Perreau-Lenz *et al.*, 2009; Spanagel, 2009). Moreover, *Per2* knock mice present a downregulation of the glutamate-aspartate transporter responsible for the hyperglutamatergic state (Spanagel *et al.*, 2005). This may be an explanatory factor in the individual variability to the risk of neurodegeneration by excitotoxicity and to the response to the pharmacological treatment with glutamatergic antagonists.

In addition, there may be a decrease in the genetic expression of most of the circadian genes in those patients who have developed a dependence disorder. This may trigger functional changes associated to different degrees of consumption depending on the subject's vulnerability (Manev & Uz, 2006), which would correlate with the rhythmic affectation observed. The first study in male alcoholic patients that has assessed this aspect has found a reduced expression of the *Clock*, *Per1* and *Per2* genes in comparison to controls (Huang *et al.*, 2010). Moreover, this study has established that after one week of abstinence the recovery of the expression of the clock genes is minimal. The consumption of morphine, heroin and cocaine also downregulates the expression of the *Per2* gene (Perreau-Lenz & Spanagel, 2008; Li *et al.*, 2009), and this may be a relevant aspect on its own in the maintenance of the consumption behaviour. *Per2* mutations increases the susceptibility of animals to the development of tumours (Spanagel *et al.*, 2005), and thus the chronic consumption of drugs affecting this gene's activity will impair the immune functions.

Circadian typology and drug consumption

Not all individuals have an identical circadian rhythmic expression. Circadian typology is an individual difference on which we have obtained much information in the last two decades. Individuals are classified into three typologies (morning-, neither- and evening-type) according to their self-assessment in specific questionnaires, of which we have validated versions in several countries. The work by Caci *et al.* (2009b) revises the most commonly used questionnaires and their psychometric characteristics. Morning-type subjects go to bed early and wake up early, and locate their best moment to carrying out their mental and physical activities in the first hours of day. In contrast, evening-type subjects go to bed and wake up late, and locate their best moment at the end of the day and even during the first hours of the night. The phase lags in circadian rhythmic functions between extreme groups range from 2 to 12h, and this has been observed both in biological and behavioural parameters (Schmidt *et al.*, 2007; Adan, 2010; Randler & Schaal, 2010). The neither-type group usually shows intermediate characteristics, and about 60% of the young adult population belong to it, whereas each extreme group represents 20% of this population respectively (Adan *et al.*, 2008).

Morning- and evening-types are different not only in their rhythmic expression, but also in personality traits and habits, and we could even talk about different life-styles (see Adan *et al.*, 2008 for a revision). The pioneering study by Adan (1994) found differences in the consumption of legal psychoactive substances (nicotine, alcohol and caffeine) among circadian typologies, the evening-type subjects being those who showed more consumption of the three substances. Subsequent works developed in different countries have confirmed this observation, and this is of special relevance for adolescent and young adult populations (Andershed, 2005; Gau *et al.*, 2007; Randler, 2008). A recent study (Prat & Adan, 2011) has also found that the evening-type subjects consume more illegal drugs (cannabis, ecstasy and cocaine) than the morning-type, and have more problems related to hazardous alcohol use and hangover. While the morning circadian typology seems to be a protection factor against the onset and maintenance of drug use, the evening typology may be considered as a risk factor. Adolescence is a critical period in regard to this, since during adolescence there is a higher frequency of evening-type subjects (Andershed, 2005; Roenneberg *et al.*, 2007).

In the initial phases of consumption, individuals who are prone to chronobiological vulnerability (evening-type) may obtain superior effects of regulation in their activation and reinforcement, and this will favour behaviour maintenance (Adan & Sánchez-Turet, 2000; Adan *et al.*, 2008; Prat & Adan, 2011). From this perspective, it has even been suggested that the onset of psychoactive substance consumption might imply in some subjects a self-medication therapy. However, the spiral of stress will appear with chronic consumption (Koob, 2006), and it may be more intense and have more dramatic consequences in the evening-type individuals. Although the association between circadian typology and drug consumption should be explained by a bio-psycho-social model, the theory of the spiral of stress may have an important role in it.

The extreme evening typology also implies a risk factor in the development of other psychopathological disorders, mainly mood disorders (Natale *et al.*, 2005; Grandin *et al.*, 2006; McClung, 2007a; Gaspar-Barba *et al.*, 2009). However, different studies have found a higher prevalence of eating disorders (Natale *et al.*, 2008; Schmitt & Randler, 2010), dysfunctional impulsivity and aggression (Adan *et al.*, 2010), attention-deficit hyperactivity disorder (Caci *et al.*, 2009a) and suicidal behaviour (Selvi *et al.*, 2011) among the evening-type subjects, when compared to the morning-type. These associations may emphasise the role of eveningness as a risk factor also for mental disorders. Circadian typology is being configured as an endophenotype in mental pathology and it clearly has a role in dual pathology, which is currently so prevalent and difficult in terms of therapeutic management. See Figure 3.

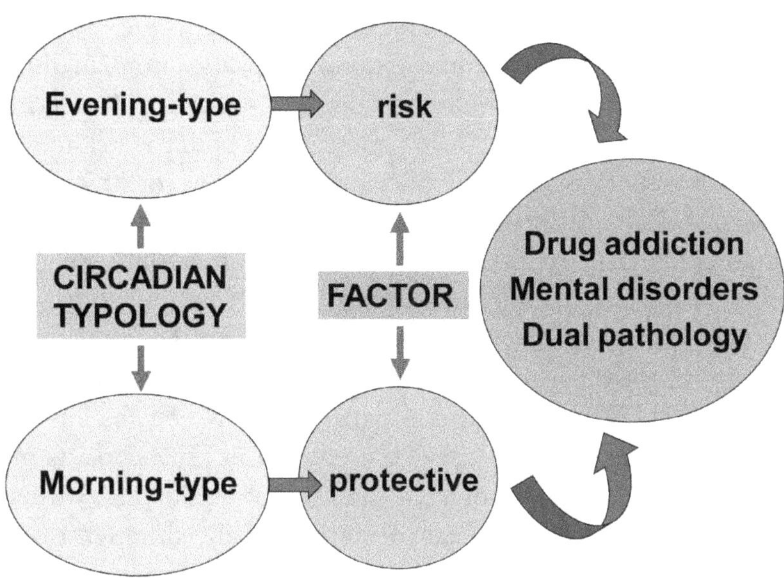

Figure 3. The individual difference of circadian typology is being configured as an endophenotype in mental pathology, including drug addiction and dual pathology.

Therapeutic strategies: time habits, light and melatonin

Preventive and therapeutic approaches to addiction should take into account the circadian rhythmic organisation, with special emphasis on redirecting the time patterns towards a better synchronisation with the light-dark cycle (Adan, 2010). In many cases it may suffice to establish regular time patterns of wake-sleep, meals and daily physical and social activity with a tendency towards a morningness pattern of functioning (Grandin *et al.*, 2006; Kosobud *et al.*, 2007). This is very helpful for patients during the phases of detox and dehabituation. Most of the professional teams working in the area of drug dependencies apply chronobiological behavioural strategies, even though they may not refer to them with this name. Moreover, it is advisable that patients follow the scheduled habits after their therapeutic release, since these promote their quality of life and constitute a protection factor for the risk of relapse (Falcon & McClung, 2009; Adan, 2010).

Exposure to morning light or light therapy may be considered as a first approach when prescribing only scheduled habits is not enough to reorganise circadian rhythmic expression. The scientific evidence available on the non-visual beneficial effects of light are unquestionable and professionals of mental health should obtain updated information in this area. Light produces melatoninergic and serotoninergic agonistic effects, with clinical benefits for mood, sleep, and circadian disorders. This favours the pineal gland to synthesise an adequate peak of night melatonin for a better night sleep (Barion & Zee, 2007) and reduces both the risk to suffer mood disorders as well as the presence of dysphoric symptomatology, which is so frequent in the phases of drug abstinence (Levi & Schibler, 2007; Adan & Prat, 2010).

For patients living in areas with adequate environmental light, it is recommended to get exposure to natural daylight from half an hour to two hours daily (direct sunlight is not necessary), preferably in the morning. The appropriate intensity of light for therapeutic effects is that of 45 minutes after sunrise (Dumont & Beaulieu, 2007). When exposure to natural light is not possible or becomes insufficient, bright light therapy may be used instead. This consists in exposure to artificial light of total spectrum at an intensity of 10,000 lux, with a standard prescription of application of at least 30 minutes daily, although this time may vary if we introduce variations in intensity. Therapeutic light eliminates ultraviolet radiation that may be harmful and has an extremely high blinking frequency in order to avoid the stroboscopic effect. Therapeutic lamps are sold in most countries and their cost is reasonable.

Bright light therapy is a safe treatment (see Table 1) and very effective to organise and direct circadian rhythmicity (Kripke *et al.*, 2007). It is also useful in

Indications	– Jet-lag and work-shifts – Change of sleep phase – Seasonal affective disorder – Major depressive disorder – Bulimia nervosa – Premenstrual syndrome – Chronic fatigue syndrome, fibromyalgia
Counter-indications	– Retinopathies – Manic or hypomanic episode
Adverse effects	– Hypomania – Irritability – Headache – Nausea – Eye irritation

Table 1. Main indications of light therapy, together with its counter-indications and possible adverse effects.

the treatment of depression, both seasonal and common (Even *et al.*, 2008), as well as in some anxiety disorders where there may be an underlying serotoninergic deficit (Terman, 2007). Table 1 summarises the main indications of light therapy, together with its counter-indications and possible adverse effects.

The administration of exogenous melatonin at the end of the day is another chronopharmacological therapeutic possibility to consider in drug addictions. The European Agency for Drug Assessment authorised its use in 2007 as a hypnotic, and it is also sold as a diet supplement in other countries where it is not acknowledged as a pharmacological drug. Melatonin has an organising effect on circadian rhythmicity (hypnotic and day activator), which involves a more conservative treatment and should be considered as a first option when compared to the benzodiazepine and non-benzodiazepine hypnotics traditionally used (Brzezinski *et al.*, 2005; Duvocovich, 2007). Melatonin also has a powerful antioxidant activity (Reiter, 2007; Paradies *et al.*, 2010), which gives it an additional beneficial effect both during the detox and dehabituation treatment as well as in dependent patients who do not stop consuming, in order to minimise the risk of neurodegeneration and the appearance of neuropsychiatric pathology (León *et al.*, 2006; Adan, 2010). For patients older than 40 or with high drug consumption, it is possible to administer melatonin without previous determinations. In young patients and especially in teenagers, the treatment should be of short duration, and it is advisable to programme previous metabolic analyses before prescription to confirm that there has been a decrease of the endogenous production of melatonin.

Melatonin's security is excellent, since no toxic dose is known despite the administration of doses from 600 to 3000 times higher than the therapeutic one. No potential for abuse has been described, and its administration may be interrupted or ended without prescription for withdrawal (Adan, 2009; Adan & Prat, 2010). Its use is counterindicated in very few circumstances and the adverse effects observed during the treatment with melatonin are not very frequent (1/1000 patients), with similar percentages to those obtained with placebo. Table 2 presents the main indications of the melatonin treatment, its counter-indications and possible adverse effects.

Strategies such as setting time habits, exposure to natural or artificial light and the prescription of melatonin, depending on each case, with the IM of reorganising the circadian rhythmic expression, may be highly beneficial in the clinical management of drug addict patients. These strategies may improve the response to treatments, avoiding the need to prescribe certain psychophar-

Indications	– Rhythm synchroniser – Hypnotic. Response in 5 to 20 days – Antioxidant / anti-inflammatory – Immunostimulant
Counter-indications	– Autoimmune disorders – Hyperprolactinemia – Systemic erythematosus lupus – Epilepsy
Precautions	– Kidney or liver failure – Pregnancy and breastfeeding – Youth under 18 years old
Adverse effects	– Sleepiness – Nausea – Tiredness, asthenia – Headaches – Dry mouth – Constipation – Abdominal pain – Irritability, nervousness – Weight increase

Table 2. Main indications of the melatonin treatment, its counter-indications and possible adverse effects.

macological drugs whose management in these patients may be complex due to their counter-indications and a higher risk of adverse reactions or development of dependence. The chronobiological strategies may be highly beneficial in the clinical management of drug-dependent patients, with the advantage that they may be used exclusively or in combination with other more traditional treatments. Moreover, the chronobiological approaches may be applied for long periods of time, even for life, since they have shown an excellent degree of security, and may also be a protective measure against relapse or against the appearance of neuropsychiatric symptoms.

Acknowledgements

Supported by a grant from the Spanish Ministry of Science and Innovation (PSI2009-12300).

References

Abarca, C, Albrecht, U & Spanagel, R (2002). Cocaine sensitization and reward are under the influence of circadian genes and rhythm. *Proceedings of the National Academy of Sciences, 99,* 9026-9030.

Adan, A (1994). Chronotype and personality factors in the daily consumption of alcohol and psychostimulants. *Addiction, 89,* 455-462.

Adan, A (2009). Melatonina: utilidad clínica en el anciano. *Informaciones Psiquiátricas, 195-196,* 21-32.

Adan, A (2010). Ritmicidad circadiana y adicción (Circadian rhythmicity and addiction). *Adicciones, 22,* 5-9.

Adan, A, Natale, V & Caci, H (2008). Cognitive strategies and circadian typology. In: Léglise, A L (Ed.). *Progress in circadian rhythms research.* 141-161. Nova Biomedical Books. New York: Nova Science Publishers, Inc.

Adan, A, Natale, V, Caci, H & Prat, G (2010). Relationship between circadian typology and functional and dysfunctional impulsivity. *Chronobiology International, 27,* 606-619.

Adan, A & Prat, G (2010). Psicofarmacología. De los mecanismos básicos a las estrategias terapéuticas. Barcelona: Marge Médica Books.

Adan, A, Prat, G & Sánchez-Turet, M (2004). Effects of nicotine dependence on diurnal variations of subjective activation and mood. *Addiction, 98,* 1599-1607.

Adan, A & Sánchez-Turet, M (1995). Smoking effects on diurnal variations of cardiovascular parameters. *International Journal of Psychophysiology, 20,* 189-198.

Adan, A & Sánchez-Turet, M (2000). Effects of smoking on diurnal variations of subjective activation and mood. *Human Psychopharmacology Clinical and Experimental, 15,* 287-293.

Andershed, K-A (2005). In sync with adolescence: the role of morningness-eveningness in adolescente. New York: Springer.

Barion, A & Zee, PC (2007). A clinical approach to circadian rhythm sleep disorders. *Sleep Medicine, 8,* 566-577.

Barnard, AR & Nolan, PM (2008). When clocks go bad: neurobehavioral consequences of disrupted circadian timing. *PLoS Genet, 4,* e1000040.

Brzezinski, A, Vangel, MG, Wurtman, RJ, Norrie, G Zhdanova, I, Be-Shushan, A & Ford, I (2005). Effects of exogenous melatonin on sleep: a meta-analysis. *Sleep Medicine Reviews, 9,* 41-50.

Caci, H, Bouchez, J & Baylé, FJ (2009a). Inattentive symptoms of ADHD are related to evening orientation. *Journal Attention Disorders, 13,* 36-41.

Caci, H, Deschaux, O, Adan, A & Natale, V (2009b). Comparing three morningness scales: age and gender effects, structure and cut-off criteria. *Sleep Medicine, 10,* 240-245.

Danel, T & Touitou, Y (2004). Chronobiology of alcohol: from chronokinetics to alcohol-related alterations of the circadian system. *Chronobiology International, 21,* 923-935.

Dumont, M & Beaulieu, C (2007). Light exposure in the natural environment: relevance to mood and sleep disorders. *Sleep Medicine, 8,* 557-565.

Duvocovich, ML (2007). Melatonin receptors: role on sleep and circadian rhythm regulation. *Sleep Medicine, 8,* S34-S42.

Even, C, Schröder, CM, Friedman, S & Rouillon, F (2008). Efficacy of light therapy in nonseasonal depression: A systematic review. *Journal of Affective Disorders, 108,* 11-23.

Falcon, E & McClung, C A (2009). A role for the circadian genes in drug addiction. *Neuropharmacology, 56,* 91-96.

Gaspar-Barba, E, Calati, R, Cruz-Fuentes, CS, Ontiveros-Uribe, MP, Natale, V, De Ronchi, D & Serretti, A (2009). Depressive symptomatology is influenced by chronotypes. *Journal of Affective Disorders, 119,* 100-106.

Gau, SS, Shang, CY, Merikangas, KR, Chiu, YN, Soong, WT & Cheng, AT (2007). Association between morningness–eveningness and behavioral / emotional problems among adolescents. *Journal of Biological Rhythms, 22,* 268-274.

Grandin, LD, Alloy, LB & Abramson LY (2006). The social zeitgeber theory, circadian rhythms, and mood disorders: review and evaluation. *Clinical Psychology Review, 26,* 679-694.

Herzog, ED (2007). Neurons and networks in daily rhythms. *Nature Reviews, 8,* 790-802.

Huang, M-C, Ho, C-W, Chen, C-H, Liu, S-H, Chen, C-C & Leu, SJ (2010). Reduced expression of circadian clock genes in male alcoholic patients. Alcoholism: *Clinical and Experimental Research, 34,* 1899-1904.

Jung-Hynes, B, Reiter, J & Ahmad, N (2009). Sirtuins, melatonin and circadian rhythms: building a bridge between aging and cancer. *Journal of Pineal Research, 48,* 9-19.

Koob, G.F. (2006). The neurobiology of addiction: a neuroadaptational view relevant for diagnosis. *Addiction, 101,* 23-30.

Kosobud, AEK, Gillman, AG, Leffel, JK, Pecoraro, NC, Rebec, GV & Timberlake, W (2007). Drugs ob abuse can entrain circadian rhythms. *The Scientific World Journal, 7 (S2),* 203-212.

Kripke, D Elliott, JA, Youngstedt, SD & Rex, KM (2007). Circadian phase response curves to light in older and young women. *Journal of Circadian Rhythms, 5,* doi: 10.1186/1740-3391-5-4

Lamont, EW, James, FO, Boiven, DB & Carmekian, N (2007). From circadian clock gene expression to pathologies. *Sleep Medicine, 8,* 547-556.

León, J, Escames, G, Rodríguez, MI, López, LC, Tapias, V, Entrena, A, Camacho, E, Carrión, MD, Gallo, MA, Espinosa, A, Tan, D-X, Reiter RJ & Acuña-Castroviejo, D (2006). Inhibition of neuronal nitric oxide synthase activity by N-acetyl-5-metoxikynuramine, a brain metabolite of melatonin. *Neurochemistry, 98,* 2023-2033.

Levi, F & Schibler, U (2007). Circadian rhythms: mechanisms and therapeutic implications. *Annual Review of Pharmacology and Toxicology, 47,* 593-628.

Li, S, Shi, J, Epstein, DH, Wang, X, Zhang, X, Bao, Y, Zhang, D, Zhang, X, Kosten, TR & Lu, L (2009). Circadian alteration in neurobiology during 30 days of abstinence in heroin users. *Biological Psychiatry, 65,* 905-912.

Liu, Y, Wang, Y, Jiang, Z, Wan, C Zhou, W & Wang, Z (2007). The extracellular signal-regulated kinase signalling pathway is involved in the modulation of morphine-induced reward by mPer1. *Neuroscience, 146,* 265-271.

Lovallo, WR (2006). Cortisol secretion patterns in addiction and addiction risk. *International Journal of Psychophysiology, 59,* 195-202.

Manev, H & Uz, T (2006). Clock genes: influencing and being influence by psychoactive drugs. *Trends in Psychopharmacological Sciences, 27,* 186-189.

McCann, UD, Peterson, SC & Ricaurte, GA (2007). The effect of catecholamine depletion by alpha-methyl-para-tyrosine on measures of cognitive performance and sleep in abstinent MDMA users. *Neuropsychopharmacology, 32,* 1695-1706.

McCann, UD & Ricaurte, GA (2007). Effects of (±) 3,4-methylenedioxymethamphetamine (MDMA) on sleep and circadian rhythms. *The Scientific World Journal, 7 (S2),* 231-238.

McClung, CA (2007a). Circadian genes, rhythms and the biology of mood disorders. *Pharmacology & Therapeutics, 11,* 222-232.

McClung, CA (2007b). Circadian rhythms, the mesolimbic dopaminergic circuit, and drug addiction. *The Scientific World Journal, 7 (S2),* 194-202.

McClung, CA, Sidiripoulo, K, Vitaterna, M, Takahashi, JS & White, FJ (2005). Regulation of dopaminergic transmission and cocaine reward by the Clock gene. *Proceedings of the National Academy of Sciences, 102,* 9377-9381.

Natale, V, Adan, A & Scapellato, P (2005). Are seasonality of mood and eveningness closely associated? *Psychiatry Research, 136,* 51–60.

Natale, V, Ballardini, D, Schumann, R, Mencarelli, C & Magelli, V (2008). Morningness-eveningness preference and eating disorders. *Personality and Individual Differences, 45,* 549-553.

Ortiz-Tudela, E, Martinez-Nicolas, A, Campos, M, Rol, MA & Madrid, JM (2010). A new integrated variable based on thermometry, actimetry and body position (TAP) to evaluate the circadian system status in humans. *PLOS Computational Biology, 6(11),* e1000996.

Paradies, G, Petrosillo, G, Paradies, V, Reiter, RJ & Ruggiero, FM (2010). Melatonin, cardiolipin, and mitochondrial bioenergetics in health and disease. *Journal of Pineal Research, 48,* 297-310.

Perreau-Lenz, S & Spanagel, R (2008). The effects of drugs of abuse on clock genes. *Drug News & Perspectives, 21,* 211-217.

Perreau-Lenz, S, Zghoul, T, Rodríguez de Fonseca, F, Spanagel, R & Bilbao, A (2009). Circadian regulation of central ethanol sensitivity by the mPer2 gene. *Addiction Biology, 14,* 253-259.

Prat, G & Adan, A (2011). Influence of circadian typology on drug consume, hazardous alcohol use and hangover symptoms. *Chronobiology International, 28,* 248-257.

Randler, C (2008). Differences between smokers and non-smokers in morningness-eveningness. *Social Behavior and Personality, 36,* 673-680.

Reinberg, A, Touitou, Y, Lewy, H & Mechkouri, M (2010). Habitual moderate alcohol consumption desynchronizes circadian physiologic rhythms and affects reaction-time performance. *Chronobiology International, 27,* 1930-1942.

Reiter, RJ (2007). Medical implications of melatonin: receptor-mediated and receptor-independent actions. *Advances in Medical Sciences, 52,* 11-28.

Rosenwasser, AM (2009). Functional neuroanatomy of sleep and circadian rhythms. *Brain Research Reviews, 61,* 281-306.

Rosenwasser, AM (2010). Circadian clock genes: non-circadian roles in sleep, addiction, and psychiatric disorders? *Neuroscience and Biobehavioral Reviews, 34,* 1249-1255.

Rupp, TL, Acebo, C & Carskadon, MA (2007). Evening alcohol suppresses salivary melatonin in young adults. *Chronobiology International, 24,* 463-470.

Sarabia, JA, Rol, MA, Mendiola, P & Madrid, JA (2008). Circadian rhythm of wrist temperature in normal-living subjects. A new candidate of new index of the circadian system. *Physiology and Behavior, 95,* 570-580.

Scaife, JC & Duka, T (2009). Behavioural measures of frontal lobe function in a population of young social drinkers with binge drinking pattern. *Pharmacology, Biochemistry and Behavior, 93,* 354-362.

Schmidt, S & Randler, C (2010). Morningness-eveningness and eating disorders in a sample of adolescent girls. *Journal of Individual Differences, 31,* 38-45.

Selvi, Y, Aydin, A, Atli, A, Boysan, M, Selvi, F & Besiroglu, L (2011). *Chronobiology International, 28,* 170-175.

Sjöholm, LK, Kovanen, L, Saarikoski, ST, Schalling, M, Lavebratt, C & Partonen, T (2010). Clock is suggested to associate with comorbid alcohol use and depressive disorders. *Journal of Circadian Rhythms, 8,* 1.

Spanagel, R (2009). Alcoholism: a systems approach from molecular physiology to addictive behaviour. *Physiological Reviews, 89,* 649-705.

Spanagel, R, Rosenwasser, AM, Schumann, G & Sarkar, DK (2005). Alcohol consumption and the body's biological clock. *Alcoholism: Clinical and Experimental Research, 29,* 1550-1557.

Tekbas, O F, Ogur, R, Korkmaz, A, Kilic, A & Reiter, RJ (2008). Melatonin as an antibiotic: new insights into the actions of this ubiquitous molecule. *Journal of Pineal Research, 44,* 222-226.

Terman, M (2007). Evolving applications of light therapy. *Sleep Medicine Reviews, 11,* 497-507.

Uz, T, Ahmed, R Akhisaroglu, M Kurtunku, M, Imbese, M, Dirim Arslam, A & Manev, H (2005). Effect of fluoxetine and cocaine in the expression of clock genes in the mousse hippocampus and striatum. *Neuroscience, 134,* 1309-1316.

Wang, X, Wang, Y, Xin, H, Liu, Y, Wang, Y, Zheng, H, Jiang, Z, Wan, C, Wang, Z & Ding, JM (2006). Altered expression of circadian clock gene, mPer1, in mouse brain and kidney under morphine dependence and withdrawal. *Journal of Circadian Rhythms, 4,* 9 doi: 10.1186/1740-3391-4-9.

Sex differences

6 Biological bases of sex differences in drug addiction

MARTA TORRENS[1,2]

[1] Addiction Programme, Institute of Neuropsychiatry
  & Addictions-Parc de Salut Mar
[2] Department of Psychiatry, Autonomous University of Barcelona, Spain

mtorrens@parcdesalutmar.cat

Abstract

In recent years gender differences in substance use disorders (SUDs) have been a focus of research. Although rates of substance abuse are higher in men than women, global studies have indicated that recently women have become increasingly more abusive of drugs and alcohol. We know that distinct gender differences, which increase addiction vulnerability for women, are observed at every phase of the addiction process: drug reinforcement process, acquisition, maintenance, and outcome. The main biological factors related to these differences are the role of neuroactive gonadal steroid hormones in craving and relapse, and sex differences in stress reactivity and relapse to substance abuse. Also, the role of co-occurring mood and anxiety, eating, and post-traumatic stress disorders and co-occurring medical disorders (HIV, hepatitis C infection) are considered in the epidemiology, natural history, and treatment of women with SUDs.

The main gender difference in the epidemiology of drug abuse and dependence, clinical aspects, such as psychiatric comorbidity and medical consequences, biological and subjective factors implicated, social matters, and specific barriers to treatment access will be reviewed.

Key words

Gender; drug addiction; comorbidity; hormones; stress response.

Introduction

Substance use disorders are chronic, relapsing disorders that affect both men and women. The clinical phenotype is the result of a complex interaction between subjective factors (such as genetic variability, psychiatric comorbidity), environmental factors (availability, family and community influences, legality) and drug-related factors (pharmacological effects, drug-induced changes in neurocircuits). Gender, as a crucial subjective factor, plays a central role in determining specific vulnerability, clinical presentation and influencing treatment outcome. Nevertheless, the majority of available data, from the early works on addiction to more recent studies, has largely neglected the role of sex differences in determining vulnerability, epidemiology and clinical issues.

Animal studies have demonstrated remarkable differences between female and male rats during all phases of addiction cycle, but especially at the transition phases. Female rats show a more robust operant behaviour in acquiring self-administration, progressing to higher amounts of substance, reinstatement of extinguished drug-seeking response (Roth *et al.*, 2004).

Craving and reward circuits also show differences concerning gender, stressing the role of the oestrous cycle in determining such variations (Carroll *et al.*, 2004). Studies conducted in humans are also bringing up increasing amounts of evidence about gender difference in addictive disorders. The principal aspects of the epidemiology of drug abuse and dependence, clinical aspects, such as psychiatric comorbidity and medical consequences, the biological and subjective factors involved, social matters, and specific barriers to treatment access will be reviewed.

Epidemiology

Differences in the prevalence and incidence rates of substance abuse between men and women have been constantly observed since the very first studies until present, with men showing significantly higher rates of substance use disorders than women (Wagner & Anthony, 2007; Gruzca *et al.*, 2008). The most recent data, however, points out a tendency towards the narrowing of this gap: if in 1980 a survey conducted on American population found a male/female rate of 5:1 for alcohol dependence (Helzer *et al.*, 1991) more recent data reports a rate of 3:1. The female population is becoming a first line challenge for treatment policy makers. Also, data from the NESARC (National Epidemiologic Survey on Alcohol and Related Conditions), the largest and most recent study on substance use disorders and other psychiatric disorders, show that if men are 2.2 times more likely than women to develop drug abuse, o women show a 1.9 times greater chance to develop a substance dependence disorder. Less conclusive data is shown regarding non-medical prescription, where women could score a higher prevalence then men, according to some studies (Simoni-Wastila *et al.*, 2004) but less according to other authors (Blanco, 2007).

When looking at women suffering from substance use disorders, one crucial phenomenon is "telescoping". Such term describes the accelerated progression, from the early onset of substance use to the development of dependence and first admission to treatment. Telescoping seems to be quite specific of female gender, since women tend to show a faster progression of disease, a more severe clinical profile at the time of admission to treatment. Moreover, women generally need less amount of substance intake and shorter time of use, compared to men, in order to progress to a severe grade of the disorder, where the severity of the clinical profile is not only determined by the addiction itself, but by higher rates of psychiatric and medical comorbidity, social problems and psychological issues. The telescoping effect was first observed and studied in alcohol use disorders, where women showed a significantly shorter time from the time of first consumption to the time of seeking treatment, together with a quicker progress from abuse to dependence on the substance (Randall *et al.*, 1999).

Men and women are found to have different pattern of substance use, as well as specific factors elicitation carving for consumption. Investigation on illicit drugs use, showed that women more often begin or maintain cocaine use in the context of or to improve intimate relationships, where men show a more peer-related pattern of use. Furthermore, female cocaine consumers were shown to develop a more severe dependence with shorter periods of abstinence (Kosten *et al.*, 1996).

Clinical features

Demographical

Women who access treatment programmes for substance use disorders have a more frequent family history of addictive disorders. This characteristic could be explained by a genetic predisposition of addictive disorders (Nelson-Zlupko *et al.*, 1995). It can also be calculated that the addictive disorder develops as a maladaptive response to some environmental stress (Lex, 1991). The relation between stress response circuits and substance use disorders will be discussed in the next section of this chapter.

A family history of disruption and over-responsibility given to women is another common trait of patients seeking help for SUDs (Nelson-Zlupko *et al.*, 1995). Women are also more likely than men to be involved in relationships with a substance-user partner (Nelson-Zlupko *et al.*, 1995), and such relationships are more frequently characterised by a higher rate of violence and abuse. Women in treatment for substance use show a prevalence of being the victims of partners' violence, ranging from 25% up to 57% (El Bassel *et al.*, 2000), where community-based studies show significantly lower values, ranging from between 1.5 and 16% (Caetano *et al.*, 2001).

Women in treatment for addictive disorders are more likely than their male counterpart to be involved in prostitution in order to support their substance use; men, on the other side, are more frequently dedicated to robbery or burglary (Kauffman *et al.*, 1997).

Medical comorbidity

Together with demographic characteristics, women also present other specific clinical traits. Overall a quicker progression to serious liver problems, hypertension, and gastrointestinal disorders is observed. As a consequence of behaviour associated with substance use, such as prostitution and more frequent sex-related risk behaviour, women experience gender-specific health issues, such as genital infections, repeated miscarriages, and premature delivery (Nelson-Zlupko *et al.*, 1995; Kauffman *et al.*, 1997).

HIV infection is a more common occurrence among female drug users than among males (Strathdee *et al.*, 2001). Female drug users report risk behaviours such as sharing needles and injecting paraphernalia, having HIV seropositive sexual partners, having sex with intravenous drug users, sex trading and not using condoms, potentially putting them at greater risk of exposure to HIV (Gilchrist *et al.*, 2011). Higher rates of HIV infection, together with other sexually transmitted infectious diseases, are found in middle aged women, where the lack of concern for pregnancy prevention leads to an easier discontinuation of barrier methods of contraception (Levy *et al.*, 2003).

Alcohol impact in medical comorbidity of women substance users has been deeply studied. Liver cirrhosis, as well as other medical consequences of alcohol intake, show a faster development, and is caused by a much smaller amount of alcohol intake compared to men (Jarque-López *et al.*, 2001). Heart diseases and breast cancer risk is found to be higher for women than it is estimated for their male counterparts. All these factors pooled determine a 50 to 100% higher rate of mortality in women compared to men who have a comparable alcohol use (Wilsnack & Bechman, 1984).

Psychiatric comorbidity

Studies conducted on the general population have highlighted different lifetime prevalence rates of various psychiatric disorders between men and women. Anxiety and mood disorders, as well as borderline personality disorder are clearly higher among the female population, whether or not they have a comorbid SUD. Data from wave 1 of the NESARC, taking into account SUD population, indicate that anxiety rates can reach as much as 29.7%, and mood disorder, namely depression, was found in 15.6% of subjects (Goldstein, 2009).

Significant differences in depressive symptoms showed by problem drinkers enhance the pivotal role of depression in substance use disorders, at least in the female population. The presence of a depressive episode may trigger a relapse in alcohol use, or else, is related to poor adherence and slower response to treatment, and leads to an worse overall clinical outcome. At the same time, alcohol-induced depressive symptoms may be particularly insidious in the case of patients with a previous history of mood disorders (Schutte *et al.*, 1997). Also, in illicit drug users, (cocaine, heroin) both the seeking and non-seeking treatment ones, women show a higher prevalence of mood disorders than men. Moreover, it has been described that such mood disorders are mostly primary rather than being substance-induced (Torrens *et al.*, 2011).

Eating disorders are estimated to have a 2-3 times higher prevalence in women than in men. Among women with SUDs, a particularly high rate of bulimia, purging subtypes, have been reported (Holderness *et al.*, 1994).

Lastly, post-traumatic stress disorder (PTSD) shows a higher prevalence in women than in men of up to 5 times more. When focusing on substance consumers, the higher chances for them to have experienced some physical or sexual abuse (from 55 to 99%) may account for a high rate of women experiencing trauma-related symptoms (Najavits *et al.*, 1997).

Specific barriers to treatment

Substance use was historically considered a problem that primarily, if not exclusively, affected men. Many studies have been conducted on population constituted mainly by men. Therefore, most of the available treatment programmes were developed according to male patient population characteristics and needs. A growing amount of data shows that the female population has specific features, and male-oriented treatment programmes may not address their needs in a satisfactory way and they may even become a barrier to access and entry treatment. If the average ratio of women entering treatment is less than one third of all patients, we have to assume that women still enter treatment programmes less than men, since the prevalence of women affected by substance use is over 30% (Brady & Ashley, 2005).

Women tend to be more frequently referred to treatment from community agencies, such as welfare, mental health providers or other health providers rather than spontaneously seeking a specific treatment for their addiction. Men, though, are twice as likely to be referred from the criminal justice system (40%, versus only 27% of women; Office of Applied studies, Substance Abuse and Mental Health Services Administration, 2006).

Specific barriers for women may include pregnancy, lack of care for pregnant women, fear of losing custody of child (Greenfield *et al.*, 2007). Fears of prosecution, voyeurism and sexual harassment have also been claimed as deterring factors (Pelissier & Jones, 2005). Child care seems to be the most critical problem for women seeking treatments: a lack of child care provided on-site, most women are likely to encounter hostility and resistance from their own families. Moreover, since the social conditions of women affected by SUDs are lower when compared to men's, they report greater problems in accessing treatment sites by public transportation (Ayyagari *et al.*, 1999). Studies performed in the USA population also detect that women, more often than men, lack an adequate health insurance coverage, which does not pay for the substance use disorders treatment (Hodgins *et al.*, 1997). Finally, the more frequent involvement in relationships with a drug-user partner has been associated with a less supportive attitude of the partner towards her access and retention in treatment (Bride, 2001).

Several studies are pointing out the growing need to develop adequate programmes, to address substance use disorders while taking care of medical issues. The high prevalence of medical comorbidity as well as specific problems, such as parenting issues and maternity care, demands the development of programmes targeting such matters, and minimising barriers to treatment for women seeking help.

As well as medical comorbidity, psychiatric disorders co-occurring in women represent a crucial element to consider, when approaching a female patient with substance use disorder. Underdiagnosed psychiatric disorders may be a first obstacle for the patient to access and remain in treatment, as well as for a successful outcome of the treatment itself.

Biological factors

Gender differences might be biologically related to neuroactive gonadal steroid hormones, as well as to neuroendocrine stress response.

Neuroactive Gonadal Steroid Hormones

Ovarian steroid hormones (e.g., oestrogen, progesterone), metabolites of progesterone, and negative allosteric modulators of the g-aminobutyric acid A (GABA-A) receptor, such as dehydroepiandrostenedione (DHEA), may influence the behavioural effects of drugs (Mello *et al.*, 2011). Progesterone attenuates the subjective response to smoked cocaine in women, but not men. The follicular phase of the menstrual cycle, in which oestradiol levels are high and progesterone is low, is associated with the greatest responsivity to stimulants (Sofuoglu *et al.*, 2004). Furthermore, in women with cocaine dependence, craving for the substance did show a positive correlation with negative moods during follicular and luteal phases. Progesterone was demonstrated to diminish stress and drug-induced craving, as well as cue-triggered anxiety (Del Rio *et al.*, 1998).

Neuroendocrine stress response

Preclinical data as well as clinical studies on the human population point out the close relationship between stress response and drug abuse, both in the motivation and in the maintenance phase of substance use (Fox & Sinha, 2009). Animal studies have brought clear support on how stress paradigms induce and maintain self-administration of opiates and alcohol (Shalev *et al.,* 2003).

The human model of coping with stress and relapse-prevention have been applied to investigate the implication of stress response circuit in drug addiction development (Marlatt & Gordon, 1985). This model presents the addiction as a result of a maladaptive response to life stressors, or else as a risk factor in subjects with poor coping capacity. Moreover, reinforcement to drug consumption can also be explained by the tension-relieving effect, as well as the "self medication" models. Overall, events that increase stress and negative moods have been shown to be strong craving inducers and predictors of drug use relapse, both in alcohol and cocaine dependent individuals (Brady *et al.,* 2006; Sinha *et al.,* 2006). Therefore, great impulse has been given to research on the hypothalamic-pituitary-adrenal (HPA) axis and its drug-induced changes.

Drug-related alterations of HPA, sympathetic adrenal medullary system (SAM) and mesolimbic dopamine (DA) together with stress and reward system pathways may bring tremendous knowledge to the pathophysiology of substance addiction disorders (Volkow et al,, 1999; Shalev *et al.,* 2002). Overlaps between reward and stress response circuits have been strongly supported by data in the literature (Sinha, 2007). Stress circuits engagement could alter central reward system balance, via alteration in the DA transmission (Piazza & Le Moal, 1997). The sustained increase of DA secretion as a result of altered circuit homeostasis may result in the increased sensitivity of stress related circuits (Koob & Le Moal, 2005).

If acute administration of alcohol and cocaine was shown to influence DA transmission, HPA activity and glucocorticoids secretion response (Adinoff *et al.,* 2003), clinical observations support the evidence of drug-related changes of stress sensitivity, especially during substance withdrawal (Sinha, 2007).

The interactions between HPA axis, stress systems and sex hormones in women is rather complex, still for a long time such interplay has been indicated to play a central role in gender variation of stress response after drug intake. Initial data seemed to suggest that oestradiol could have an excitatory role on HPA, where progesterone would be responsible for an inhibitory effect. Such data raised interest in the importance of the hormonal variation of stress response induced by drug administration, as well as craving and relapse vulnerability (Mc Cormick & Marheuws, 2007). Further studies have come to the conclusion that the oestradiol excitatory effect is rather a result of the lack of progesterone inhibiting acute stimulatory effects (Justice & de Wit, 2000). Progesterone may indeed mask or else attenuate subjective effects of cocaine and amphetamines both in healthy and in female cocaine dependent subjects, while during the luteal phase of MC. greater "high" effects were reported with smoked cocaine (Evans *et al.*, 2002).

Gender differences in stress response and correlated changes in stress-systems has been studied since the early 70s, when the first data emerged about an impaired catecholamine response to stressors in females compared to men (Frankenhaeuser *et al.*, 1978). Further clinical data confirmed that men consistently had a higher heart rate, higher blood pressure and greater HPA sensitivity compared to matched female subjects, when challenged with standardised experimental stressors (Kirschbaum *et al.*, 1999). Interestingly, despite such enhanced physiological stress response, men report a significantly lower rate of distress to the challenge.

Gender differences in stress-systems alterations have been investigated, despite multiple methodological difficulties. Few agreements have been reached, although we are still missing detailed conclusions.

1. Women with substance use disorder present higher emotional sensitivity then men to stress systems variations, especially if triggered by acute drug administration (Fox & Sinha, 2009).
2. They show a stronger emotional response after stress as well as after drug cue stimuli exposure (Fox & Sinha, 2009).
3. Evidence has been put forward showing that women with alcohol and cocaine dependence show a significant imbalance in their HPA axis response to stress. An altered cortisol response to ACTH stimulation was detected, and a blunted cortisol response to stress in SUD female subjects could be involved in relapse vulnerability (O'Malley *et al.*, 2002).
4. Hormonal changes and fluctuations correlated to the menstrual cycle can also influence stress systems adjustments in women with SUD.

Mood and anxiety, as well as other negative emotional statuses show a consistent positive correlation with craving induction in alcohol dependent women (Fox *et al.*, 2007; Sinha *et al.*, 2008). Similarly, cocaine craving is found to be strongly enhanced by stress-related anxiety and sadness (Fox *et al.*, 2008).

Conclusions

Gender differences in substance use and dependence is now a well-established fact. Despite still showing higher prevalence in the male population, a growing incidence of substance use disorders in females, as well as the identification of clinical specific characteristics, demand the development of gender-specific research and treatment planning.

Women show different patterns of substance use, faster and easier progression to a severe state of the disease, as well as more frequent a problematic medical and psychiatric comorbidity.

Because of specific clinical features and social issues, women still have greater difficulties in accessing treatment programmes, and overall show poorer outcomes.

Further investigation and knowledge on the biological basis of gender differences in response to drug intake, as well as stress induced relapse vulnerability is a major challenge in order to design specific treatment and prevention strategies for women.

Acknowledgments

Financial support was received from the Instituto de Salud Carlos III FEDER (Red de Trastornos Adictivos-RTA RD06/001/1009). I would like to thank Dr Paola Rossi for her helpful comments and editing assistance.

References

Adinoff, B, Ruether, K, Krebaum, S, Iranmanesh, A & Williams, M J (2003). Increased salivary cortisol concentrations during chronic alcohol intoxication in a naturalistic clinical sample of men. *Alcohol and Clinical Experimental Research, 27,* 1420–1427.

Ayyagari, S, Boles, S, Johnson, P & Kleber, H (1999). Difficulties in recruiting pregnant substance abusing women into treatment: problems encountered during the cocaine alternative treatment study. *Health Services Research, 16,* 80-81.

Blanco, C, Alderson, D, Ogburn, E, Grant, B F, Nunes, EV, Hatzenbuehler, ML & Hasin, DS (2007). Changes in the prevalence of non-medical prescription drug use and drug use disorders in the United States: 1991-1992 and 2001-2002. *Drug and Alcohol Dependence, 90,* 252-260.

Brady, KT, Waldrop, AE, McRae, AL, *et al.* (2006). The impact of alcohol dependence and posttraumatic stress disorder on cold pressor task response. *Journal of Studies on Alcohol, 67,* 700-706.

Brady, TM, Ashley, OS (Eds.) (2005). Women in substance abuse treatment: results from the Alcohol and Drug Services Study (ADSS). Rockville,MD: *Substance Abuse and Mental Health Services Administration, Office of Applied Studies*; DHHS Publication, No. SMA 04-3968, Analytic Series A-26.

Bride, BE (2001). Single-gender treatment of substance abuse: effect on treatment retention and completion. *Social Work Research, 25,* 223-232.

Caetano, R, Nelson, S & Cunradi, C (2001). Intimate partner violence: dependence symptoms and social consequences from drinking among White, Black and Hispanic couples in the United States. *American Journal on Addiction, 10,* 60-69.

Carroll, ME, Lynch, WY, Roth, ME, Morgan, AD & Cosgrove, KP (2004). Sex and estrogen influence drug abuse. *Trends in Pharmacological Sciences, 25,* 273-279.

Del Rio, G, Velardo, A, Menozzi, R, *et al.* (1998). Acute estradiol and progesterone administration reduced cardiovascular and catecholamine responses to mental stress in menopausal women. *Neuroendocrinology, 67,* 269-274.

El-Bassel, N, Gilbert, L, Shilling, R, Wada, T (2000). Abuse and partner violence among women in methadone treatment. *Journal of Family Violence, 15,* 209-228.

Evans, SM, Haney, M & Foltin, RW (2002). The effects of smoked cocaine during the follicular and luteal phases of the menstrual cycle in women. *Psychopharmacology, 159,* 397-406.

Fox, HC, Berquist, KL, Hong, KI & Sinha, R (2007). Stress-induced and alcohol cue-induced craving in recently abstinent alcohol dependent individuals. *Alcohol and Clinical Experimental Research, 31,* 395-403.

Fox, HC, Hong, KA, Siedlarz, KM & Sinha, R (2008). Enhanced sensitivity to stress and drug/alcohol craving in abstinent cocaine dependent individuals compared to social drinkers. *Neuropsychopharmacology, 33,* 796-805.

Fox, HC & Sinha, R (2009). Sex differences in drug-related stress-system changes: implications for treatment in substance-abusing women. *Harvard Review of Psychiatry, 17,* 103-119.

Frankenhaeuser, M, von Wright, MR, Collins, A, von Wright, J, Sedvall, G & Swahn, CG (1978). Sex differences in psychoneuroendocrine reactions to examination stress. *Psychosomatic Medicine, 40,* 334-343.

Gilchrist, G, Blazquez, A, & Torrens, M (2011) Psychiatric, behavioural and social risk factors for HIV infection among female drug users. *AIDS and Behavior, 15,* 1834-1843.

Goldstein, RB (2009). Comorbidity of substance use with independent mood and anxiety disorders in women: results from the National Epidemiologic Survey on Alcohol and Related Conditions. In: Brady KT, Back SE, Greenfield SF, editors. *Women and addiction: a comprehensive handbook.* 173-192. New York: Guilford Press;

Greenfield, SF, Brooks, AJ, Gordon, SM, *et al.* (2007). Substance abuse treatment entry, retention, and outcome in women: a review of the literature. *Drug and Alcohol Dependence, 86,* 1-21.

Grucza, RA, Norberg, K, Bucholz, KK, *et al.* (2008). Correspondence between secular changes in alcohol dependence and age of drinking onset among women in the United States. *Alcohol and Clinical Experimental Research, 32,* 1493–1501.

Helzer, JE, Burnam, A & McEvoy, LT (1991). Alcohol abuse and dependence. In: Robins L.N. & Regier D.A. (Eds.). *Psychiatric disorders in America: the epidemiological catchment area study.* 81-115. New York: The Free Press.

Hodgins, DC, Ed-Guebaly, N & Addington, J (1997). Treatment of substance abusers: single or mixed gender programs? *Addiction, 92,* 805-812.

Holderness, CC, Brooks-Gunn, J & Warren, MP (1994). Co-morbidity of eating disorders and substance abuse: review of the literature. *International Journal of Eating Disorders, 16,* 1-34.

Jarque-Lopez, A, Gonzalez-Reimers, E & Rodríguez, F (2001). Prevalence and mortality of heavy drinkers in a general medical hospital unit. *Alcohol and Alcoholism, 36,* 335-338.

Justice, AJ & de Wit, H (2000). Acute effects of d-amphetamine during the early and late follicular phases of the menstrual cycle in women. *Pharmacology Biochemistry & Behavior, 66,* 509-515.

Kauffman, SE, Silver, P & Poulin, J (1997). Gender differences in attitudes toward alcohol, tobacco, and other drugs. *Social Work, 42,* 231-241.

Kirschbaum, C, Kudielka, BM, Gaab, J, Schommer, NC & Hellhammer, DH (1999). Impact of gender, menstrual cycle phase, and oral contraceptives on the activity of the hypothalamuspituitary-adrenal axis. *Psychosomatic Medicine, 61,* 154-162.

Koob, GF & Le Moal, M (2005). Plasticity of reward neurocircuitry and the "dark side" of drug addiction. *Nature Neuroscience, 8,* 1442-1444.

Kosten, TR, Kosten, TA, McDougle, CJ, *et al.* (1996). Gender differences in response to intranasal cocaine administration to humans. *Biological Psychiatry, 39,* 147-148.

Levy, JA, Ory, MG & Crystal, S (2003). HIV/AIDS interventions for midlife and older adults: current status and challenges. *Journal of Acquired Immune Deficiency Syndromes, 33,* S59-S67.

Lex BW. (1991). Gender differences and substance abuse. *Advances in Substance Abuse, 4,* 225-296.

Marlatt, GA & Gordon, JR (1985). *Relapse prevention: maintenance strategies in the treatment of addictive behaviors.* New York: Guilford.

McCormick, CM & Mathews, IZ (2007). HPA function in adolescence: role of sex hormones in its regulation and the enduring consequences of exposure to stressors. *Pharmacology Biochemistry & Behavior, 86,* 220-233.

Mello, NK, Knudson, IM, Kelly, M, Fivel, PA & Mendelson, JH (2011). Effects of progesterone and testosterone on cocaine self-administration and cocaine discrimination by female rhesus monkeys. *Neuropsychopharmacology, 36,* 2187-2199.

Najavits, LM, Weiss, R & Shaw, S (1997). The link between substance abuse and posttraumatic stress disorder in women: a research review. *American Journal on Addiction, 6,* 237-283.

Nelson-Zlupko, L, Kauffman, E & Dore, MM (1995). Gender differences in drug addiction and treatment: implications for social work intervention with substance-abusing women. *Social Work, 40,* 45-54.

O'Malley, SS, Krishnan-Sarin, S, Farren, C, Sinha, R & Kreek, MJ (2002). Naltrexone decreases craving and alcohol self-administration in alcohol-dependent subjects and activates the hypothalamopituitaryadrenocortical axis. *Psychopharmacology, 160,* 19-29.

Office of Applied Studies, Substance Abuse and Mental Health Services Administration. (2006). Treatment Episode Data Set (TEDS) highlights-2005 national admissions to substance abuse treatment services: 1995–2005. Rockville (MD): SAMHSA; Available at: *http://oas.samhsa.gov/teds2k5/TEDSHi2k5.htm*

Pelissier, B & Jones, N (2005), A review of gender differences among substance abusers. *Crime Delinquency, 51,* 343-372.

Piazza PV, Le Moal M. (1997) Glucocorticoids as a biological substrate of reward: physiological and pathophysiological implications. *Brain Research Review, 25,* 359-372.

Randall, CL, Roberts, JS, DelBoca, FK, Carroll, KM, Connors, GC, Mattson, ME (1999). Telescoping of landmark events associated with drinking: a gender comparison. *Journal of Studies on Alcohol, 60,* 252-260.

Roth, ME, Cosgrove, KP & Carroll, ME (2004). Sex differences in the vulnerability to drug abuse: a review of preclinical studies. *Neuroscience & Biobehavioral Reviews, 28,* 533-546.

Schutte, KK, Seable, JH & Moos, RH (1997). Gender differences in the relations between depressive symptoms and drinking behavior among problem drinkers: a threewave study. *Journal of Consulting and Clinical Psychology, 65,* 392-404.

Shalev, U, Grimm, JW & Shaham, Y (2002). Neurobiology of relapse to heroin and cocaine seeking: a review. *Pharmacological Reviews, 54,* 1-42.

Shalev, U, Marinelli, M, Baumann, MH, Piazza, PV & Shaham, Y (2003). The role of corticosterone in food deprivation-induced reinstatement of cocaine seeking in the rat. *Psychopharmacology, 168,* 170-176.

Simoni-Wastila, L, Ritter, G & Strickler, G (2004). Gender and other factors associated with the nonmedical use of abusable prescription drugs. *Substance Use and Misuse, 39,* 1-23.

Sinha, R, Fox, HC, Hong, KA, Bergquist, KL, Bhagwagar, Z & Siedlarz, KM (2008). Enhanced negative emotion and alcohol craving, and altered physiological responses following stress and cue exposure in alcohol dependent individuals. *Neuropsychopharmacology, 33,* 796-780.

Sinha, R (2007). The role of stress in addiction relapse. *Current Psychiatry Reports, 9,* 388-395.

Sinha, R, Garcia, M, Paliwal, P, Kreek, MJ & Rounsaville, BJ (2006). Stress-induced cocaine craving and hypothalamic-pituitary-adrenal responses are predictive of cocaine relapse outcomes. *Archives of General Psychiatry, 63,* 324-331.

Sofuoglu, M, Mitchell, E & Kosten, TR (2004). Effects of progesterone treatment on cocaine responses in male and female cocaine users. *Pharmacology Biochemistry & Behavior, 78,* 699-705.

Strathdee, SA, Galai, N, Safaiean, M, *et al.* (2001) Sex differences in risk factors for HIV seroconversion among injection drug users: a 10-year perspective. *Archives of Internal Medicine, 161,* 1281-1288.

Torrens, M, Gilchrist, G, Domingo-Salvany, A, psyCoBarcelona Group. (2011). Psychiatric comorbidity in illicit drug users: substance-induced versus independent disorders. *Drug and Alcohol Dependence, 113,* 147-156.

Volkow, ND, Fowler, JS & Wang, GJ (1999). Imaging studies on the role of dopamine in cocaine reinforcement and addiction in humans. *Journal of Psychopharmacology, 13,* 337-345.

Wagner, FA & Anthony, JC (2007). Male-female differences in the risk of progression from first use to dependence upon cannabis, cocaine, and alcohol. *Drug and Alcohol Dependence, 86,* 191-198.

Wilsnack, SC & Bechman, LJ (Eds.) (1984). *Alcohol problems in women: antecedents, consequences, and intervention.* New York: Guilford Press.

7 Female polydrug abuse and psychopathology – Gender differences: An overview

EDLE RAVNDAL

Norwegian Centre for Addiction Research (SERAF)
University of Oslo, Norway

edle.ravndal@medisin.uio.no

Abstract

The literature focusing on female substance abuse and psychopathology is scarce, and several methodological problems have to be considered. Different sample characteristics, diagnostic criteria and assessment procedures are main factors that cause problems in drawing final conclusions. The prevalence of Axis I and II disorder are by far more significant in clinical samples/ reviews compared to normal population studies. In a literature review of different treatment populations, females had a higher prevalence of psychiatric symptoms than males, but calculating the median value, there were no differences between females and males as to the total prevalence of psychiatric symptoms. However, in several other treatment studies of female substance abusers the prevalence of depression, anxiety disorders, post-traumatic stress disorders (PTSD) and eating disorders are significantly higher than among substance-abusing males. Very few studies have examined personality disorders (PD) and gender differences among substance abusers. In a literature review there was a tendency towards more PDs among women than among men. Altogether the prevalence of antisocial PD was significantly higher among males than among females, while no gender difference was found for borderline PD.

According to female-specific theories, women's focus on relationships is seen as natural and necessary - rather than pathologised as dependence or lack of a sense of self. The relational perspective in understanding female substance abuse and psychopathology is therefore of utmost importance for treatment and recovery. There are also important physical and biological gender differences that are of great importance in understanding female substance abuse and psychopathology.

Key words

Substance abuse; drug abuse; female; psychopathology; gender.

Introduction

In literature concerning substance use, there are many different definitions of the substances being used and the degree of dependence.[1] Alcohol use, drug use, substance use, poly-substance use, and polydrug use are among the most used terms. As for indications as to the *degree* of dependence, terms like substance/drug use, misuse, abuse, and addiction are the most common. However, upon reading the literature, the use of these terms is not always based on the same definitions, making it quite difficult to compare different studies that seem to be based on more or less similar populations.

The aim of the present literature review is to look at gender differences in psychopathology among polydrug abusers. However, many studies presenting substance use/abuse populations seem to have materials with quite similar drug abuse patterns as studies using the term polydrug abusers. These studies are therefore also included in the review. In addition, some studies of female alcohol abuse have been included in order to research whether there are clear cut differences between females using legal substances such as alcohol versus females using illegal substances such as opiates, amphetamines, cannabis, etc.

---

[1] Literature search was performed using bases such as Medline, Psychlit, Embase and ISI (the National Library on Addictions, the Norwegian Institute of Alcohol and Drug Research).

In this literature review I have chosen to use the term *substance abuse* (that may also include alcohol abuse) most of the time, since this term seems to be the most used in the literature at hand.

Undertaking a literature review of gender differences concerning substance abuse and psychopathology is quite demanding with regard to methodological problems. Firstly, the prevalence of Axis I and Axis II disorders may vary according to certain *sample characteristics* such as age, setting and primary substance at use. For example, it is well known that non-maintenance clients in inpatient settings, compared to non-maintenance clients in outpatient settings, have more severe substance abuse problems and more psychiatric co-morbidity. Therefore it may be assumed that inpatient clients have a higher prevalence of both Axis I and II disorders than outpatients. However, for clients in maintenance treatment this difference in substance abuse history and psychopathology between in- and outpatients does not necessarily exist.

Secondly, *diagnostic criteria,* which depend on the chosen classification system, the time-frame that is employed when setting diagnosis, and the use of exclusion criteria, may vary a lot.

Finally, *assessment procedures* may have an effect on the observed prevalence rate. For example some authors argue that self-report instruments overestimate the prevalence of PDs more than interview methods, leading to higher reported prevalence rates (Hunt *et al.,* 1992; Widiger *et al.,* 1987). However, others researchers contend that even if the two methods will diagnose a certain amount of PDs, they will probably identify somewhat different dimensions of the same underlying disorder because of the different approaches used (Torgersen & Alnæs, 1990, Butler *et al.,* 1991).

In almost all studies, setting, the primary substance of use, and assessment methods are reported on. However, information concerning some of the other factors, like gender, time-frame and the use of exclusion criteria, are provided by far fewer studies.

In fact, most studies on alcohol and drug dependence pay little or no attention to gender differences. In addition, co-morbid DSM-IV Axis I and II disorders in substance abusers have mostly been studied in separate samples. There is also limited knowledge about the relationship between gender and personality disorders (PD) in different subtypes of substance abusers (Landheim *et al.,* 2003).

With this background, considering all the methodological weakness, I will try to present the main characteristics of female substance abusers as to both Axis 1 and Axis II disorders. Sometimes an explicit comparison will be made with male substance abusers, and sometimes not.

However, not only mapping Axis I and II disorders may present different problems among females and males. Women's more basic way of behaving and relating to others, also seems to be of utmost importance when trying to understand their substance abuse problems and how to help them when they seek treatment (Beyer & Conahan, 2002). In the same line, it is also important to take into consideration that women's biological and genetic reactions to different substances may be quite different compared to men.

Psychiatric co-morbidity and gender difference

Large-scale, national studies using community samples show some consistent gender differences in the overall co-occurrence of psychiatric disorders (Regier *et al.*, 1988; Kessler *et al.*, 1994; Grant *et al.*, 2004). Anxiety and affective disorders are most likely to co-occur in women while substance disorders, conduct disorders, and antisocial personality disorders are those most likely to co-occur in men (Kessler *et al.*, 1997).

Prevalence of psychiatric symptoms among substance abusers in the general population

Data from the National Co-morbidity Survey (NCS), collected in 1994 have been analysed to derive specific gender differences and similarities in psychiatric co-morbidity among the problem-drinking community subgroup. The majority of people in the NCS community sample with an alcohol disorder had at least one psychiatric disorder as well. Furthermore, the co-occurrence was stronger among women than in men (Kessler *et al.*, 1997). The lifetime prevalence of alcohol abuse was 6.4 percent among women and 12.5 percent for men. Lifetime alcohol dependence rates were 8.2 percent and 20.1 percent, respectively. Over the course of a lifetime, drug dependence co-occurred with alcohol dependence in 34.5 percent of women and 29.5 percent of men. Furthermore, larger portions of women than men with alcohol abuse or dependence reported prior anxiety disorders, affective disorders and drug disorders. The presence of prior psychiatric disorders was predictive of alcohol dependence, especially among women. Lifetime co-occurrence was positively associated with the persistence of alcohol dependence in both women and men.

Prevalence of personality disorders among substance abusers in the general population

There are few studies from the general population that show the prevalence of personality disorders (PD). The Epidemiological Catchment Area Study (ECA-study) shows that 14% of persons with an alcohol disorder had an antisocial PD, while the prevalence was somewhat higher for persons with other substance disorders (18%). Another population study from the USA indicated that among persons with an alcohol disorder, 29% had at least one PD, compared to 48% among persons with a drug abuse disorder. Antisocial, histrionic and dependent PD was the most common both among alcohol abusers and drug abusers (Grant *et al.*, 2004).

There are relatively few studies from the general population that show the prevalence of psychiatric disorders among substance abusers. In general, existing studies show a high prevalence of both psychiatric symptoms and PD among persons with substance abuse, which is far higher than among persons without substance abuse. Furthermore, drug abusers have a higher prevalence of psychiatric symptoms and PDs than alcohol abusers. Most studies show that the more serious the substance abuse is, the more serious the psychiatric disorders. Female substance abusers also have more psychiatric symptoms than males.

In general, persons with the most serious substance abuse, and most psychiatric disorders are more prone to seek treatment (Berkson's fallacy). Hence, the prevalence of psychiatric co-morbidity is higher in studies of clinical populations than in general population studies.

Prevalence of psychiatric symptoms among substance abusers in treatment

In a review of 16 studies that researched psychiatric symptoms among alcohol abusers and/or drug abusers in treatment, gender differences were reported in eight (Landheim, 2007). The 16 chosen studies were based on well-known diagnostic instruments, included 100 persons or more and were cross-checked with two relevant literature reviews (Bradizza *et al.*, 2006; Hintz & Mann, 2005). Most of the studies had researched life-time prevalence of psychiatric symptoms. In six of the studies, females had a higher prevalence of psychiatric symptoms than males, but when calculating the median value, there were no differences between females and males with regard to the total prevalence of psychiatric symptoms. In samples with females the prevalence varied between 33-85% (median: 69%), while in samples with males the corresponding percentages were 16-84% (median: 70%).

However, several separate studies have shown significant differences in psychopathology between women and men who seek help for substance dependency (Brady *et al.*, 1993; Magura *et al.*, 1998). In Brady *et al.*'s (1993) descriptive study of 100 inpatient substance abusers, women were significantly more likely to have another current Axis I disorder in addition to substance abuse. The finding is consistent with the Epidemiological Catchment Area (ECA) study of the general population, which found that Axis I diagnoses were twice as prevalent in women (Regier *et al.*, 1988). Women had almost twice the number of current anxiety disorders as men, particular panic disorder (18 percent versus 10 percent) and post-traumatic stress disorders (PTSD) (46 percent versus 24 percent). These rates are substantially higher than the ECA data of the general population of women. No significant differences were found in the rates of affective disorders between female and male substance abusers, which contrasts the findings in the ECA study in which major depression was twice as common in women as in men (Weissman & Klerman, 1977). In addition, the majority of addicted men experienced the onset of depression after the onset of substance abuse, indicating a more substance-induced condition in men. For both women and men, social phobia and PTSD predated the onset of substance dependence in the majority of cases, which would support a self-medication hypothesis.

The findings from the BioMed II IPTRP project, with a sample of 828 inpatients in 30 different therapeutic communities in nine European countries (De Wilde *et al.*, 2004; De Wilde *et al.*, 2006), are in line with the American literature in the field. In this study, using the EuropASI, women were more likely to report depression, problems in understanding, concentrating or remembering, and were prescribed more medication than their male counterparts. They also reported more serious thoughts of suicide and had attempted suicides more often than men. They also had a more serious history of sexual abuse.

Brady *et al.* (1993) found more pronounced gender differences within primary alcoholics. Female alcoholics had substantially more anxiety and affective disorders than males, the ratios of which are consistent with the ECA data. Panic disorder was significantly more likely to predate alcoholism in women, supporting the use of alcohol to self-medicate. In contrast, within the primary cocaine dependent group, no significant gender differences in psychopathology were found between genders. Use of cocaine was not found to precipitate depressive episodes that outlasted intoxication and withdrawal, thereby minimising any gender differences. There were no differences in Axis II diagnoses between genders.

Landheim *et al.* (2003) show in their study of poly-substance abusers and pure alcoholics seeking treatment, that among women poly-substance abusers the prevalence of PTSD is significantly higher than among pure alcoholics (38% vs. 17%) and that female poly-substance abusers have significantly more PTSD than male poly-substance abusers (38% vs. 21%).

Magura *et al.* (1998) studied a sample of 212 methadone patients who were dually addicted to opiates and cocaine. Similar to the findings in the National Comorbidity Survey (Kessler *et al.*, 1994), women addicts were more likely than men to present concurrent mood and anxiety disorders. Methadone-dependent women with an antisocial PD were likely to continue their opiate abuse and were less likely to have a concurrent alcohol use disorder.

In a study of treatment-seeking opiate abusers, life-time psychiatric comorbidity (in particular, major depression, social phobia, eating disorders) was more than twice as common in women as in men (Brooner *et al.*, 1997).

A high frequency of PTSD among female poly-substance abusers is found in several both clinical and epidemiological studies (Helzer *et al.*, 1987; Cottler *et al.*, 1992; Brady *et al.*, 1998). In a longitudinal, national study in the USA, Kilpatrick *et al.* (1997) demonstrated that the use of illicit drugs was strongly associated with both sexual and physical assaults in women. In the ECA study, Cottler *et al.* (1992) found that female gender and the use of cocaine or opiates were the strongest predictors of PTSD. This shows the importance of identifying and focusing on the treatment of PTSD in many female substance abusers.

Patients seeking detoxification and dual diagnosis inpatient treatment were studied by Westreich *et al.* (1997). Females more often had an affective disorder, while men more often were admitted with a diagnosis of schizophrenia than women. Women were also more often diagnosed with psychosis, substance-induced hallucinations and borderline PD. Furthermore, the higher percentage of women in detoxification with previous psychiatric treatment seems also to suggest that women were directed to psychiatric services rather than to addiction services. Women also reported to be fearful of treatment due to the belief that they could lose their children or there would be inadequate care for the children. The findings of Westreich *et al.* (1997) replicate the results of an earlier study of dually diagnosed outpatients (Comtois & Ries, 1995), which also found that women more often were diagnosed with affective disorders and men with schizophrenia.

Prevalence of personality disorders (PD) among substance abusers in treatment

There are considerable differences in the prevalence of PDs among substance abusers in treatment. As mentioned before, these variations are mostly due to different characteristics of the samples, use of different diagnostic instruments and use of different time windows in treatment when making the diagnosis. Even if the prevalence rates are very varying in the different studies, in general the average rate is quite high (median: 61%), and most studies show more PDs in samples of drug abusers than among alcohol abusers (Landheim, 2007). There are also very few studies that have examined PD and gender differences.

Verheul *et al.* (1995) summarised 52 studies that researched the total prevalence of PD and the prevalence of antisocial and borderline PD among substance abusers in treatment. Twelve of the studies looked at gender differences, but only three studies researched the prevalence of all PDs. These three studies showed a tendency towards more PDs among women than among men. Altogether more men than women had an antisocial PD (median: 39% vs. 19%), while no gender difference was found for borderline PD.

A Norwegian study examined gender differences in the prevalence of symptom disorders and PDs among substance abusers seeking treatment (n=260) (Landheim *et al.*, 2003). The main findings were that major depression, PTSD and eating disorders were significantly more prevalent in women than in men. Female poly-substance abusers differed significantly from all other substance abusers by suffering more often from major depression, simple phobia, PTSD, and borderline PD. Male poly-substance abusers more often presented antisocial PD and less often Cluster C disorders than all other substance abusers The conclusion of the study as to PD is that they found rather minor gender differences, and that the primary substance of abuse is a more important variable than gender for explaining differences in the prevalence and type of Axis II disorders. By contrast, gender, and not primary substance of abuse, seems to be the most important factor in the prevalence and type of Axis I disorders.

Relational perspectives on gender and treatment

Relational perspective

In the 1970s, the psychological and social development of females began to be studied by progressive feminists like Miller (1976) and Gilligan (1982) and their colleagues at the Stone Center at Wellesley College (www. wellesley.edu/WCW) in the US. Their qualitative research suggested that female development occurs in the context of relationships, with mutually empathic and giving relationships being both a source and a goal of development. This contrasts traditional developmental theories that ignored or pathologised much of women's experiences by studying males and generalising their experiences to females. According to the female-specific theories, women's focus on relationships is seen as natural and necessary - rather than pathologised as dependence or lack of a sense of self.

According to Miller (1976), women's use of substances is an attempt to repair and re-establish destructive relationships. The substances become a remedy to endure untenable relations, and substance abuse develops through vicious circles where the substances deteriorate the quality of the relationship, which again result in an even bigger intake of substances. Miller (1990) describes this as the "depressive spiral", where dysfunctional relationships provoke feelings of contempt, confusion and exhaustion. Addiction, according to Miller, is the woman's answer to the wish, the need and loss of taking part in meaningful relationships.

According to Gilligan (1982) the primary task of moral development of girls and women is to achieve a balance between self-nurture and care of others, not separation and autonomy. This balance fosters a heightened awareness and appreciation of self. This feminist view of development gives significant weight to contextual influences from the media and peers, and the significant changes in expectations and negative influences that girls face when they transition into puberty, often increase their vulnerability to drug and alcohol use and mental illness.

Dysfunctional families of origin

It is suggested that female substance abusers are more likely to come from dysfunctional families of origin. There are higher rates of mental illness, alcoholism, drug dependence, and depression in early family life of substance-abusing females than in families of substance-abusing males (Straussner, 1985). On the other hand, other studies indicate that males have experienced just as much emotional and physical problems in their families of origin as females, but it is more that the meaning of these adverse circumstances is experienced and talked about in a different way among males (Biong & Ravndal, 2007). Most studies show, however, that sexual abuse both in the family of origin, and by other people in the surroundings of these families, is far more frequent among female substance abusers than among male substance abusers (Gil-Rivas *et al.*, 1997; Melberg *et al.*, 2003). Women typically enter treatment with higher rates of post-traumatic stress disorders, depression and other mental health disorders than males (Gil-Rivas *et al.*, 1997).

Women typically indentify significant life events connected to family issues as precipitating factors to their addiction when entering treatment. Such events may be miscarriage, loss of contact with their children, infidelity, separation, and divorce and the like. It is detrimental to their connection to treatment when women are chastised for blaming their addiction problems on these events. Rather it is important to empathise with the impact of these precipitants in the process of explaining how they contribute to the promotion of the disease process.

Primary motivators for women to enter treatment are physical and emotional concerns as well as family issues, while men are most influenced by job and legal problems (Blume, 1997; Ravndal, 2008).

Partners

Women who lack or who have lost significant relationships are at most risk for substance abuse problems (Ravndal, 1982; Wilsnack *et al.*, 1986). An interesting finding is that women who were living/cohabitated with their partners were more likely to be heavy drinkers than those who were married (Wilsnack *et al.*, 1986). Several explanations may be possible, one being that couples who do not get married, but just live together, are living according to more non-traditional values, hence the female drinking pattern may be different. It might also be that cohabitation, in contrast to being married, is an expression of a more emotionally difficult relationship, where alcohol consumption helps relieve emotional problems and less satisfying relationships.

More important is the finding that women's drinking pattern is highly correlated with those of their significant others, and more so for women than for men. This is a finding that is repeated in many studies both in Europe and the US. Research shows that most addicted women begin their use under the influence of a significant male in their lives (Hser *et al.*, 1987; Ravndal, 2008). In contrast, males are more likely to begin using substances in the context of male peer relationships. Addicted women who enter treatment are more likely than addicted men to have an addicted partner, whose use patterns these women parallel (Dahlgren & Willander, 1989; Ravndal, 2008). Women are also more likely to be divorced or separated, and describe their existing relationships as less happy and supportive (Schilit & Gomberg, 1987; Dahlgren & Willander, 1989).

It is also important to recognise that women who seek treatment experience more blame and opposition from families and friends and report greater conflicts with them than men do (Beckman & Amaro, 1986).

The relational model in addiction treatment

Covington (1999) who is a pioneer in integrating the relational development theory into addiction treatment, has conceptualised the process of addiction and recovery as a spiral. As the addiction progresses, it constricts the woman's life until she is totally focused on the drugs. The dependence on the substances becomes the primary relationship in the woman's life to the exclusion of self-care and participation in other relationships and activities. Recovery is a process of transformation that allows her to expand her sphere of focus to encompass healthy relationships and other positive activities that promote her self-esteem. Understanding the impact of relationship history has significant implications on the understanding of women's addictive behaviour (Ravndal & Vaglum,1994). According to Covington (1999) women may use substances to alter themselves to fit into their available relationships (i.e. managing addiction in a partner, engaging in sex, coping with violence). Imbalances of power or responsibilities can significantly decrease a woman's self-esteem. Substances may provide energy, a sense of power, and relief from confusion, compensating for what the relationship is not providing.

When women in treatment are asked what the substances did for them, they are typically able to state what attracted them to the substances and how it helped them to cope. It is very easy for women to conceptualise their relationship with a substance. In a therapeutic community (TC) in Norway (Veksthuset/Phoenix House, Oslo), the women in the re-entry phase typically worked a lot with their grief in the process of giving up their favourite drug in special women's groups. Their wording and reactions were heart-breaking and were very similar to saying a final farewell to their most beloved boyfriend (Ravndal, 1987-1990).[2] Because of this strong relationship association, women with coexisting mental disorders need to have the ability to acknowledge the positive things that the substance did for them in order to more fully grieve the need to let go. Focusing solely on the consequences of their drug use may not get at their alliance with the substance.

As mentioned earlier in this paper, most addicted women date the onset of their heaviest use to some stressful event. To ignore or discourage them from talking about the meaning of this event, because it would foster self-pity instead of self-responsibility, ignores the contextual factors that are so important to women. Although there is more interest and understanding in the mental health field to acknowledge precipitating events and understanding the meaning of their impact, the psychopharmacological interventions foster the primacy of a medical model, which focuses on the management of symptoms and does not necessarily address contextual variables.

It is interesting that relational theory is supported by the philosophy of twelve-step-based addiction treatment for women, but it also calls for change (Covington, 1999). Twelve-step meetings and the TC model of treatment have always prioritised making connections, and have even elevated the value of relationships by emphasising their spiritual nature, thus in many ways fostering a feminist approach. However, in an attempt to simplify the process, guidance may be imposed in ways that ignore women's unique problems and issues in early recovery and their need for less hierarchical, more collaborative relationships with treatment providers. Also, women's relationship focus is not always sensitively addressed through traditional treatment addiction approaches.

Another issue is that recovering women who struggle in their attempts to balance care for self with others, are often viewed as being relationship dependent or co-dependent, when in reality their struggle with priorities is well within the realm of normal for women. Therefore women's focus on relationships can be used to enhance motivation for recovery. Women can be counselled on how they sacrifice too much of themselves in order to mould themselves to fit into relationships with persons who are unwilling or unable to change without pathologising their relationship desires and commitment (Ravndal, 1982; Ravndal & Vaglum, 1994; Collins, 1993; Favorini, 1995; Lossius, 2008).

Physical and biological gender differences

There are also important physical and biological gender differences that are of great importance in understanding female substance abuse and psychopathol-

---

[2] Written notes from participant observations in women's groups at Veksthuset 1987-1990.

ogy. Most often gender, psychopathology, physiology and biology are tied together in intrinsic patterns that have to be understood and dealt with in order to give female substance abusers adequate and professional help. Below follows the most important factors concerning physiology and biology among female substance abusers.

Physical differences

Biological differences in how women metabolise alcohol make it more likely that they will develop physical consequences more rapidly, even with a lower intake. This has primarily been attributed to alcohol being more dilute in the bodies of men who have more water and less fat cells, but lately also to the fact that women have less of the stomach enzyme alcohol dehydrogenase, which begins the metabolism of alcohol (Frezza *et al.*, 1990). Much less alcohol is digested and therefore more of it goes directly to body tissues. Therefore, it is not surprising that women are likely to react more intensely to a given dose of alcohol and that the effects are less predictable (Blume, 1997). Due to women's proportion of fat and less water than men, which increases with age, benzodiazepines and barbiturates have longer half-lives, and marijuana takes longer to clear (Barry, 1986). Altogether the physical effects of alcohol have a more severe course and more rapid onset in women, probably due to the increased chronic concentrations in their systems (Blume, 1997).

"Telescoped development"

For women abusing alcohol, there are fewer years between landmark symptoms and progression to a later stage of illness. This has been termed the "telescoped effect" of the progression of the disease in women (Piazza *et al.*, 1989). Some contend that this syndrome is particularly pronounced for women who are depressed before the onset of their alcohol abuse (Smith & Cloninger, 1981). Analyses of data from the Epidemiological Catchment Area (ECA) nationwide study in the US confirm the rapid development of alcohol dependence in women, but conclude that this rapid accrual of alcoholic symptoms in women is independent of both psychiatric co-morbidity and the amount of alcohol consumption (Lewis *et al.*, 1996).

Fertility, sex and promiscuity

Alcohol and drugs interfere with women's fertility and can exacerbate gynae-cological disorders (Blume, 1997). The presence of premenstrual dysphoria has been associated with increased quantity and frequency of alcohol and marijuana use, and women with diagnosable premenstrual syndrome have higher rates of alcohol abuse and dependence (Tobin *et al.,* 1994). Unsafe sex, associated with trading sex for drugs, or relationships with addicted partners, is related to increases in sexually transmitted diseases. Sexual dysfunction, such as lack of desire, inability to orgasm, and painful intercourse, can cause women to use alcohol or drugs to cope, or these problems may be consequences of addiction. A subjective sense of needing substances in order to perform sexually may lead many newly recovering women to avoid sexual relations, despite research that indicates the quality of sexual relations is likely to improve (Blume, 1997).

Contrary to popular opinion, research indicates that alcohol-dependent women are not necessarily more promiscuous under the influence of alcohol. Wilsnack *et al.* (1986) demonstrate from findings in their representative population studies from the US that 60 percent of female drinkers were likely to experience sexual aggression by someone else who had been drinking. In the research summarised by Blume (1997), 16 percent of alcohol-dependent women reported that they were raped during their drinking history, and more of them were likely to experience violence from their spouses. Stigmatisation of female substance abusers has always existed. Despite research dispelling the stereotype of increased promiscuity, substance-abusing women typically internalise the shame society and cultural, moralistic norms are placing upon them.

Pregnancy

The impoverished environment often associated with illegal drug use, as well as the stigma associated with such use while pregnant, are other big issues for female sub-stance users. Even if the foetal alcohol syndrome (FAS), connected with too much alcohol use during pregnancy, is by far a much bigger problem in all normal, repre-sentative populations than the consequences of heroin addiction to unborn babies (NAS), it is the smaller group of drug-abusing women who become pregnant that get by far most negative attention and moralistic condemnation. Research shows that it is the use of the legal drug, alcohol, that is by far the most frequent and direct cause of birth defects such as for example mental retardation, physical abnormalities and neurological impairments. However, for all substance-abusing females, the shame of not living up to the expected female values of being the good and caring mother, has typically prevented many addicted women to seek treatment in due time. Unresolved maternal grieving of abortion, or of the effects of addiction on infants, and/or loss of custody are significant treatment issues that can contribute to depression and behavioural management problems in addicted women (Raskin, 1992).

Across all socio-economic groups, addiction has severe effects on maternal-infant bonding that can have lifelong ramifications. The shame, guilt, loss and fear of separation from their infants that addicted mothers feel can create significant barriers to treatment entry and less than optimal cooperation and compliance within the different treatment systems.

Conclusions

The literature focusing on female polydrug abuse and psychopathology is scarce, and several methodological problems have to be considered. Different sample characteristics, diagnostic criteria and assessment procedures are main factors which cause problems in drawing final conclusions. The prevalence of Axis I and II disorder also varies a lot between normal population studies and clinical samples/reviews. In general, persons with the heaviest substance abuse and more psychiatric disorders are more prone to seek treatment. Hence, the prevalence of psychiatric co-morbidity is higher in studies of clinical populations than in general population studies. In a literature review of different treatment populations, females had a higher prevalence of psychiatric symptoms than males, but calculating the median value, there were no differences between females and males as to the total prevalence of psychiatric symptoms. In samples with females, the prevalence varied between 33-85%, while in samples with males the corresponding percentages were 16-84%. However, in several other treatment studies of female substance abusers the prevalence of depression, anxiety disorders, post-traumatic stress disorders (PTSD) and eating disorders are significantly higher than among substance abusing males. Very few studies have examined personality disorders (PD) and gender differences among substance abusers. In a literature review there was a tendency towards more PDs among women than among men. Altogether the prevalence of antisocial PD was significantly higher among males than among females, while no gender difference was found for borderline PD.

According to female-specific theories, women's focus on relationships is seen as natural and necessary - rather than pathologised as dependence or lack of a sense of self. The relational perspective in both understanding female substance abuse and to enhance motivation for recovery is of great importance.

There are also important physical and biological gender differences that are of great importance to understand female substance abuse and psychopathology. Most often gender, psychopathology, physiology and biology are tied together in intrinsic patterns that have to be understood and dealt with in order to give female substance abusers adequate and professional help. De Wilde *et al.*(2006) propose, because of a much worse profile in various areas of functioning when entering treatment, female substance abusers may require a gender-adapted set of therapeutic interventions at the moment they enter treatment.

References

Barry, PP (1986). Gender as a factor in treating the elderly. NIDA Research Monograph 65, 65-69.

Beckman, L & Amaro, H (1986). Personal and social difficulties faced by women and men entering alcoholism treatment. *Journal of Studies on Alcohol*, 47, 135-145.

Beyer, E & Conahan, JA (2002). Females with dual diagnoses. Implications for specialized clinical approaches. In: O'Connell, D & Beyer, E (Eds.). *Managing the Dually diagnosed Patient.* 99-151. Binghamton, NY: The Haworth Press, Inc.

Biong, S & Ravndal, E (2007). Young men's experiences of living with substance abuse and suicidal behaviour: Between death as an escape from pain and the hope for a life. *International Journal of Qualitative Studies on Health and Well-being*, 2, 246-259.

Blume, SB (1997). Women: Clinical aspects. In: Lowinson, JH, Ruiz, P, Millman, RB & Langrod, JG (Eds.). *Substance abuse: A comprehensive textbook.* 645-654, 3rd edition, Baltimore: Williams & Wilkins.

Bradizza, CM, Stasiewicz, PR & Paas, ND (2006). Relapse to alcohol and drug use among individuals diagnosed with co-occurring mental health and substance use disorders: a review. *Clinical Psychology Review*, 26, 162-178.

Brady, KT, Dansky, BS, Sonne, SC & Saladin, MS (1998). Post-traumatic stress disorder and cocaine dependence: Order of onset. *American Journal of Addiction*, 7, 128-135.

Brady, KT, Grice, DE, Dustan, L & Randall, C (1993). Gender difference in substance use disorders. *American Journal of Psychiatry*, 150, 1707-1711.

Brooner, RK, King, VL, Kidorf, M, Schmidt, CV & Bigelow, GE (1997). Psychiatric and substance use comorbidity among treatment-seeking substance opioid abusers. *Archives of General Psychiatry*, 54, 71-80.

Butler, SF, Gaulier, B & Haller, D (1991). Assessment of axis II personality disorders among female substance abusers. *Psychological Reports*, 68, 1344-1346,

Collins, B (1993). Reconstruing co-dependency using self-in-relation theory: A feminist perspective. *Social Work*, 38, 470-476.

Comtois, KA & Ries, RK (1995). Sex differences in dually diagnosed severely mentally ill clients in dual-diagnosis outpatient treatment. *American Journal on Addictions*, 4, 245-253.

Cottler, JB, Compton, WMD, Mager, D, Spitznagel, EL & Janca, A (1992). Post-traumatic stress disorders among substance abusers from the general population. *American Journal of Psychiatry*, 149, 664-670.

Covington, S (1999). *Helping women recover: A program for treating addiction*. New York: Guilford Press.

Dahlgren, E & Willander, A(1989). Are special treatment facilities for female alcoholics needed? A controlled 2-year follow-up study from a specialized female unit (EWA) versus mixed male/female treatment facility. *Alcoholism: Clinical and Experimental Research*, 13, 499-504.

De Wilde, J, Broekaert, E & Rossel, Y (2006). Problem severity profiles of clients in European therapeutic communities: Gender differences in various areas of functioning. *European Addiction Research*, 12, 128-137.

De Wilde, J, Soyez, V, Broekaert, E, Rossel, Y, Kaplan, C & Larsson, J (2004). Problem severity profiles of substance abusing women in European therapeutic communities: Influence of psychiatric problems. *Journal of Substance Abuse Treatment*, 26, 243-251.

Favorini, A (1995). Concept of co-dependency: Blaming the victim or pathway to recovery? *Social Work*, 40, 827-830.

Frezza, M, DiPadova, C, Pozzato, G, Terpin, M, Baroona, E & Lieber, CS (1990). High blood alcohol levels in women: The role of decreased gastric alcohol dehydrogenase activity and first-pass metabolism. *New England Journal of Medicine*, 12, 871-878.

Gil-Rivas, V, Fiorentine, R, Anglin, D & Taylor, E (1997). Sexual and physical abuse: Do they compromise drug treatment outcomes? *Journal of Substance Abuse Treatment*, 14, 351-358.

Gilligan, C (1982). *In a different voice. Psychological theory and women's development*. Cambridge, MA: Harvard University Press.

Grant, BF, Stinson, FS, Dawson, DA, Chou, SP, Ruan, WJ & Pickering, RP (2004). Co-occurrence of 12 month alcohol and drug use disorders and personality disorders in the United States: Results from the National Epidemiologic Survey on alcohol and related conditions. *Archives of General Psychiatry*, 61, 361-368.

Griffin, ML, Weiss, RI, Mirin, SM & Lang, U (1989). A comparison of male and female cocaine abusers. *Archives of General Psychiatry*, 46, 122-126.

Helzer, JE, Robins, JN & McEvoy, L (1987). Post-traumatic stress disorders in the general population : Findings of the epidemiologic catchment area survey. *North England Journal of Medicine*, 317, 1630-1634.

Hintz, T & Mann, K (2005). Comorbidity in alcohol use disorders: Focus on mood, anxiety and personality. In: Stohler, R & Rössler, W (Eds.). *Dual Diagnosis. The evolving conceptual framework*, 65-91. Bibliotheca Psychiatrica No. 172. Basel: Krager.

Hser, Y, Anglin, M & McGlothlin, W (1987). Sex differences in addict careers: I. Initiation of use. *American Journal of Drug Abuse*, 13, 33-57.

Hunt, C & Andrews, G (1992). Measuring personality disorders: A review of issues and research methods. *Archives of General Psychiatry*, 149, 1645-1653.

Kessler, RC, Crum, RM, Warner, LA, Nelson, CB, Schulberg, J & Anthony, JC (1997). Lifetime co-occurrence of DAM-III-R alcohol abuse and dependence with other psychiatric disorders in the National Comorbidity Survey. *Archives of General Psychiatry*, 54, 313-321.

Kessler, RC, McGonagle, KA, Zhao, S, Nelson, CB, Hughes, M, Eshleman, S, Wittchen, HU & Kendler, KS (1994). Lifetime and 12-month prevalence of DSM-III-R psychiatric disorders in the US. Results of the National Comorbidity Study. *Archives of General Psychiatry*, 51, 8-19.

Kilpatrick, DG, Acierno, R & Resnick, HK (1997). A 2-year longitudinal analysis of the relationships between violent assaults and substance use in women. *Journal of Consulting Clinical Psychology*, 65, 834-847.

Landheim A (2007). Psychiatric disorders among patients in the substance abuse field: Prevalence and association to the long-term outcome of substance abuse. Doctoral Thesis, Department of Behavioural Sciences in Medicine, Faculty of Medicine, University of Oslo.

Landheim, A, Bakken, K & Vaglum, P (2003). Gender differences in the prevalence of symptom disorders and personality disorders among poly-substance abusers and pure alcoholics. *European Addiction Research*, 9, 8-17.

Lewis, CE, Bucholz, KK, Spitznagel, E & Shayka, JJ (1996). Effects of gender and comorbidity on problem drinking in a community sample. *Alcoholism: Clinical and Experimental Research*, 20, 466-476.

Lossius, K (2008). Kvinner, alkohol og behandling (Women, Alcohol and Treatment). In: Duckert, F, Lossius, K, Ravndal, E & Sandvik, B (Eds.). *Kvinner og alkohol.* (Women and Alcohol). 107-143. Oslo: Universitetsforlaget.

Magura, S, Kang, SY, Rosenblum, A, Handelsman, L & Foote, J (1998). Gender differences in psychiatric comorbidity among cocaine-using opiate addicts. *Journal of Addictive Diseases*, 17, 49-61.

Melberg, HO, Lauritzen, G & Ravndal, E (2003). *Hvilken nytte, for hvem og til hvilken kostnad? En prospektiv studie av stoffmisbrukere i behandling.* (Which use, for whom and at what cost? A prospective study of drug abusers in treatment). SIRUS report no. 4. Oslo: National Institute for Alcohol and Drug Research.

Miller, JB (1976). *Toward a new psychology of women.* Second edition. Boston: Beacon Press.

Miller, JB (1990). Connections, disconnections and violations. Work in progress no. 33. Wellesley, MA: Stone Center, Working Paper Series.

Piazza, NJ, Vrbka, JL & Yeager, RD (1989). Telescoping of alcoholism in women alcoholics. *International Journal of Addictions*, 24, 19-28.

Raskin, VD (1992). Maternal bereavement in the perinatal substance abuser. *Journal of Substance Abuse Treatment*, 9, 149-152.

Ravndal, E (1982). *Hvordan kvinner selv kan mestre sine alkoholproblemer.* (How females themselves can cope with their alcohol problems). SIFA-report no.54. Oslo: National Institute for Alcohol and Drug Research.

Ravndal, E (2008). Kvinner og alkohol (Women and Alcohol). In: Duckert, F, Lossius, K, Ravndal, E & Sandvik, B (Eds.). *Kvinner og alkohol.* (Women and Alcohol). 37-66. Oslo: Universitetsforlaget.

Ravndal, E & Vaglum, P (1994). Treatment of female addicts: The importance of relationships to parents, partners and peers for the outcome. *The International Journal of the Addiction*, 29, 115-125.

Regier, DA, Boyd, JH, Burke, JD, Rae, DS, Myers, JK, Kramer, M, Robins, LN, George, LK, Karno, M & Locke, BZ (1988). One month prevalence of mental disorders in the US. *Archives of General Psychiatry*, 45, 977-986.

Regier, DA, Farmer, ME, Rae, DS, Locke, BZ, Keith, SJ, Judd, LL *et al.* (1990). Comorbidity of mental disorders with alcohol and other drug abuse. Results from The Epidemiological Catchment Area (ECA) Study. *Journal of the American Medical Association*, 264, 2511-2518.

Schilit, R & Gomberg, E (1987). Social support structures of women in treatment for alcoholism. *Health and Social Work*, 12, 187-195.

Smith, EM & Cloninger, CR (1981). Alcoholic females: Mortality at twelve-year follow-up. *Focus on Women*, 2, 1-3.

Straussner, S (1985). Alcoholism in women: Current knowledge and implications for treatment. *Alcoholism Treatment Quarterly*, 5, 139-155.

Tobin, MB, Schmidt, MD & Rubinow, DR (1994). Reported alcohol use in women with premenstrual syndrome. *American Journal of Psychiatry*, 151, 1503-1504.

Torgersen, S & Alnæs, R (1990). The relationship between the MCMI personality scales and DSM III, axis II. *Journal of Personality Assessment*, 55, 698-707.

Verheul, R, Van den Brink, W & Hartgers, C (1995). Prevalence of personality disorders among alcoholics and drug addicts: an overview. *European Addiction Research*, 1, 166-177.

Weissman, MM & Klerman, GL (1977). Sex differences and the epidemiology of depression. *Archives of General Psychiatry*, 34, 98-111.

Westrich, L, Guedj, P, Galanter, M & Baird, D (1997). Differences between men and women in dual-diagnosis treatment. *American Journal on Addictions*, 6, 311-317.

Widiger, TA & Frances, A (1987). Interviews and inventories for the measurements of personality disorders among alcoholics admitted to an alcoholism rehabilitation setting. *Clinical Psychological Review*, 7, 49-75.

Wilsnack, SC, Wilsnack, RW & Klassen, AD (1986). *Epidemiological research on women's drinking 1974-84. Women and Alcohol: Health-related issues.* 1-68. NIAAA, Research Monograph no. 16. Washington DC: Department of Health and Human Services.

8 The impact of motherhood on recovery – Lessons we can learn from the treatment journeys of mothers with problematic substance misuse issues

KAREN BIGGS

Phoenix Futures
London, England

Karen.biggs@phoenix-futures.org.uk

Abstract

Many researchers and service providers are looking to writing on recovery capital to give them some insight into how to deliver and design services that build on and sustain positive recovery capital and reduce the negative recovery capital of those accessing treatment.

In this study we sought to understand what impact being a mother had on recovery. Using the recovery capital model we have tracked the progress of mothers entering treatment with and without their children. We have used data collected during their progress through treatment to compare the outcomes achieved.

Parental problem drug use can, and does, cause serious harm to children. Effective treatment of the parent can have major benefits for the child. If motherhood does generate some positive recovery capital, we owe it to the children of the drug-using population to understand it better.

Our study suggests that being a mother in recovery sets you apart from non-mothers in a number of ways. Firstly, your motherhood can act as both an incentive and disincentive to access treatment. The added complexity of being a mother and needing drug treatment explains the contradictory views from mothers about accessing our treatment provision. Secondly, mothers outperform non-mothers in their health gains from treatment. Regardless of whether their children are in treatment with them or not, the mothers in our study made the biggest improvement in both residential and non-residential treatment.

Key words

Motherhood; recovery; recovery capital; health gains; treatment.

Introduction

Many studies have pointed to the impact gender has on treatment but there is less information about the impact parenthood has on recovery. Non residential treatment can, and is often accessed by parents who still maintain responsibility for their children. However, there is less opportunity in the UK for parents to access residential treatment whilst still maintaining primary caring responsibility for their children.

A central plank of the new UK Drug Strategy introduced in December 2010, is to support services to work with individuals to develop their recovery capital. The strategy defines recovery capital as the resource that is necessary to start and sustain recovery from drug and alcohol dependence.

Many researchers and service providers are looking to writing on recovery capital to give them some insight into how to deliver and design services. These services must build on and sustain positive recovery capital, whilst reducing the negative recovery capital of those accessing treatment.

In this study we sought to understand the impact motherhood has on an individual's recovery. Using the recovery capital model we have tracked the progress of mothers entering treatment with and without their children. We have used data to compare their progress through treatment and the outcomes achieved. We have endeavoured to understand whether motherhood impacts women's progression through treatment.

This study does not look at the experience of fathers moving through treatment. It is however, our opinion that this is certainly a topic worthy of study.

Recovery Capital

The concept of recovery capital is important for recovery services providers. It allows us to understand what positive and negative attributes groups of people wanting to address their substance misuse may have.

Granfield & Cloud (1999) define recovery capital as "the breadth and depth of internal and external resources that can be drawn upon to initiate and sustain recovery from AOD [alcohol and other drug] problems".

By developing a better understanding of the resources people bring with them to formal treatment we can ensure that our treatment services are responding to those negative and positive attributes to enhance the possibility of recovery. By understanding recovery capital we shift our "… focus from the pathology of addiction to a focus on the internal and external assets required to initiate and sustain long term recovery" (White & Cloud, 2008).

This study seeks to understand how the concept of recovery capital can be applied to mothers in treatment using the TOP scores as indicators of personal recovery capital. Personal recovery capital includes: physical recovery capital such as physical health and also human capital including self-confidence and sense of meaning and purpose (White & Cloud, 2008).

Using the concept of recovery capital applied to the study of mothers experience through treatment allows us to understand how mothers respond differently to treatment. This is important if we are to offer the best treatment options possible for mothers wanting to address their substance misuse.

A woman's treatment journey in the UK

Most mixed gender treatment options in the UK are dominated by men. In the UK there are limited women-only treatment options available; which are fewer still for women entering residential treatment with their children. It is no surprise therefore that a recent report by the National Treatment Agency detailing the numbers of women in treatment in the UK showed that women make up 27% of the treatment population and 2% of them enter residential treatment (NTA, 2010). Moreover, this report revealed that 61% of women entering the UK treatment system are mothers; half of them have parental responsibility for their children. The report comments on the apparent contradictory view in the treatment sector that parenthood is both an incentive and disincentive to treatment. Mothers are fearful of accessing treatment due to the risk of having their children taken from them. Conversely, they are incentivised to address their substance misuse through a desire to be a better parent. Whilst the report highlights that men and women who are parents derive greater benefits from treatment than non-parents, it shows little understanding of why that might be the case. This study seeks to test that claim. We aim to understand what, if any, recovery capital mothers have that enhances their recovery journey.

Keeping children safe

The sad reality is that there are between 250,000 and 350,000 children of problem drug users in the UK – about one for every problem drug user. Parental problem drug use can, and does, cause serious harm to children. The effective treatment of parents can have major benefits for their children. The number of affected children is only likely to decrease when the number of problem drug users decreases (ACMD 2003). It is therefore paramount that we ensure that services for parents deliver the greatest potential for recovery. If motherhood does generate some positive recovery capital, we owe it to the children of the drug-using population to understand it better.

The study

The study mapped the progress of women in 3 treatment settings: adult-only residential services, family residential services and non-residential services. A national outcome tool was used to measure women's progress through treatment and their resulting health gains.

All residential services were treated using a Therapeutic Community model. The length of the programme for women in the family and adult services was consistent. There were some differences in the programme delivery between the family and adult services to accommodate child care responsibilities. The non-residential services were community-based programmes that allowed men and women to access the programme whilst living at home.

The national outcome tool used was TOP (Treatment Outcome Profile). In the UK, the National Treatment Agency (a special health authority within the NHS) introduced the Treatment Outcome Profile tool in 2007. This is a mandatory nationally utilised clinical tool to measure treatment outcomes in England. The Psychological Health, Physical Health and Quality of life of the client are measured on a scale of 0 to 20 during a key work session. The client is asked to self-score their current health in these 3 domains. Progress is tracked through key stages of the recovery journey.

This study has split the cohort into three groups: mothers entering treatment with their children, mothers entering treatment without their children and non-mothers.

The data was analysed to compare the TOP scores of clients as they enter the treatment episode, against the score upon their departure. Comparisons have been made between the entry level scores of women in each of the groups, and also the progress made by the women within the residential and non-residential settings.

In this study we tracked the treatment journeys of 100 women entering the 3 treatment settings over a 12 month period between 01/01/2010 and 01/01/2011.

The study also drew on the personal treatment journeys of women themselves. These anecdotes were collected through a survey of a further 43 women who are currently undergoing treatment in 3 different treatment settings.

Findings

Mothers in our study were more likely to complete a residential programme than non-mothers. However their chances of completion were increased by 40% if their children were with them during their residential treatment.

This initial look at the completion levels of mothers and non-mothers would suggest that mothers undergoing intensive treatment with their children do better than non-mothers and mothers without their children. However, we need to look closer at the outcome scores to understand the treatment gains being made through these treatment episodes.

Psychological Health Gains

In the residential provision mothers who did not have their children living with them reported the lowest entry score for psychological health. The anecdotal evidence provided by this group suggests that their substance misuse had resulted in the loss of parental responsibility for their children. This had a noticeable impact

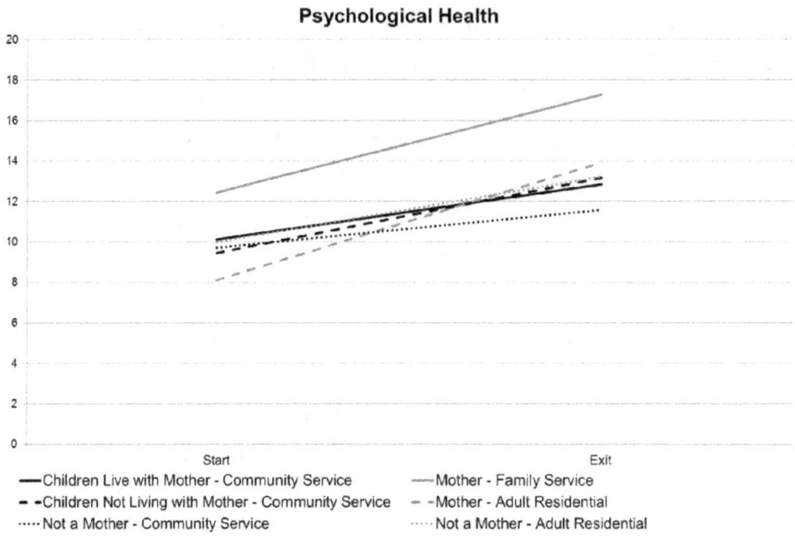

Figure 1. Psychological Health gains for women in the 3 groups across residential and non-residential provision. This chart shows the comparable psychological health gains of mothers and non-mothers as they progress through the treatment journeys. Mothers entering residential treatment with their children show the highest levels of psychological health at the start and end of the treatment episode. Mothers without their children start treatment with the lowest levels of psychological health but make the largest gains through their treatment episode.

on their psychological health. However, this group made the biggest improvement through treatment in this domain. They overtook non-mothers who entered treatment with higher scores.

Mothers entering residential treatment with their children reported better psychological health scores on entry and at completion than the other 2 groups. Having said this, the improvement made through treatment was less marked than the improvement made by non-mothers.

Similarly, in the community services mothers experienced more positive gains through treatment than non-mothers.

Women nationally showed a 24% improvement in psychological health as reported by the NTA from 2008-9 performance figures (NTA, 2010). Our mothers compare very favourably to the national average. Mothers in our residential services with their children improved by 40%. Our mothers in residential treatment without their children reported a 72% increase in their psychological health. Non-mothers in community services showed the lowest improvement and finished with the lowest psychological health scores of 20%, which is lower than the national average.

So, in relation to psychological health gains our study indicates that mothers do better than non-mothers regardless of whether they have their children with them. The improvements made by mothers in our residential provision outperform the national women's average scores.

The improvements that mothers in residential treatment without their children make are marked. This group get the best benefit from residential provision of all groups included in our study.

Physical Health Gains

Mothers who no longer have their children with them enter treatment with the lowest score in this health domain across residential and non residential settings. Despite this, their improvement through treatment is the most marked at 80%. Indeed, they finish treatment with the highest physical health score. This compares with a 38% improvement in physical health for non mothers in a residential setting.

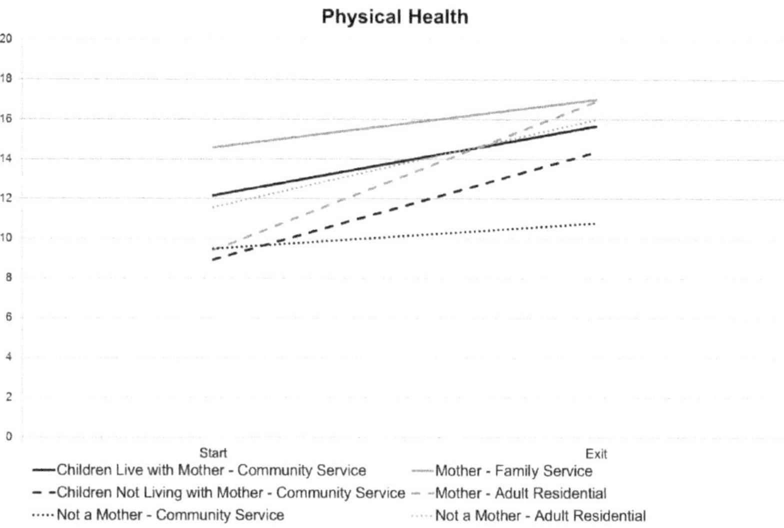

Figure 2. Physical Health gains for women in the 3 groups across residential and non-residential provision. This chart shows the comparable physical health gains of mothers and non-mothers as they progress through the treatment journeys. Again mothers entering treatment with their children show the highest levels of physical health at the beginning and at the end of the treatment episode. Mothers accessing residential treatment without their children make the most significant health gains. All women, whether mothers or non-mothers achieve more physical health gains in residential services than community services. This is attributable to the nature of the care delivered in these treatment settings.

Mothers in a community setting who do not live with their children also make significant improvements in their physical health, demonstrating a 62% improvement.

The overall health outcomes are lower for all women in community services compared with those in residential services. Women in community services report the poorest physical health scores upon completion.

Clearly, the nature of residential treatment provision, including the provision of greater care and support for the client, would result in increased physical health improvements. The national average physical health improvement score according to NTA figures was 19%. However, the marked difference in scores between mothers and non-mothers in the same setting is noteworthy.

Quality of Life Improvements

At the start of treatment, mothers in residential treatment who no longer have their children with them report the lowest quality of life scores compared to any

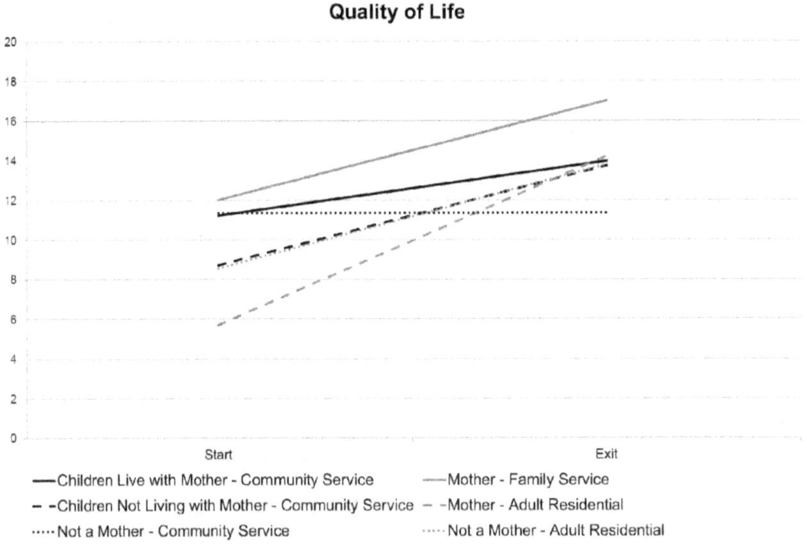

Figure 3. Quality of life gains for women in the 3 groups across residential and non-residential provision
This chart shows the comparable quality of life improvements of mothers and non-mothers as they progress through the treatment journeys. Mothers accessing residential treatment with their children start and end treatment with the highest self-reported quality of life scores. Mothers accessing residential treatment without their children start with the lowest scores but make the most improvement. Non-mothers report the lowest quality of life scores on exiting this treatment episode.

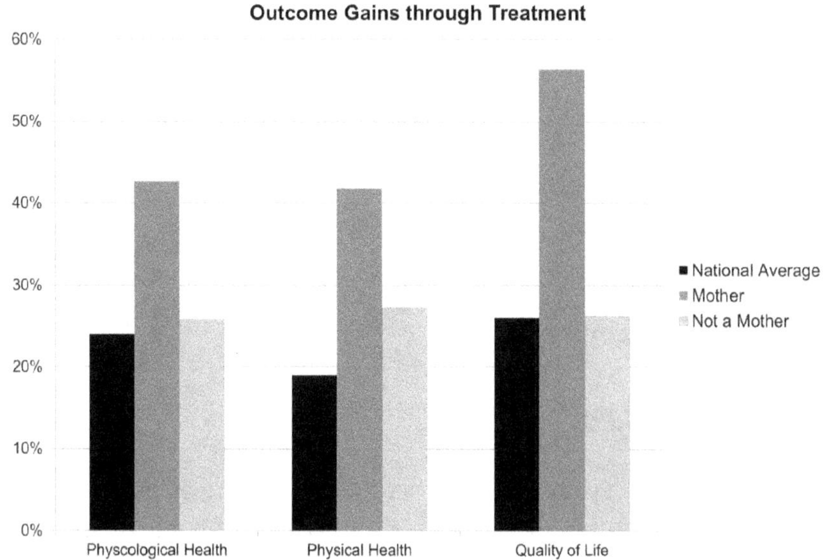

Figure 4. Comparable improvement for mothers and non-mothers across the 3 health domains. In all 3 health domains across all treatment settings, mothers make the most improvement through their treatment episode. The biggest disparity in the improvement made by mothers and non-mothers is in the quality of life domain.

other group in the study. Their average self-score is 6, compared to mothers entering treatment with their children with a score of 12. However, they report the highest improvement in physical health gains at 149%.

The highest entry and exit scores for this domain are mothers who enter residential treatment with their children.

The national average for improvement in quality of life scores for women in 2008-9 was 26%.

Trends across the 3 health domains

Mothers who access residential treatment without their children enter with the lowest scores in 2 domains. It is these women who make the most marked improvement. They overtake all groups in health scores, except for women in residential treatment with their children.

Mothers entering residential treatment with their children report the highest entry and exit scores in all domains. They still make significant improvements throughout their treatment; far outperforming the national average improvements score for women in each health domain.

Mothers in community services show similar improvements and outperform non-mothers in each domain.

Non-mothers in community services exit with the lowest scores in each domain.

Clues to a mother's recovery journey

Does motherhood give you recovery capital?

The mothers in our study showed a different experience of our treatment than the non-mothers. The differences between reported health gains amongst mothers and non-mothers in the same treatment setting suggest an inherent difference between these groups.

The fact that non-mothers scored less than mothers in all domains in all settings again indicates that mothers have an advantage over non-mothers. This remains an advantage, regardless of whether they have their children with them or not.

Women that are able to maintain parental responsibility for their children report higher recovery capital than those mothers who no longer have parental responsibility. Safeguarding processes are established to ensure that the most chaotic mothers would lose access to their children. The comparable completion rates between mothers and non-mothers would tell us that maintaining custody of your children is a powerful external motivator to change. Conditions placed on women entering treatment with their children act as a powerful incentive to stay in treatment. It is understandable that women who have lost custody of their children report lower scores in the 3 health domains, either as a result of losing their children or as a contributing factor to the loss of their children. However the significant improvements made by mothers who do not have their children with them over that of non-mothers suggest that motherhood does give you added recovery capital.

For the women in our sample, it would seem that motherhood at best is positive recovery capital and at the very least enhances your responsiveness to treatment once you have entered formal treatment.

What did the women tell us?

During the study we took anecdotal evidence from 43 mothers through a written survey. 81% of the women were still in treatment either with or without their children across the residential and community settings.

The purpose of the survey was to collect evidence from women about their experience of the treatment system as mothers. Furthermore, it sought to better comprehend the impact women believed motherhood to have had on their recovery.

When asked why they entered treatment, 88% of all women in the survey said that their children were a motivating factor for them accessing treatment. This concurs with reports that state that motherhood acts as an incentive to treatment.

When asked what impact being a mother had on their treatment, 81% said that being a mother was a barrier to treatment. Key barriers to treatment were: that disclosure would lead to their children being placed into care and secondly, accessing practical assistance with childcare during treatment. This sheds some light on the often contradictory claims that motherhood is both an incentive and a disincentive to treatment. Clearly women are disincentivised from entering treatment if they fear their children will be taken away from them. However, if they can enter treatment with their children they do well, and if they enter treatment without their children they do even better. Looking at the evidence collected from mothers in our study leads to an appreciation that motherhood can simultaneously be an incentive and a disincentive, however contradictory this may appear.

Being a mother remained an important part of the women's identity throughout recovery, regardless of whether they had their children with them or not. Mothers in our survey often defined recovery in maternal terms, for example, talking about being a "drug-free mum". One mother said accessing treatment with her child has helped her "to get insight into drug use and bond with my child and for him to have a drug-free mum".

Whilst mothers reported that being a mother was an important part of their recovery not all had positive experiences of the treatment system as a mum: "I have two kids, one is in care and one lives with his Dad. All through my treatment I'm asked loads of questions about myself and no one has asked me if I am a mum. They ask me if I have parental responsibility for any children which I don't, so that makes me think they don't think of me as a mum".

What is the impact of motherhood on recovery?

Our findings suggest that being a mother in recovery sets you apart from non-mothers in a number of ways.

Firstly, your motherhood can act as both an incentive and disincentive to accessing treatment. The complexity of being a mother accessing treatment explains the contradictory views about the accessibility of our treatment provision. Motherhood is neither an incentive nor a disincentive, it is both; this adds a layer of complexity to the recovery processes that non-mothers do not experience.

For treatment providers and commissioners of recovery systems this makes the task of understanding how best to deliver services to mothers more complex. However complex though, it is important that commissioners of recovery systems and providers of services find effective ways to reduce the disincentive of being a mother and increase the incentives for this group to access recovery services.

Secondly, mothers outperform non-mothers in the health gains from treatment. Regardless of whether their children are with them or not, the mothers in our study made the biggest improvement in both residential and non-residential treatment.

If motherhood does provide additional motivation as this study suggests, treatment services need to respond to this. Services must ensure they are maximising on this recovery capital as women enter treatment and take steps to improve the retention of women in services when their children are not present.

When women have been deemed by the system to have failed as mothers, their motherhood should still be an important element of their treatment. By maximising on this recovery capital we are ensuring our mothers the best chance of recovery and their children the best hope of a reunited, safe family. Clearly the treatment experience is just an element of someone's recovery journey. To get an accurate picture of the impact of motherhood on recovery we need to follow the progress of these groups of women through their recovery journey post treatment. It is our aim to do a 1-year follow up project with this group.

Further work is also needed to understand the impact of fatherhood on recovery. It was not possible to extend this study at this stage, however our experience tells us that there are increasing numbers of fathers progressing through treatment and becoming primary carers of their children. By looking at fathers' experience we could start to develop a clearer picture of the recovery capital of parenthood itself.

The subject of parental substance misuse is fraught with moral judgement and emotion. Whilst those of us responsible for delivering recovery services focus primarily on those with the addiction we cannot effectively do our jobs if we do not understand the impact recovery has on those closest to the problem drug user. When we look at the recovery capital of mothers we are of course trying to understand which intrinsic factors will help improve the recovery process. We are doing that so that we can give those seeking recovery the best possible chance of success. The impact of that change in people reaches far beyond the individual seeking recovery. It extends to their family, friends neighbours and the larger community in which they live. When that person seeking recovery is a mother, the impact of their recovery is more far-reaching. The impact of having a mother with an addiction is devastating and the damage to that child can be far-reaching. For this reason it is essential for all involved in recovery services to ensure they know how best to engage mothers in the recovery process and work with them to sustain that recovery.

Whilst the findings in this study are not conclusive, they do provide some important evidence to suggest further study into the comparative recovery experience of mothers would give us better knowledge about how to support those seeking an end to their substance misuse.

Acknowledgments

The research and analysis for this study was carried out by Ruby Newton, Tom Westall and Natalie Wood. I would like to thank the women who took part in this study for their bravery and honesty and the staff and service users who attended a focus group to review the findings of the work and help me reach my conclusions.

References

Advisory Council on the Misuse of Drugs Report (2003). Hidden Harm: Responding to the needs of children of problem drug users.

Granfield, R & Cloud, W (1999). Coming Clean: Overcoming Addiction without treatment. New York: New York University Press.

NTA (2010). Women in Drug Treatment; what the latest figures reveal. March 2010 National Treatment Agency Report.

White, W & Cloud, W (2008). Recovery Capital: A primer for addictions professionals. Counselor, 9(5), 22-27.

Therapeutic communities

9 Quality of life in therapeutic communities for substance abuse[1]

ERIC BROEKAERT

Department of Orthopedagogy
Ghent University, Belgium

Eric.broekaert@Ugent.be

Abstract

This chapter attempts to provide a basic insight into what "quality of life" means to the therapeutic community for substance abusers. For this, we will start with a definition of the therapeutic community. We situate the background of the therapeutic community, go into the practical functioning of the therapeutic community, its "daily" philosophy reinsertion and the central question of recovery. In this line, we seek a definition of quality of life, look at the background of quality of life and the philosophy, the practical aspects and qualitative demands for positive recovery. It is found that the concept of quality of life is set amongst powerful contradictions in science, religion and philosophy. Because quality of life is so essential for therapeutic communities and for recovery from substance abuse, it is proposed that a definition is needed in this (therapeutic community) context.

---

[1] This text is based on the conference presentations at the 4th World Federation Genoa Institute, 2010 and the 10th ISQOLS International Conference, Bangkok, 2010. Understanding quality of life and building a happier tomorrow, and the Ewodor Symposium_Drug Dependence: Treatment generalities and specificities. Barcelona, 2011.

Key words

Therapeutic communities; quality of life; recovery.

Introduction

It is the goal of this chapter to provide a deeper insight into the quality of life in therapeutic communities for substance abuse. Quality of life is an important concept for therapeutic communities. However it is seldom researched. This concept not only provides a basis for measuring success, but also to go deeper into the subjective interpretation of residents concerning their wellbeing in Therapeutic Communities. For this we will describe the specificity of the therapeutic community and its approach to quality of life. We will try to demonstrate that quality of life has to be defined in context, in this case in the TC context. This is necessary because quality of life is a concept set amidst powerful contradictions in science, religion and philosophy. Doing so, we hope to come to a definition that provides space for the essential characteristics of a therapeutic community, such as the development of human potential, the survival of addiction and striving for the recovery of substance abusers. It is also the hope of the author that this chapter will contribute towards more attention being given to this concept and its powerful possibilities for the worldwide therapeutic community movement

The therapeutic community for substance misuse

The "drug-free, hierarchic, conceptual, therapeutic community for addictions or therapeutic community for substance abuse" is commonly defined as: A TC is a drug-free environment in which people with addictive (and other) problems live together in an organised and structured way in order to promote change and make a drug-free life possible in outside society. The TC forms a miniature society in which residents, and staff - in the role of facilitators- fulfil distinctive roles and adhere to clear rules, all designed to promote the transitional process of the residents. Self-help and mutual-help are pillars of the therapeutic process in which the resident is the protagonist who is mainly responsible for achieving personal growth, a more meaningful and responsible life, and upholding the welfare of the community. The programme is voluntary in the sense that the resident will not be held in the programme by force or against his/her will (Ottenberg, 1993).

The current Therapeutic Community goes back to the Synanon movement of the late fifties. It was founded by Charles (Chuck) Dederich (a recovered alcoholic) and influenced by Moral Rearmement (a movement that was striving for basic Christian values), Alcoholics Anonymous, the utopian hippy lifestyle of the sixties, humanistic psychology (with leading figures such as Rogers and Maslov), and the romantic and idealist philosophy of W.R. Emerson (the power of love as a basis for the organisation of society). In essence, the Synanon movement was part of humanistic existentialism and strived for the drug-free development and psychic growth of the drug abuser. From Synanon California, the movement spread over America, Europe and gradually the rest of the world. The TC movement broke with Synanon because of its demand for life-long engagement.

Synanon itself dissolved and the therapeutic community movement blossomed. In Europe the TC for substance misuse became influenced by the already existing democratic therapeutic communities of Maxwell Jones (influenced by psychoanalysis and with an accent on social learning) (Broekaert *et al.*, 2000). In the end Synanon became a religious cult and was dissolved. The existing therapeutic communities were grouped into the World Federation of Therapeutic Communities and regional organisations such as the European Federation of Therapeutic Communities. The EFTC possesses a scientific body: The European Working group in Drugs Oriented Research. It supports the International Journal of Therapeutic Communities.

The functioning of a therapeutic community is built on social interaction and the creation of a milieu. It creates a transitional space of experience, where a strict daily structure and a hierarchy of resident functions are brought into balance with the expression of emotions that leads to a process of identification. The milieu is based on safety and acceptance of one another. For this no physical violence nor drugs can be tolerated in "the house", the residents work and act in different departments such as service crew, kitchen and cooking, creative energy, sports and leisure and so on (Broekaert, 2001). They follow a routine of house meetings, seminars, working activities encounter and emotional groups. In the groups negative behaviour is put into question. The confrontation of negative behaviour in an atmosphere of dialogue leads to the expression of emotions in which young residents identify with the stories, experiences and TC values of older residents and staff. This process of identification reflects the educational character of the therapeutic community. Or to put it in other words: The essence of the therapeutic community consists of methodical meaning in full interaction in educational context order to reach recovery (Broekaert *et al.,* 2004).

Every day, the philosophy of the therapeutic community is discussed during the morning meeting and further explored in feelings and action during the rest of the day. This philosophy is concrete and refers to self-reliant ego-development. The philosophy of Daytop New York reads as follows "I am here: because there is no refuge, finally, from myself. Until I confront myself in the eyes and hearts of others, I am running. Until I suffer them to share my secrets, I have no safety from them. Afraid to be known, I can know neither myself nor any other; I will be alone. Where else but in our common ground, can I find such a mirror? Here, together, I can at least appear clearly to myself, not as the giant of my dreams, nor the dwarf of my fears. But as a person, part of the whole, with my share in its purpose. In this ground, I can take root and grow. Not alone anymore, as in death, but alive to myself and to others" (Richard Bauvais in: O'Brien, 1993). Other communities may have a slightly different philosophy, but in essence the message is the same.

Since the rupture with Synanon in the mid sixties, therapeutic communities such as Daytop, Odyssey and Phoenixhouse New York, actively strived for reinsertion into society. After a phase of introduction, acceptance and treatment, integration into society follows. Most therapeutic programs have halfway houses and rooms in villages and cities at their disposal. During those different phases the TC tries to attain its ultimate goal of recovery. This whole therapeutic process normally takes more than a year, but recovery itself takes a whole lifetime. Recovery is seen as the pursuit and realisation of a "normal" life without the use of illegal drugs. Even if substance abuse is mostly seen as a chronic mental illness, TC proves through many examples that recovery can be reached. Even if a drug-free life is the goal, the therapeutic community accepts the use of adapted psychotropic medication. In recent years some therapeutic communities have also integrated the use of methadone in their programmes, but surrounded with psychotherapeutic care and relational support.

Quality of life

A univocal definition of quality of life is almost impossible. "Life" is a complex phenomenon and is approached in philosophy, ideology, arts and science from different and almost opposite positions. Within philosophy, soberness can be described in terms of hedonism or virtue (Stoa versus Dyonisius). In arts, fine arts, as well the beauty or ugliness of life can be at the centre of the expression (Delvaux versus Bosch). Within science, life can be researched in a global or reductionist way, (phenomenology versus empiric analytic approaches).

The multi-dimensional concept "quality of life" needs a definition in context (De Mayer *et al.*, 2010). This means that we will have to search for a proper definition of "Quality of life in the context of the therapeutic community", within its philosophy and functioning.

The concept of quality of life is a relatively new concept. It did gain momentum in "Disability Studies". The "Disability Studies" form a Postmodern reaction towards "Special education". Postmodernism is firstly a reaction against modernism. Philosophers such as M. Foucault (1973), G. Deleuze (1983), J. Derrida (1995), and J.F. Lyotard (1984) reacted against the all-explaining theories of Hegel and existentialism. They embraced the radical value critical viewpoints of F. Nietsche (Groot, 2003). They grouped into two streams: post-constructionalism and post-structuralism. The first sees man (in social interaction) as an active constructor of his world, the second concentrates on the critical societal aspects of the structures that determine us. They do not consider a person from the point of view of a handicap (mental retardation, deafness, physical handicap), or a disorder (behaviour or emotional disorder), but seek civil rights, emancipation, inclusion and self-advocacy for all people. They do not look for the great theory, but approach people from their own stories. As they also embrace scientific research, there is a living tension between subjectivity and objectivity. Where the pioneer of "quality of life in disability studies, R. Shallock (1996) embraces a rigorous scientific approach, others accentuate the subjective experiences of people (Roets *et al.*, 2004).

As it becomes clear that the concept of quality of life is set amidst powerful contradictions, it might seem fair to go into the consequences of this. If we consider contradictions as "thesis" and "anti-thesis", the integration of these contradictions may lead to a new synthesis that might be the start of a process of integration, in which the synthesis is confronted again with a new anti-thesis. The above mentioned integration can be discussed in terms of transition towards a new stage of conceptualisation, in this case a better understanding and knowledge of quality of life. Going back to our examples: the confrontation between Stoa and Dyonisius can lead to a good personal equilibrium in values, the one between Delvaux and Bosch to a better taste of fine arts, the one between evidence-based knowledge and practical-based evidence towards a combination of qualitative and quantitative based research studies. This new transition is part of an alternative combination of diverse choices and responsibilities taken upon the attainment of a better situation: a higher quality of life: I made the choice to also look to Delveaux's statement as well as Bosch's. This freedom and responsibility of choosing to reach a better condition in life is a human prerogative and a project for man. It is the antipode of choosing one system that should represent the absolute truth and the proponent of scientific doubt (Broekaert *et al.*, 2010).

The Dutch pedagogue, W. Ter Horst, described the basic forms of educational acting (my translation and formulation): The touching (the person is responsible for his own action), taking care of (providing comfort), the meal (the real place for dialogue), the game (creativity), the move (looking for extending one's horizon), work (looking for action), learning (searching for insight), language (expression), rituals (searching for deeper meaning) (Ter Horst, 1980). These basic forms can provide a framework or categorisation for quality of life. However, the concretization in daily life is up to the individual and her/his field of social interaction and the limitations set by society and law. For the person, quality of life means an acceptable and enjoyable fulfilment of these categories. The practice of quality of life lies in a free choice of meaningful action and intention. Intention is seen as a stochastic action in which actor and goal form a unity. In this sense, quality of life surpasses mono-centric visions and absolute value systems, but remains within the obligations of society (for example: the destruction of an experimental setting to look for knowledge on genetically modified crops may not be destroyed by fundamental action groups that seem to know "in advance" what the results of this research should be. But the action groups have full rights to express their opinions orally and without violence).

For a long time, methadone treatment and harm reduction were seen as an antipode to therapeutic community treatment. Nowadays the integration of treatment systems prevails (Broekaert *et al.*, 2003). This means that some TCs also use methadone and psychotropic medication if needed to cure people. J. De Maeyer (2010) carried out research within the scope of her PhD Dissertation: The "Quality of life among opiate-dependent individuals after starting methadone maintenance treatment". She researched 159 methadone users who had been taking methadone for at least 5 years, by means of the Lancashire Quality of Life Profile, Brief System Inventory and the Addiction Severity Index. There seems to be a positive appreciation of quality of life, but not only health-related solutions are the foremost. More psycho-social support is requested. Attention has to be paid to the relationship with family and friends.

In conclusion: the multi-dimensional concept of quality of life covers much more than recovery itself. It broadens the umbrella to a diversity of ways of coping with addiction. The subjective feeling of happiness and living an acceptable life is part of the concept. This conclusion once again supports the position of searching for methods that go alternatively together and complete each other above the prevalence of fixed contradictions. The therapeutic community disposes of a multitude of psycho-social interventions, and methadone/harm reduction can promote health and diminish dangers towards society. It also has to be mentioned that most addicts went through a lot of different treatment systems during their career, which highlights the importance of case management throughout the system (Vanderplasschen *et al.*, 2004).

Quality of life in the therapeutic community

By the early eighties, G. Deleon and colleagues started the discussion on quality of life in the therapeutic community. Thus, sophisticated indices are needed to capture the extent and diversity of individual change. In addition to psychological dimensions, a portrait of the "health or adaptation, of the successful individual must include social drug use and quality-of-life variables" (Deleon, 1982). They stress the need to research psychological, social drug, and quality of life variables in the broader context of measuring the success of the therapeutic community. This is logical as therapeutic communities have to permanently prove their reason of existence in a sector dominated by medical approaches. The pursuit of a high quality of life is not only an important goal of the therapeutic community but also sets it apart from the other approaches such as methadone and medication.

It is also clear that Deleon and colleagues search for objective approaches of quality of life. Much later, with an editorial on "Addiction" entitled "What future for the Therapeutic Community in the field of addiction?", there is a plea to put more accent on quality of life research in order to guarantee the survival of the TC (Broekaert, 2006). "They (TCs) saw, in comparison to other residential approaches, the effectiveness of their treatment first and foremost as a collection of good practices that enhance the quality of life. This is in contrast to the findings of some meta-analyses that, from a TC point of view, suffer from statistical problems" (Broekaert, 2006). In essence, this discussion is part of the evidence-based medicine versus practice-based evidence. Unfortunately evidence-based medicine is seen as the golden standard, and brings in a hierarchical order between approaches, which is in contrast to the principle of equal standing between treatment approaches with their own identity and of a different nature (Broekaert *et al.*, 2010).

However, it is still rare for us to find almost no scientific studies on quality of life in TCs. A study on quality of life in the Czech Republic shows that there is no difference in quality of life in the TC population than the control group (Doležalová, 2006). An interesting Spanish study evaluates a test for quality of life for substance abuse and saw positive results for reliability and validity (Lozano, 2007). A Belgian study reveals a better situation in all life areas of the Addiction Severity Index, except for physical condition. There was a strong decrease in the severity of misuse: 6.52 to 2.40 and very positive results for the general psycho-social situation considering the time spent in the programme (Soyez *et al.*, 2009).

In 1994, M. Picchi wrote an important essay: His "progetto per l'Uomo (project mankind)" which sees the therapeutic community as a school for life. It describes the principles upon which a human approach towards the cure of substance abusers can be based, and was further established and developed in Italy, Spain and Latin America. This human basis sees the struggle of life and positive values as the cornerstone for further development. It is not only the search for wellbeing that is at stake, but also responsible human action.

However, beside these objective and necessary aspects of quality of life, there is also a need for a more subjective position. Residents who enter a therapeutic community and throughout treatment express an active interest in survival and rebirth from addiction, "to be reborn is our ultimate reality..." (residents Last Renaissance s.d.). During the time in the programme this hope of survival is tested during daily activities and encounter groups. It goes together with painful and joyful moments. It proves that the subjective fulfilment of quality of life cannot be univocal understood. Later, anxieties concerning reinsertion, the way to cope with family and old friends, and the pride of overcoming said anxieties; these difficulties colour the picture. Once back in society there is often still the daily responsibility of not relapsing. This process is actively supported by interaction with peers and staff. So quality of life in a therapeutic community can hardly be described as a personal expression of the most inner experiences but as part of an educational process of social interaction. Good examples of this phenomenon can be found in the writings of residents on their situation.

"The programme was very important to me because I learned to recognise my feelings. This was the heaviest task for me. In fact I only knew two feelings, namely anger and joy. But other feelings such as pain, shame or sorrow were unknown to me. I was working on this during emotional groups" (resident of "De Kiem"- Belgium – my translation from the Dutch p. 19.); "The process of falling down and getting up is bearable, it is indeed a process and one of a transitory nature" (resident of "De Kiem"- Belgium – my translation from the Dutch, p. 15).

Conclusions

If we combine the above mentioned aspects on quality of life - which involves objective and subjective aspects of quality of life - the ever-present social educational aspects of pedagogy, and the striving of TCs for recovery, we could come to the following definition on quality of life: "The energy and power of a person in interaction with peers, which enables him or her to survive addiction, to realise growth in different life areas, to experience happiness in order to reach recovery". This definition includes tension between aspirations, striving for meaningful goals and action towards an accent on behaviour, facts to be analysed through comparison and seeking random-based experiments and significant correlative results. When further researching this question, we come into the field of interest between "evidence-based research" and "practice-based research as evidence". This is however an old question. It is the question mark between the phenomenon of the logic of action and behavioural objectivity. The first is concerned with meaningful life and interpretation, the other with observable behaviour and random experiments. It is the opinion of this author of this chapter that "these two" can "go together alternatively". It is in the tension of a dialogue between the quality of life based on the internal relationship and of the one based on "facts". This tension between counterparts can lead to a new transition and an advanced vision of quality of life in the TC for substance abusers.

References

Broekaert, E (2001). Therapeutic communities for drug users: Description and overview. In Rawlings, B & Yates, R (Eds.), *Therapeutic communities for the treatment of drug users*. Pp. 29-42. London/Philadelphia: Jessica Kingsley Publishers.

Broekaert, E (2006). What future for the Therapeutic Community in the field of addiction? A view from Europe. *Addiction*, 101(12), 1677–1678.

Broekaert, E, Autrique, M, Vanderplasschen, W *et al.* (2010). The Human Prerogative': A Critical Analysis of Evidence-Based and Other Paradigms of Care in Substance Abuse Treatment. *Psychiatric Quarterly*, 81(3), 227-238.

Broekaert, E & Vanderplasschen, W (2003). Towards the integration of treatment systems for substance abusers: report on the second international symposium on substance abuse treatment and special target groups. *Journal of Psychoactive Drugs*, 35(2), 237-345.

Broekaert, E, Vanderplasschen, W, Temmerman, I, Ottenberg, D & Kaplan, C (2000).

Retrospective study of similarities and relations between the American drug-free and the European therapeutic communities for children and adults. *Journal of Psychoactive Drugs*, 32(4), 407-417.

Broekaert, E, Vandevelde, S, Schuyten, G, Erauw, K & Bracke, R (2004). Evolution of encounter group methods in therapeutic communities for substance abusers. *Addictive Behaviours*, 29(2), 231-244.

De Maeyer, J, Vanderplasschen, W & Broekaert, E (2010). Quality of life among opiate-dependent individuals: A review of the literature. *International journal of drug policy*, 21(5), 364-380.

De Maeyer, J, Vanderplasschen, W, Lammertyn, J, van Nieuwenhuizen, C, Sabbe, B & Broekaert, E (2010). Current quality of life and its determinants among opiate-dependent individuals five years after starting methadone treatment. *Quality of Life Research* (Epub ahead of print).

Deleon, G, Wexler, K & Jainchill, N (1982). The therapeutic community: Success and Improvement Rates 5 Years after Treatment. *The International Journal of the Addictions*, 17(4), 703-747.

Deleuze, G (1983). *Nietzsche and philosophy*. New York: Columbia University Press.

Derrida, J (1995). *On the name*. Chicago: Stanford University Press.

Doležalová, P (2006). Kvalita života drogově závislých v terapeutických komunitách [The Quality of Life of Drug Addicts in Therapeutic Communities]. Adiktologie, 6(1), 12-25.

Foucault, M (1973). *Madness and civilization*. New York: Vintage Books.

Groot, G (2003). *Vier ongemakkelijke filosofen. Nietzche, Cioran, Bataille, Derrida [Four philosophers uncomfortable. Nietzche, Cioran, Bataille, Derrida]*. Amsterdam: Sun.

Lozano, ÓM, Rojas, A, Pérez, C, Apraiz, B, Sánchez, F, Marín, YA (2007). Test para la evaluación de la calidad de vida en adictos a sustancias psicoactivas (tecvasp): estudios de fiabilidad y validez. *Trastornos Adictivos*, 9, 97-107.

Lyotard, JF (1984). *The postmodern condition: a report on knowledge*. Minneapolis, MN: University of Minnesota Press.

O'Brien, WB (1993). *You can't do it alone*. New York: Simon and Schuster.

Ottenberg, D, Broekaert, E & Kooyman, M (1993). What cannot be changed in a therapeutic community? *Special Education Ghent*, 2, 51-62.

Picchi, M (1994). *Un progetto per l'Uomo*. Associazione. Centro Italiano di solidarietà. Roma.

Resident TC DeKiem Driemaandelijks tijdschrift van De Kiem v.z.w. jaargang 18 (4) 2010.

Resident TC De Kiem Driemaandelijks tijdschrift van De Kiem v.z.w. jaargang 19 (1) 2011.

Residents TC Last Renaissance. Part of the philosophy of TC Last Renaissance. Washington.S.D.

Roets, G, Van de Perre, D, Van Hove, G, Schoeters, L & De Schauwer, E (2004). One for All - All for One! An account of the joint fight for human rights by Flemish Musketeers and their Tinker Ladies. *British Journal of Learning Disabilities 32*, 54-64.

Schallock, R (1996). *Quality of life, volume & conceptualization and measurement*. Washington. American association on mental retardation.

Soyez, V , Broekaert, E (2009) De psychosociale situatie van bewoners van "De Kiem" voor en na de behandeling. Tijdschrift "De Kiem" p.10-13.

Ter Horst, W (1980). *Algemene orthopedagogiek: proeve van een theorie-concept*. Kampen: Kok.

Vanderplasschen, W, Rapp, RC, Wolf, J & Broekaert, E (2004). The development and implementation of case management for substance use disorders in North America and Europe. *Psychiatric Services*, 55, 913-922.

10 The essential elements of treatment: a European therapeutic communities perspective

Ilse Goethals

Department of Special Education
Faculty of Psychology and Educational Sciences
Ghent University, Belgium

ilse.goethals@ugent.be

Abstract

Both adaptation and innovation have been the keys to survival for therapeutic communities (TCs) for addiction in Europe since their introduction in the 1970s. Although history clearly shows that the TC approach is flexible enough to be implemented for a variety of populations in different cultures and in various settings, little is known about the constant challenge to uphold what is essential in treatment. In this study we will highlight the core characteristics of European TC treatment and investigate whether traditional and modified TC programmes remained faithful to the essential elements of the classic TC model as outlined by De Leon (1995a; 2000). To answer previous questions, the "Therapeutic Community Scale of Essential Elements Questionnaire (SEEQ)- short version" was used. The European TCs that were found eligible for this study (n = 19) were members of the European Federation for Therapeutic Communities (EFTC). Overall, we found relatively high mean scores on each of the six SEEQ dimensions indicating that the TCs in this European sample largely adhere to the basic elements outlined in De Leon's classic TC model. Regarding the cluster differences, the results indicate that the traditional TCs scored significantly higher than the modified TCs on three SEEQ dimensions (n = 6) and eight SEEQ domains (n = 27). The findings clearly indicate that in Europe, the "modified" programmes are more eclectic than the "traditional" programmes.

Key words

Therapeutic communities; substance abuse treatment; traditional; modified; democratic; hierarchical; questionnaire.

Introduction

The therapeutic community mentioned in the title refers to the drug-free concept-based therapeutic community for the treatment of addiction that originated at Synanon in the United States. Since its conception in the 1950s, this treatment modality has spread all over the United States leading to TCs such as Daytop and Phoenixhouse (Broekaert *et al.,* 2006).

In Europe, the American Drug-free TC became part of a longstanding tradition of milieu-therapy, different schools of therapy and a large diversity of European cultures and ideologies (Broekaert *et al.,* 2006). It was studied from a historical (Broekaert *et al.,* 2000), national (Yates, 2003) therapeutic (Ottenberg, 1984) and research perspective (Ravndal, 2003). Historically it was linked to the new school movement, the TCs for children, the Maxwell Jones democratic TC and the Northfield experiments (Broekaert *et al.,* 2000). From a therapeutic point of view, the European TC was, due to its milieu-therapeutic background, influenced by psychoanalysis. There was abhorrence towards behaviour modification techniques such as wearing signs and shaving heads (Broekaert *et al.,* 2000). More than in the United States, professionals took over from ex-addicts (Kooyman, 2001; Yates, 2003), softened the method, and replaced harsh confrontation in groups by more dialogue (Broekaert *et al.,* 2004). In their research efforts the European therapeutic community researchers extensively looked to the knowledge and experience of American researchers, but soon established their own identity within the European Working Group on Drugs Oriented Research (EWODOR) (Broekaert *et al.,* 2002). The research traditions were mostly based on phenomenological descriptive (case) studies and quasi-experimental research (Ravndal, 2003; Soyez *et al.*, 2004). Only during recent years has the importance of evidence-based experimental designs been more generally acknowledged (Autrique *et al.*, 2008).

Despite these deserving efforts to the global study of the TC approach and theory (Kooyman, 1992), evidence of what is really essential in European TC treatment does not exist. It is however well documented that during the last couple of decades the TCs in Europe, as in the United States, have modified their approach to keep up with the demands of society. Many European governments cut funds and insisted on "new management" with emphasis on efficiency, continuity of care and collaboration between the different treatment systems. Most TCs displayed flexibility and modified aspects of their approach to the new management style by creating more complex, but unique treatment settings for different populations and with varied durations of stay (Broekaert, 2006b; Soyez *et al.*, 2004).

The large diversity of TC programmes that exists since the eighties due to these modifications has urged European TCs and members of the EFTC to define what is essential and basic to the TC approach and philosophy (De Leon, 1995). A first effort was made at the European Scientific Institute in De Haan, Belgium in 1991. The members of this institute started the discussion with the following question: "if there is nothing constant but change in a TC, what cannot be changed without losing the essential goals and striving of our movement" (Broekaert, *et al.*, 1993). The main conclusions of this meeting were to uphold the TCs quality of care through regular revisions and evaluations of their programme, recruit adequately trained staff members, and to abide with the standards and goals of the EFTC. Also, treatment should primarily be directed towards recovery of drug abuse and ultimately promote a drug-free life in society (Broekaert *et al.*, 1993).

More recently, in the UK, the quality network "community of communities"[1] created service standards for European TCs for addiction. Those standards represent developing views on the central elements of TC practice and were primarily developed as an audit and evaluative system for the TCs in the field of mental health (Haigh & Tucker, 2004). From 2006 until 2007, the service standards where piloted by ten European TCs for addiction. However, the results of this research have not yet been published.

The aim of the present study is to address previously mentioned research gaps using the abbreviated version of the "Therapeutic Community Scale of Essential

---

[1] http://www.rcpsych.ac.uk/clinicalservicestandards/centreforqualityimprovement/communityofcommunities/servicestandards/addictiontcs.aspx

Elements Questionnaire (SEEQ)" (Melnick & De Leon, 1999). In essence, the SEEQ identifies and codifies the core characteristics of a drug-free hierarchical concept based TC approach. The two main research questions are: (1) Do European TCs have a common agreement on what is essential and important in TC treatment? (2) Do traditional as well as modified TCs remain faithful to the essential elements of the classical TC model, outlined by De Leon (1995a, 2000).

Method

Research Sample

With the support of the EFTC president we administered the SEEQ to the directors of the TCs that are members of the European Federation of Therapeutic communities (EFTC) (n = 38). A total of 24 programmes responded. However, outpatient programmes, halfway-houses, and TC programmes with stays of less than six months (n = 5) were excluded from the study. The 19 remaining programmes varied in the expected duration of stay from 6 months to 2 years. Of those 19 TCs, 8 were identified by the authors as modified (4 programmes served special target groups and 4 programmes had duration of stay between 6 - 10 months).

The population of the TCs were predominantly Caucasian (93%), adult (63%) and male (73%). Their treatment mostly focuses on clients with heroin problems (48.4%) and polydrug misuse (31.7%) followed by cocaine- (15.2%) and alcohol problems (10.7%). On average 24% were referred by the courts.

Research instrument

The SEEQ is based on the theoretical framework of the TC treatment model as described by De Leon in 1995. It was further refined with the help of an advisory group, a selected group of 11 TC experts and 1 well experienced researcher. After several extensive reviews by all the members of this group, the SEEQ ultimately entailed 135 likert-type items organised around 6 broad dimensions and 27 domains.

These dimensions represent the different components of TC treatment whilst the domains highlight the modalities' distinctive philosophy and treatment elements. Ratings per item go from 0 = "not important" to 4 = "Extremely important".

For this study we used the short version of the SEEQ (Melnick *et al.*, 2000). The adaptation of the original form comprised the consolidation of the different items per domain into one statement. For example, the 2 items belonging to the domain "Role of the Family" were comprised of the following statement: "Where appropriate, the family is included in the treatment plan".

The SEEQ can be used as a framework for TC programmes, giving allowance for programme-specific exceptions. It can also be used as a utility for programme evaluation, research, development of TC-oriented programme protocols and staff training (Melnick & De Leon, 1999). A disadvantage perhaps is that the SEEQ has not yet been validated. However, applications of the SEEQ in published research revealed rather promising results. In a first study, the data from a survey of 59 TC programmes that were members of the Therapeutic Communities of America (TCA) (Melnick & De Leon, 1999), demonstrated a high degree of adherence to the essential elements of a TC as outlined by De Leon (1995a; 1995b; 2000) but also showed slight divergence of beliefs between traditional TC programmes and modified TC programmes. In a second study, using an abbreviated form of SEEQ, the results of 19 American TCs that participated in the Drug Abuse Treatment Outcomes Study (DATOS) supported earlier findings by confirming differences in SEEQ scores between programmes previously identified as traditional and modified TCs (Melnick *et al.*, 2000). In a third study, Dye and her colleagues (2009) examined the extent to which modified TCs were able to retain the underlying core technology of the TC using 49 items of the SEEQ. For a total of 380 self-identified TCs they concluded that certain modifications to the traditional TC model are possible without losing the TC model's core technology. However, modifications of the structure or to the intensity of the TC programming did have a significant impact on adherence to the TCs' core characteristics (Dye *et al.*, 2009).

Data Analysis

For the first research question we computed the percentage of the maximum possible score represented by the means. This percentage equates the various scales for the number of domains and expresses the degree to which scores can be considered high or low.

One way analysis of variance for independent groups (ANOVA) was used was to test whether the mean scores of the European traditional TCs on the dimensions and domains of the SEEQ differed significantly from the mean scores of the modified European TCs.

	Number of domains	Cronbach's alpha	M	SD	% of maximum
The TC Perspective	4	.75	13.47	2.04	84
Treatment Approach and Structure	5	.75	17.42	1.92	87
Community as Therapeutic Agent	7	.78	22.37	3.47	80
Educational and Work Activities	3	.85	9.89	2.23	82
Formal Therapeutic Elements	4	.78	13.05	2.37	82
TC Process	4	.77	13.84	1.64	87
TOTAL	27	.78	90.04	13.67	84

Table 1. Overall concordance (N=19).

Results

The percentages in table 1 indicate a fairly high degree of adherence between the participating European TCs as to the essential elements of a traditional TC model. The total SEEQ scale had a mean score (M = 90.04) that represents 84% of the maximum possible score of 108 (4 x 27). The dimensions showing the strongest agreement were *"Treatment Approach and Structure"* and *"Treatment Process"*. Both dimensions achieved a mean score of 87% of the maximum possible score. The dimension demonstrating the least agreement (80% of the maximum mean score) was "Community as Therapeutic Agency".

Comparisons between traditional and modified TCs in Europe show significant differences on 3 SEEQ dimensions and 8 SEEQ domains. More specifically, traditional TCs rated the dimensions "TC Perspective" (F (1,18) = 11,3; p = 0.004), "TC treatment approach and structure" (F = 9,1; p = 0.008) and "TC process" (F = 9,8; p = 0.006), higher than the modified TCs. With respect to the SEEQ domains, the traditional TCs more strongly emphasised "the view of the addictive disorder" (F(1,18) = 7,7; p = 0.023) and "the view of the addict" (F (1,18) = 5,8; p = 0.027). In comparison to the modified TCs, they also paid more attention to "formal educational activities" (F (1,18) =4,9; p = 0.040) and to the "roles and functions of clients" (F (1,18) = 5,6; p = 0.029). In addition, traditional TCs more strongly agreed on the importance of "peers as gate keepers" (F (1,18) = 5,0; p = 0.040) and "peers' mutual self-help" (F (1,18) = 4,8; p = 0.044) as critical components of the recovery process. Finally, traditional

	Traditional TC		Modified TC	
	M	**SD**	**M**	**SD**
View of the addictive behaviour	3.6	0.50	2.8	0.89
View of the addict	3.5	0.69	2.5	1.20
View of recovery	3.8	0.40	3.3	1.16
View of right living	3.5	0.52	3.5	0.53
The TC perspective	**3.6**	**0.34**	**3.0**	**0.48**
Agency organisation	3.7	0.47	3.5	0.53
Agency approach to treatment	4.0	0.00	3.9	0.35
Staff roles and functions	3.6	0.50	3.0	0.93
Client role and functions	3.7	0.47	3.1	0.64
Healthcare	3.3	1.00	2.6	0.74
The Agency: Treatment approach and structure	**3.7**	**0.30**	**3.2**	**0.35**
Peer as gate keepers	3.5	0.52	3.0	0.53
Mutual help	3.5	0.69	2.8	0.71
Enhancement of community belonging	3.6	0.67	3.4	0.74
Contact with outside community	3.8	0.77	3.0	0.76
Community/clinical management: privileges	3.2	0.75	2.4	1.31
Community/clinical management: sanctions	3.5	0.69	3.4	0.74
Community/clinical management: surveillance	3.1	0.83	2.9	0.99
Community as Therapeutic Agent	**3.4**	**0.42**	**3.0**	**0.54**
Formal educational elements	3.5	0.82	2.3	1.30
Therapeutic educational elements	3.5	0.69	3.3	0.46
Work as therapy	3.8	0.60	3.0	1.36
Educational and Work Activities	**3.6**	**0.47**	**2.9**	**0.90**
General therapeutic techniques	3.4	0.67	3.1	0.35

Continues

Continuation

Groups as therapeutic agents	3.5	0.52	2.9	0.83
Counselling techniques	3.5	0.69	2.9	0.99
Role of the family	3.5	0.52	3.0	1.07
Formal Therapeutic Elements	**3.5**	**0.44**	**3.0**	**0.67**
Stages of treatment	3.5	0.69	3.1	0.99
Introductory period	3.7	0.65	3.3	0.46
Primary treatment stage	3.5	0.52	3.1	0.64
Community re-entry period	3.8	0.40	3.3	0.71
TC Process	**3.7**	**0.36**	**3.2**	**0.32**

Table 2. Responses to the Survey of Essential Elements Questionnaire (SEEQ) by type of TC.

TCs assigned greater importance to "frequent group activities" that reinforce community norms (F (1,18) = 4,66; p = 0.46) and to "the re-entry phase" where they prepare clients for a life in the outside community (F (1,18) = 5,0; p = 0.04).

Discussion

The results show that the European TCs in our research sample share a fairly common belief on what is essential in treatment. Overall, we found relatively high mean scores on each of the six SEEQ dimensions indicating that the TCs in this European sample largely adhere to the basic elements outlined in De Leon's classic TC model. The strongest agreement was found for the dimensions *"Treatment Approach and Structure"* and *"Treatment Process"*. This result illustrates that the daily structure and activities, the participation of both staff members and residents, the preoccupation with health care issues, and the different stages of incremental learning are the core characteristics of European TC treatment. The dimension receiving the lowest average score was "Community as Therapeutic Agent" thus indicating that European TCs have a slightly different perspective on the therapeutic advantage of peer support, mutual help and the use of behaviour modification techniques for the clinical progress of residents.

Despite the relatively high level of overall agreement, univariate data-analysis also revealed significant differences between traditional and modified TCs on several key dimensions of the SEEQ. For instance, European modified programmes are less convinced about the TC perspective on recovery than the traditional programmes. The belief that "drug abuse" is not the problem but a symptom of underlying psychological and behavioural disorders is less pronounced in modified TCs. In the dimension "TC treatment approach and structure", modified TCs put significantly less emphasis on the "roles and functions of clients" such as the expectation of clients to function as members of the community, reinforce community values and to serve as role models. In the dimension "Community as Therapeutic Agent", the differences between modified and traditional programmes focused on the importance of "peers as gate keepers" and "peers' mutual self-help" as critical components of the recovery process indicating a reduced role of the peer community in the European modified TCs. In the fourth dimension, "Educational and Work Activities", modified TCs scored significantly lower on "educational activities" such as seminars in special topics, academic training and/or vocational training. Concerning the dimension "Formal Therapeutic Elements", significant differences were found for the domain "frequent group activities", showing that modified TCs in Europe put less emphasis on group activities that reinforce community norms and encounter negative behaviours. Finally, in the dimension "TC Process", modified TCs assigned less importance to "the re-entry phase" thus indicating that not all residents are being prepared for a life in the outside community.

Summarising these differences, we notice that European modified TCs put less emphasis on "community as method", which is in fact the quintessential element of TC treatment according to De Leon (2001). They also have a different perspective on recovery and on the use of behavioural confrontation techniques. Comparing these results with the results of an American study (Melncik *et al.,* 2000) it becomes clear that the adaptations of the classic TC model to special populations or to programmes with alternate durations of stay, have had a more profound impact in Europe. The abandonment of "community as method" as their primary treatment element points towards the idea that most of the European modified TCs in our study sample are in reality "TC-oriented" programmes (Goethals *et al.,* 2011). An additional explanation for the differences found in this study might reflect their own unique historical development. As mentioned in the introduction, the early European TCs for addiction were influenced by psychoanalysis and humanistic psychology. They implemented alternative therapeutic methods, supported family involvement and depended more on professional staff than on ex-addicts. In all probability, contemporary modified TCs in Europe still rely more on psychoanalysis, thus exercising individual therapy in addition to group therapy (Haigh and Lees, 2008). In encounter groups the focus could have moved from mutual confrontation towards a more balanced and respectful dialogue (Broekaert *et al.*, 2004). Furthermore, a stronger reliance on professional staff and family in treatment might have reduced the importance of "self-help" and "mutual help". However, what is more difficult to explain is the different perspective on recovery. Perhaps, and for reasons of survival, some TC programmes admit clients that are on methadone maintenance treatment, which is in essence incompatible with a drug-free TC ideology. Changes in TC ideology might also be connected to the more recent advances in neurosciences. Viewing addiction as a chronic, relapsing brain disease might explain the re-occurring relapses and therefore be more in agreement with the clinical experience of staff members in TCs.

Notwithstanding the differences, an average score of "very important" to "extremely important" on five SEEQ domains and nineteen SEEQ dimensions supports the idea that regardless of their origin, TCs in Europe share a fairly common perspective on what is essential in treatment.

The current study also provides proof that the SEEQ can help European TCs determine their fidelity and uphold the quality of their care. On one hand, the instrument allows programmes to clearly specify the elements of the TC model that have been implemented as intended, while on the other hand it creates the ability to modify certain components in order to adapt to different populations and settings without abandoning "community as method". For European TC researchers, the SEEQ presents an opportunity to generalise findings based on the similarity of elements. Yet, it does not provide evidence of programme effectiveness. More comprehensive assessments of the typical components of the TC model and the analysis of what actually occurs during treatment is needed to determine which elements of the TC programme are effective in producing positive outcomes.

There are a number of other limitations to consider when interpreting the results. First, this study relies on a small sample size that might have caused statistical non-significance in the remaining domains and dimensions of the SEEQ. The readers should also be aware that the designation of the European programmes as traditional or modified was identified by the first author based upon the TCs' length of stay and the population served. Another factor that might have influenced the statistical significance in this study is the difference in professional affiliation of the respondents who actually filled out the SEEQ. Fifteen surveys were completed by the programme's director and four with the help of a senior staff member. Secondly, the SEEQ only provides quantitative data on the essential elements of the TC treatment while a qualitative study might give more detailed information on the specificity of the modifications. In addition, the items of the abbreviated survey do not capture subtle differences between programmes. For example: the SEEQ item representing the use of confrontational and behavioural modification techniques might be graded as extremely important by both the European and the American traditional TCs while in reality the European TCs have a different idea on the intensity of confrontations.

References

Autrique, M, Vanderplasschen, W, Broekaert, E & Sabbe, B (2008). The Drug-Free Therapeutic Community: Findings and Reflections in an Evidence-Based Era. *Therapeutic Communities: The International Journal for Therapeutic and Supportive Organisations*, 29(1), 5-15.

Broekaert, E, van der Straten, G, D'Oosterlinck, F & Kooyman, M (1999). The Therapeutic Community for ex-addicts: a view from Europe. *Therapeutic Communities: The International Journal for Therapeutic and Supportive Organizations*, 20, 255-266.

Broekaert, E, Vanderplasschen, W, Temmerman, I, Ottenberg, D & Kaplan, C (2000). Retrospective study of similarities and relations between the American drug free and the European therapeutic communities for children and adults. *Journal of Psychoactive Drugs*, 32, 407-417.

Broekaert, E, Vandevelde, S, Vanderplasschen, W, Soyez, V & Poppe, A (2002). Two decades of "research-practice" encounters in the development of European therapeutic communities for substance abusers. *Nordic Journal of Psychiatry*, 56, 371-377.

Broekaert, E, Vandevelde S, Schuyten, G, Erauw, K & Bracke, R (2004). Evolution of encounter group methods in therapeutic communities for substance abusers. *Addictive Behaviors*, 29, 231-244.

Broekaert, E, Vandevelde S, Soyez, V, Yates, R & Slater, A (2006a). The third generation of therapeutic communities: the early development of the TC for addictions in Europe. *European Addiction Research*, 12, 1-11.

Broekaert, E (2006b). What future for the Therapeutic Community in the field of addiction? A view from Europe. *Addiction*, 101, 1677-1678.

De Leon, G (1995a). Therapeutic communities for addictions: A theoretical framework. *International Journal of the Addictions*, 30, 1603-1645.

De Leon, G (1995b). Residential therapeutic communities in the mainstream: Diversity and issues. *Journal of Psychoactive Drugs*, 27, 3-15.

De Leon G, (2000). The therapeutic community. *Theory, Model, and Method*. New York: Springer.

De Leon, G (2001). Therapeutic communities for substance abuse: developments in North America (pp. 79-104). In Rawlings, B. & Yates, R. (Eds.). *Therapeutic communities for the treatment of drug users*. London: Jessica Kingsley Publishers.

Dye, MH, Ducharme, LJ, Johnson, JA, Knudsen, HK & Roman, PM (2009). Modified therapeutic communities and adherence to traditional elements. *Journal of Psychoactive Drugs*, 43, 275-283.

Goethals, I Soyez, V, De Leon, G, Melnick, J & Broekaert, E (2011). Essential elements of treatment: A comparative study between European and American TCs for addiction. *Substance Use & Misuse, 46*: 1023-1031.

Haigh, R & Lees, J (2008). Fusion TCs: Divergent histories, converging challenges. *Therapeutic Communities*, 29, 347 - 374.

Haigh, R & Tucker, S (2004). Democratic development of standards: A quality network of therapeutic communities. *Psychiatric Quarterly,* 75, 263-277.

Kooyman, M (1992). The therapeutic community for addicts: *intimacy, parent involvement and treatment outcome.* Rotterdam: Universiteitsdrukkerij. Erasmusuniversiteit.

Kooyman, M (2001). The history of therapeutic communities: a view from Europe. In Rawlings, B & Yates, R (Eds.). *Therapeutic communities for the treatment of drug users.* London: Jessica Kingsley Publishers.

Melnick, G & De Leon, G (1999). Clarifying the nature of therapeutic community treatment: A survey of essential elements. *Journal of Substance Abuse Treatment,* 16, 307- 313.

Melnick, G, De Leon, G, Hiller, ML & Knight, K (2000). Therapeutic community: diversity in treatment elements. *Substance Use and Misuse,* 35, 1819- 1847.

Ottenberg, DJ (1984). Therapeutic community and the danger of the cult phenomenon, Paper presented at the third generation of therapeutic communities. Proceedings of the first European Conference on milieu therapy, Eskilstuna.

Ravndal, E (2003) Research in the concept-based therapeutic community - its importance to European treatment research in the drug field. *International Journal of Social Welfare,* 12, 229-238.

Soyez, V, Tatrai, H, Broekaert, E & Bracke, R (2004). The implementation of contextual therapy in the therapeutic community for substance abusers: a case study. *Journal of Family Therapy,* 26, 286-305.

Yates, R (2003). A brief moment of glory: the impact of the therapeutic community movement on the drug treatment systems in the UK. *International Journal of Social Welfare,* 12, 239-243.

11 MECETT, the journeymen model transferred to staff training in TC's

GEORGE VAN DER STRATEN

Therapeutic Communitie Trempoline
Belgium

georges.straten@gmail.com

Abstract

Since 1960, TCs have spread from country to country, not based on academic training, but through travel and knowledge exchange between the teams. As for residents of TCs, peer exchange is at the heart of the improvement process of teams. Since 1974, Georges van der Straten has travelled throughout Europe visiting many TCs; he brought best practices back and implemented them in the TC he manages. These trips and exchanges are also an opportunity to observe differences in social and political environments of TCs and stimulate strategic thinking and a continuous process of quality improvement. The quality approach is indispensable in the context of TCs, because residential centres are expensive and in countries that are reducing the "public health" budget, only dynamic TCs that will be able to demonstrate their cost-benefit ratio will survive. The purpose of international benchmarking is the continuous improvement of quality of care and work efficiency. Models and methods found abroad can strengthen the long-term financial security of TCs. Travelling is an accelerator of innovation and creativity, but is even more so in terms of professional motivation. Therefore, benchmarking should be accessible to all members of organisations throughout their lives. After a meeting with the French organisation of journeymen "Les Compagnons du Devoir", G. van der

Straten has transferred this model of learning by transferring it to the world of TCs (ECEtt network). This method can now benefit many other professional sectors.

Key words

Journeymen; learning; network; quality; ECEtt.

From a therapy for addicted persons to an innovative learning method

The MECETT method of skills management is the result of long-term experience in therapeutic communities (TC) for drug addicted people. It resorts to the "self help group" approach, which means a dynamic of mutual help among drug addicted people so that each participant (resident in treatment) succeeds to change his way of thinking, of living and of behaving and learns how to solve the problems of everyday life through relationships to his fellows, rather than using chemicals or other ways, whose long-term impact is negative for oneself and the community. TCs have a vision of change based on a continuous interaction between responsibility and solidarity and on a fundamental belief in the learning potential of people, whatever their situation. Their motto is "you alone can do it, but you can't do it alone". The TC movement is an international network whose know-how has been transferred worldwide, from team to team, through visits and exchanges.

Georges van der Straten, the leader of a Belgian CT, met the movement of the "Compagnons du Devoir" and intended to transfer the model of the journeymen apprenticeship to TC staff members. He created the ECEtt network so that teams of TCs could benefit from a life-long learning system through travel and improve the quality in all the network's TCs. Over five years, various ECEtt projects were conducted with the support of the European Union, and this approach has become a new method of management of quality improvement available to many working environments in the public or private as well in the profit or non-profit sectors. Learning and changing happens as much through the effort to meet others, to listen and learn from their experience as through welcoming them, talking to them and sharing one's own experience.

New challenges for TCs

Therapeutic communities for drug addicted people emerged in the 60s in the U.S. and this model was transferred to Europe during the 70s. At that time, therapeutic communities were the only specialist treatment offered to help drug addicts because legislation limited the duration of substitution treatment to several months. Since the proliferation of drug abuse, black market, criminality and the increase of HIV, this has posed major problems for security and public health. Governments therefore changed their priorities: "stabilisation of addiction" became a priority instead of the "rehabilitation" prospect for drug addicts. The government asked the medical profession to take charge of the heroin addicts through substitution. In most countries, laws have been amended so that substitution could be a chronic treatment (10 years or more). Despite this policy change, therapeutic communities have continued to grow slowly but became a small face of the overwhelming majority represented by substitution treatments, harm reduction and other medical-pharmaceutical approaches. In 2008, for a sample of 8 European countries (Great Britain, Spain, France, Italy, Belgium, Greece, Poland and Bulgaria), 37,000 addicts appealed to therapeutic communities compared to 680,000 to substitution treatment (which must be added to clients of other pharmacological treatments and harm reduction).

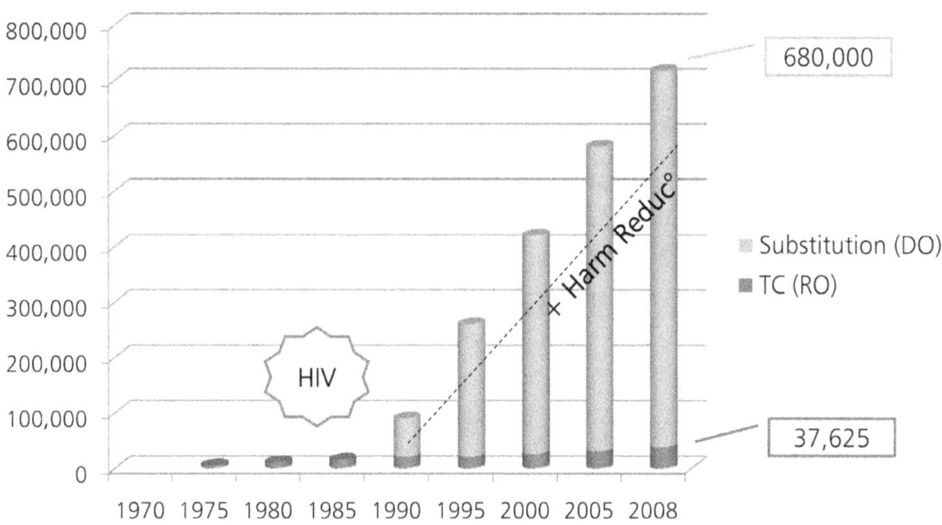

Figure 1. Recovery and disease oriented approaches in EU.

But this explosion in the number of substitution treatment is not uniform in all countries. There are significant differences across countries in the distribution of patients in substitution treatment and those in therapeutic communities. France accounted for almost one extreme where everything was oriented to medical approaches and virtually nothing to therapeutic communities. In contrast, in Poland, almost all efforts were directed towards rehabilitation through therapeutic communities and access to substitution treatment was virtually non-existent. Greece represented an intermediate case where about 50% of addicts were in substitution treatment and 50% were in therapeutic communities. In this general context, where patients in substitution treatment were 19 times more frequent than patients in therapeutic communities, and because the cost of 1 year-long residential treatment in TCs is much higher than the cost of outpatient treatment, TCs had to take their fate into their own hands and show their effectiveness.

Learning through travel and networking

The history and development of therapeutic communities was done by travel and transfer. As in the Alcoholics Anonymous movement, therapeutic communities have developed by travelling to observe what was practiced in countries where the first therapeutic communities have emerged and TC professionals have met regularly at international conferences (EFTC, WFTC, Euro-TC, etc.). Increasing pressure issues on cost/benefit and competition with other treatment models have prompted TC leaders to stick together and work with university researchers in order to objectify the effectiveness of TC outreach. Each therapeutic community has had to adapt to its local context, its national environment. To accomplish this coping strategy, it is inspiring to visit colleagues who live in other socio-economic or socio-political contexts. This has led Georges van der Straten (director of the Trampoline therapeutic community in Belgium) to regularly visit colleagues in a dozen countries in Europe. This was an opportunity to observe not only best practices and opportunities that appeared in some contexts, but also to identify threats to some therapeutic communities according to their socio-political context. Returning home, he could better anticipate potentially adverse developments of situations and identify pitfalls and ways to avoid them, and also strengthen the approach and enrich his own centre with what is practiced abroad and prepare to cope with future risks in his own environment.

Trip	Model of origin	Tools introduced in TC Trempoline	Year
1986	« Accoglienza » : CeIS Roma	Residential **Welcome phase** (Accueil)	1988
1986	« Coinvolgimento Familiare » : CeIS Roma	**Family Service**	1988
1986	« Gruppo Solidarietà » : CeIS Roma	Mutual help **groups for parents** (Solidarité)	1988
1978	« TC concept » USA → Ghent + Netherlands,	TC based on the self-help method	1989
1978	« Reentry phas » : USA + Ghent + Netherlands,	**Reentry** house (RS)	1991
1987	« Casa del Sole » : Rome, Modena, Madrid	**Staff training** + prevention (Re-Sources)	1994
1997	« Cooperative B » : CeIS Mestre-Venice,	**Vocational training** (CIIP)	1998
1997	« Ulysse » : CeIS Venice,	**Groups for relapsed** residents (Horus)	1999
1999	« Casa Mimosa » Modena + « Villa Emma » Venice	Program for **mothers + children** Kangourou	2000
1996	EWODOR, Research CeIS-Modena,	**Research** Service (R&D)	2002
2000	« ROIS » De Leon → Warsaw EFTC	**Integrated System** network (WaB)	2003
2001	Research U-Ghent & TC's Kethea & De Sleutel,	Europ-ASI follow-up	2004
2000	« Compagnons du Devoir » Cologne & Paris	**Learning through travel** (ECEtt)	2004
2001	« ITP » Coolmine, Dublin,	**Individual Treatment Plan**	2006
2000	Proyecto Hombre, CoC and Phoenix-Futures	Control of **Quality** process	2009
2009	« Winadd » CEID Bordeaux,	Patients data registration **software** WINAdd	2010

Figure 2. Copy and adapt.

"Copy and adapt"

After 35 years of experience and travelling through the therapeutic communities, he claims that 80% of what has been put in place at Trampoline has been transferred from abroad. He stresses the concept of "copy and adapt" and not "copy and paste." Models of inspiration for Trampoline mainly came from Italy, the Netherlands, the United States, Spain and Greece.

The meetings with colleagues and the search for best practices are not only an opportunity to discover expertise, but also to make surprising discoveries that we call "Aha! Experiences". Whether countries with therapeutic communities are doing well or badly, in both cases, unexpected facts and conversations can raise awareness of opportunities and new ways of thinking, seeing and developing pro-creativity and innovation. Almost all the services in his TC were marked by best practices and "Aha! Experiences" seen abroad.

The journeymen of "Compagnons du Devoir"

In 2000, Georges van der Straten went to Cologne for a two-day training course at the "Compagnons du Devoir" (French network of journeymen). This is how he discovered the learning method of journeymen. He was struck by the similarity between the principles and values of companionship and those of TCs and support groups for addicts. The learning process is among the journeymen, as in TCs: the existence of a home network with shared values, everyday-life community, pragmatic learning, transfer of the experience of seniors to juniors, the exchange of experiences among peers, the role of elders as role models and the centrality of the learner as the main actor.

Being a member of the Companions or of a TC is being part of a network of peers who wish to solve similar problems, where each trainee is invited to ask himself the question "What is my problem?", "What do I want to learn?". Everyone is invited to define his personal goal, the problem he wants to solve and which assistance he requires, but everyone is also asked to be supportive and help others in their learning efforts. In this context, the learner can begin to meet peers and experts, exchange with them and see how they can solve the problems they are facing.

The ECEtt network

The ECEtt network was then able to start operating and the European Union helped it to develop. The 2006-2008 ECEtt-Pilot project, funded by the Leonardo da Vinci agency, has accurately described how to build a knowledge exchange process that would be effective for the traveller and his team of belonging and for skills development throughout life. Over the years, the ECEtt network became a platform for knowledge exchange that includes more than 700 possible internship sites in Europe.

Exchange of best practices fosters quality services

Each partner can visit others and welcome them according to their needs. Everyone then brings home the best practices he deems appropriate and shares his findings with his team and the ECEtt network. Throughout this process, the quality of all services is growing and this helps them to become stronger and to cope with challenges and threats in their environment: hyper-complexity, continuous change, reductions in departmental budgets, etc.

After work had been carried out to describe the exchange process and after measuring the results achieved in the context of the 2006-2008ECEtt-Pilot, the Leonardo da Vinci Agency urged managers of the ECEtt network to enter into a

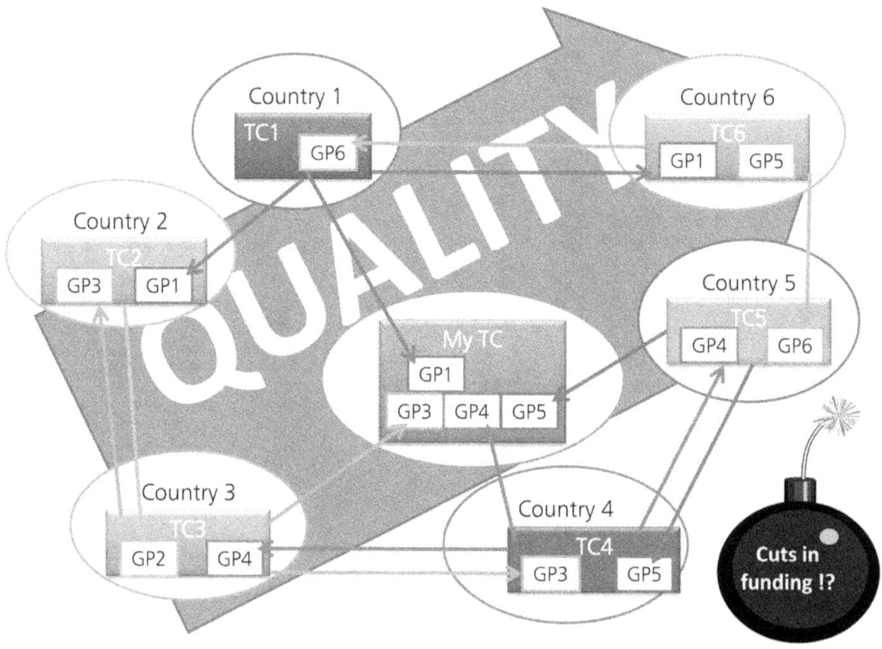

Figure 3. Exchange of best practices.

new stage: the transfer of the process of knowledge exchange to other professions. This is the purpose of the "ECEtt-Transfer of Innovation" project for 2009-2011.

The network "addiction"

The ECEtt network is based on three pillars. The first pillar is the ECEtt method (MECETT), that is to say a training process by means of the journey that cuts across all the professional networks: addictions, social work, prevention and other trades. The first pillar is managed by a central office, in Belgium, which coordinates several helpdesks, distributed in different countries: Spain, Italy, Greece, Poland, Bulgaria, France and Belgium.

The second pillar consists of a referential of expertise, that is to say, a database that includes all the possible training sites in the "addiction" network. This referential of expertise includes the list of possible internship sites that have signed an agreement with ECEtt and a list of expertise and best practices that can be found in all these internship places. The ECEtt network includes large national organisations, as well as smaller organisations working in the field of addiction.

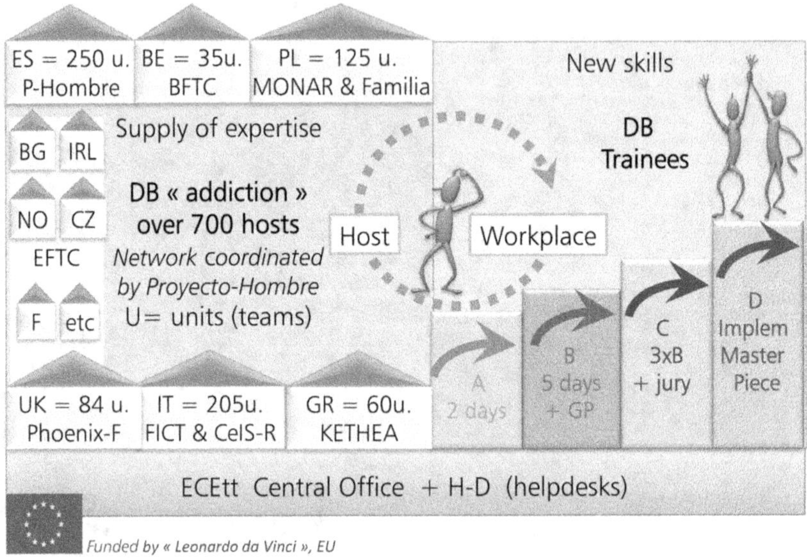

Figure 4. ECEtt Network: Addiction.

Large organisations are MONAR (Poland) that includes over 125 organisations, Proyecto Hombre (Spain), which includes 250 training sites, Phoenix Futures (UK), which includes 84 training sites, the CEIS-Formazione and FICT (Italy) including a total of 205 units or course places, Kethea (Greece), which includes 60 places. In addition, many smaller therapeutic communities, part of the EFTC (European Federation of Therapeutic Communities) and the EFTC are also members of the ECEtt network. Proyecto Hombre Madrid coordinates the database of expertise in addiction, which encompasses more than 700 training sites.

The third pillar consists of the trainees. In all member organisations, some staff members want to explore best practices and improve their skills. Any member of these teams may submit a request to ECEtt to discover, in the ECEtt network, places that have experience in and answers to the problems these teams encounter.

From two days to five years

Each candidate trainee addresses their application to the helpdesk speaking his language. This helpdesk will seek internship places that have the expertise and skills researched by the trainee and will ask him which type of traineeship matches the best: a two-day "A" trip, on their own or with team members, or a "B" traineeship

(5 days with writing and validation of a best practice. Some will go further and make several trips and carry out an implementation project of a best practice that will be presented to the "C" jury. Finally, "D" trainees will start the implementation of best practice in their workplace. This implementation will be presented as a main piece of work to a "D" jury. From here, he may be considered an "ECEtt Journeyman".

The role of helpdesks is to help trainees to match the demand and supply of expertise and to support the trainees during their knowledge-exchange project, from their workplace to other places of expertise across Europe.

The ECEtt learning method is very flexible: it can range from a commitment of a two-day trip to a learning process spanning five years. For example, an individual can go on his own for a single trip to a single host, and not go further than that, or he can go beyond that and may make other "A" trips together with several of his colleagues, in the same area of expertise. He can also add a "B" traineeship (five days) after which he will write up a best practice. Some trainees will accumulate a minimum of fifteen days visiting three different hosts and bring back three best practices that they will present to the "C" jury. Subsequently, those who are certified by the jury can have support for two or three years to implement a best practice in their workplace.

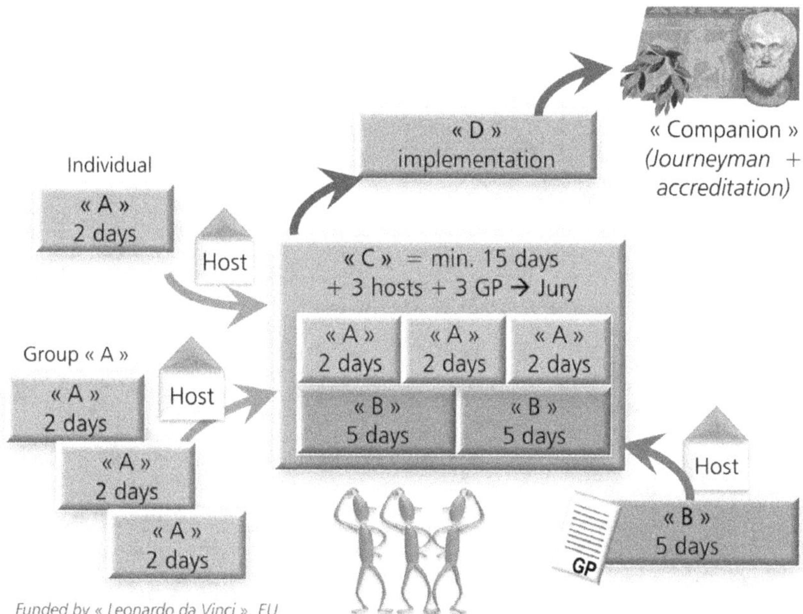

Figure 5. From two days to five years.

The whole process, from training to implementation

The ECEtt learning process is a perspective of improving the quality in Deming's "Plan, Do, Check, Act" model. Each trainee starts his learning project with a problem he can observe in his workplace. He will follow a learning process until he implements a best practice that aims at quality improvement. The entire learning process is built on the objective of "quality". Very often, it starts from the observation of quality issues at the client level.

When a team is faced with , quality problems at the client level over several years, there is probably a skills problem within the team. Some team members may put themselves in question, seek solutions and contact the ECEtt network. From there, the team members can make several trips to various training sites in Europe to research best practice, writing best practices and, from there, they can return to their team, share their findings and propose to change internal work processes. The implementation of best practice continues, often through the organisation of a new "A" journey, with several team members visiting the workplace where the best practice is under control. The team can then build an operational plan for implementation, train team members and implement and measure changes and outcomes. After anything from a year and a half to five years, depending on the

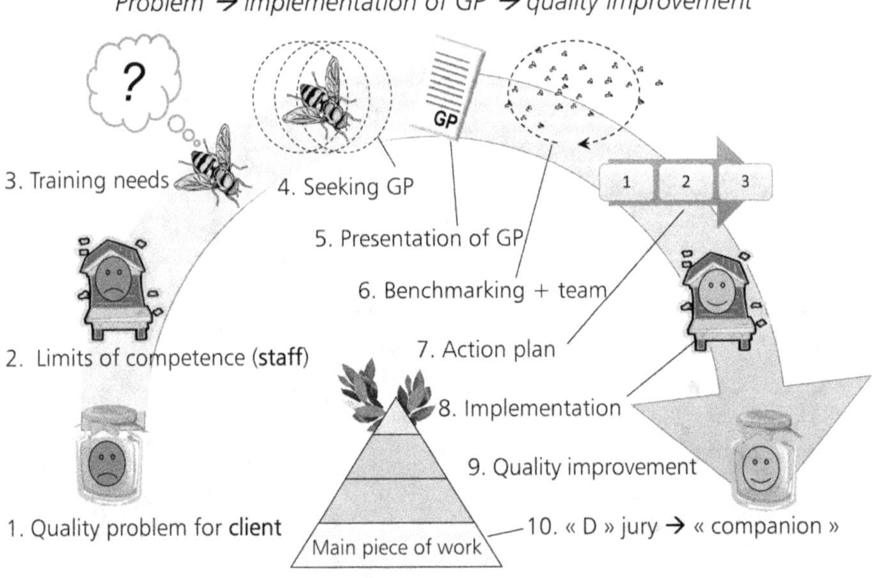

Figure 6. Plan, Do, Check, Act.

ambition of the implemented best practice, the trainee presents his main piece of work to the "D" jury, with the outcome measure, before and after the implementation of the best practice.

Tools to travel abroad

A feature of the "journeymen apprenticeship" (MECETT) is that the primary responsibility of the training process is in the hands of the learner and not the trainer. ECEtt has developed a toolkit that is available to all candidate trainees. The toolkit includes the ECEtt Handbook, which contains general travelling rules and a personal "travel file" in which each trainee will build his project, step by step.

The toolkit also includes the addresses of all the helpdesks in English, French, Polish, Italian, Greek, Spanish and Bulgarian. The tools of the toolkit are available on the e-learning platform (see website www.ecett.eu) which was developed by CeIS-Formazione and the University of Bologna. The e-learning platform includes the catalogue of hosts and the referential of expertise, as well as lists of best practices, newsletters, evaluations tools, follow-up, forums of discussion, etc. In collaboration with the University of Bologna, these training courses will be credited with ECTS points.

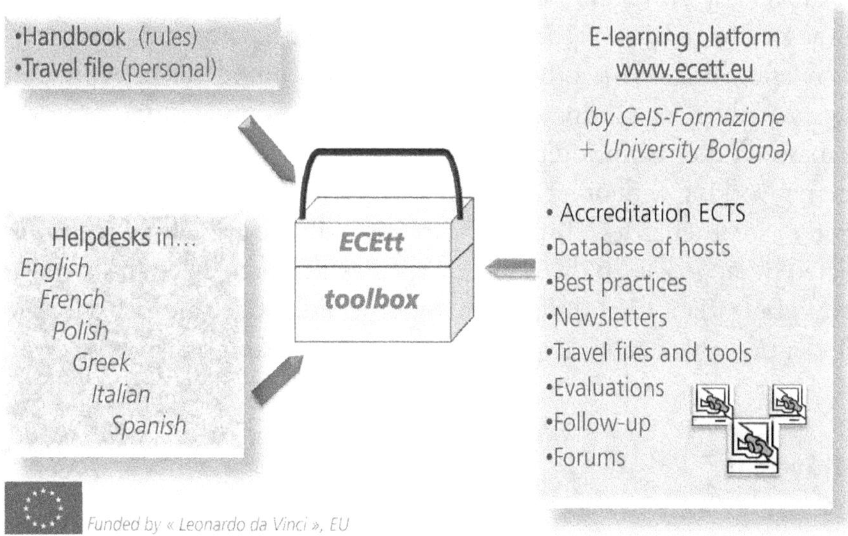

Figure 7. Tools to travel abroad.

Language → / Institutions cities → / List of expertise	French	Spanish	Italian	Polish	Greek	Bulgar	English	Other	Out EU
	1.Trempoline : B 2.Phénix : Be 3.APTE : Fr 4.CEID : Fr	PH 1.Madrid 2.Galicia 3.Catalunya	FICT 1.Modena 2.Venezia 3.Etc.	MONAR 1.Warsaw 2.Gdansk 3.Krakow	KETHEA 1.Athens 2.Thess 3.Herakl	1.Solidar. 2.CNT 3.Butterfly 4.Etc.	1.Coolmine IRL 2.Phoenix London 3.Phoenix Sheffield 4.Etc.	1.De Kiem Be 2.De Sleutel Be 3.Parnassia NL 4.Terval. : Fi	1.Daytop 2.Beirut 3.Etc.
Before TC									
EX 1 : Intake session (De Leon)	1,2,3	1,2,3,4,5	1,2,3,4,5	1,2,3,4	1,2,3	1	1,2,3	1,2,3	1,2,3
EX 2 :	1,2,3	1,2,3,4,5	1,2,3,4,5	1,2,3,4	1,2,3	1	1,2,3	1,2,3	1,2,3
GP 1 : Reorientation	1	3		2	3			1	1
GP 2 : Etc.			1,2,3	1,2,3,4,5	1,2,3,4,5	1,2,3,4	1,2,3	1	1,2,3
TC programs									
EX 1 : Encounter group (De Leon)	1,2,3	1,2,3,4,5	1,2,3,4,5	1,2,3,4	1,2,3	1	1,2,3	1,2,3	
EX 2 :	1,2,3	1,2,3,4,5	1,2,3,4,5	1,2,3,4	1,2,3	1	1,2,3	1,2,3	
GP 1 : Art therapy			1,2,3	1,2,3,4,5	1,2,3,4,5	1,2,3,4	1,2,3	1	1,2,3
GP 2 : Gender groups		1,2,3	1,2,3,4,5	1,2,3,4,5	1,2,3,4	1,2,3	1	1,2,3	
Reintegration									
EX 1 : Relapse prevention		1,2,3	1,2,3,4,5	1,2,3,4,5	1,2,3,4	1,2,3	1	1,2,3	1,2,3
EX 2 : Etc .	1,2,3	1,2,3,4,5	1,2,3,4,5	1,2,3,4	1,2,3	1	1,2,3	1,2,3	1,2,3
GP 1 : Vocational training	1	3		4				1,2,3	1
GP 2 : Etc.		1	3		2	3		1	
Networking									
EX 1	1,2,3,	1,2,3,	1,2,3	1,2,3					
GP1		1,2,3	1,2,3,4,5	1,2,3,4,5	1,2,3,4	1,2,3	1	1,2,3	
Etc...									

Figure 8. Catalogue of expertise and hosts (managed by P-Hombre).
Orientation of trainees according to expertise and languages.

Catalogue of hosts and referential of expertise

The "catalogue of hosts" and the "referential of expertise" for the "addiction" sector are coordinated by Proyecto Hombre in Madrid. This referential of expertise guides trainees according to the expertise they are looking for and the languages they know.

This referential covers two types of data: a list of hundreds of experiences and techniques used before, during or after a rehabilitation programme. In addition to the database of expertise in addiction, some databases may include networking with families, networking with other services and specific target groups that need help in addiction or in other areas. This list of expertise will include a list of centres, which are ordered by language. So there are centres in which French, Spanish, Italian, Polish, Greek, Bulgarian, English or other languages are spoken and for each language, we can identify which training place can offer which kind of expertise or practice.

The "Travel File"

The "Travel File" is the main learning tool in the hands of each trainee student. This is a personal notebook for the intern in which step by step, he comes across all the documents necessary for success in the learning project. The first part deals with his CV and his objectives, namely: "What is driving this traineeship?". The following step will be negotiations with the host, that is to say the dates, the potential cost for housing, food and "languages solutions". This part 2 also foresees a schedule of the training organised by the host, according to the objectives and motivations described by the trainee. This schedule will resume all the details, hour by hour, from the moment the trainee arrives at the place of internship until he leaves.

The third part, after the course, will include an assessment of the student's satisfaction with regard to his internship (3a) and gathers 4 "strong ideas" that he will share with his team (3b) and a description of the place of internship (3c). In the case of "B" and "C" trainees, that is to say those who stay for five days on site, are also asked to write a best practice (3d) or a description of the skills needed for that best practice (3e). The travel file also includes travel budgets, a ledger of all expenses incurred during the trip, the costs of booking flights and hotels and, finally, any certifications for travel grants or academic courses.

The "travel file" is modelled on the Europass, so that each trainee can build his own résumé showing all his internships and his life-long learning process, country after country, using documents on European models.

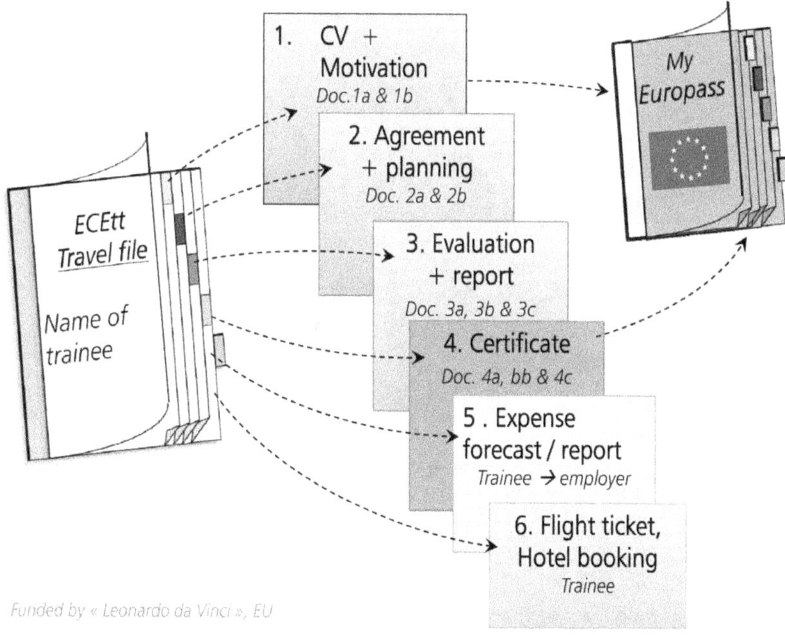

Figure 9. The "Travel file".

Helpdesks, trainees, hosts, etc.

The role of helpdesks is to help students and hosts. These helpdesks are helped in this by tutors who are generally ECEtt alumni who know the method and can communicate in English, in addition to their mother tongue.

These tutors work in partner institutions of the ECEtt network and can act as an intermediary or "ambassador", and to explain to their team members how to use the ECEtt network, how to go in search of best practices abroad and can also explain to hosts how their team should welcome a foreign trainee who comes looking for best practices. All helpdesks and tutors coach trainees and hosts in the flow of information and in the exchange of expertise across the network.

Follow-up of trainees for 6 months

Each helpdesk will follow the interns in their country during the whole process of the internship, which is approximately six months. These include three months of preparation before the course and three months of follow-up work after the course. Each trainee is assisted by his helpdesk every fifteen days, based on his

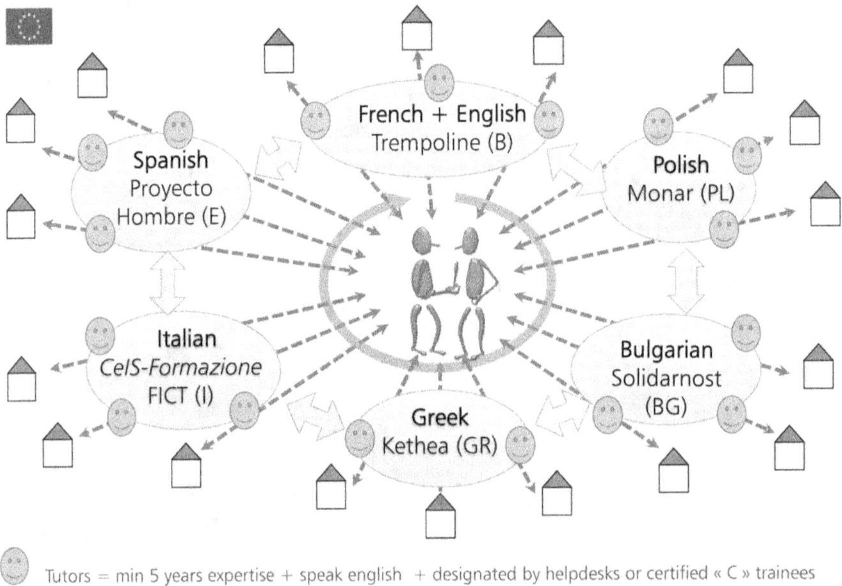

Figure 10. Trainees and hosts are coached bu helpdesks and tutors (in seven languages).

"travel file". Each "travel file" document is linked to a deadline upon which the document must have been completed. The CV should reach the helpdesk at least 90 days before the course and the course objectives should reach the helpdesk sixty days before the course.

The internship agreement must be signed between the host and the intern forty-five days before the course. Budget details must be settled one month before the course. The trainee must receive his schedule ten days before departure. After the internship, the intern has fifteen days to draw up his evaluation documents and financial records. He has thirty days to share, the "strong ideas" he has brought back from his internship with his team and his employer. The helpdesk questions the trainee regularly and helps him to solve the problems he faces, be it financial problems, language problems or other communication problems with the host. The helpdesk will also monitor the student after the internship so that his best practice might be validated.

Validation of best practices

Each trainee freely chooses one professional technique upon which he wants to write a "best practice". The report is based on thirty questions about best prac-

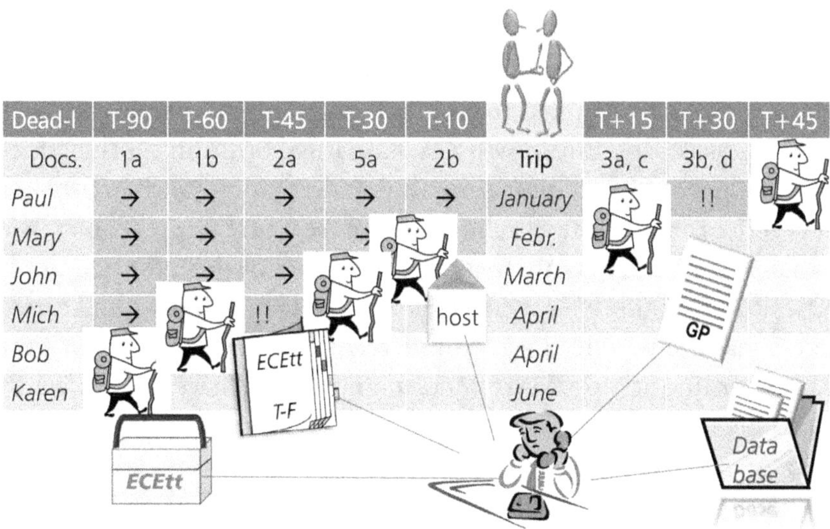

Figure 11. Helpdesks follow trainees over six months.

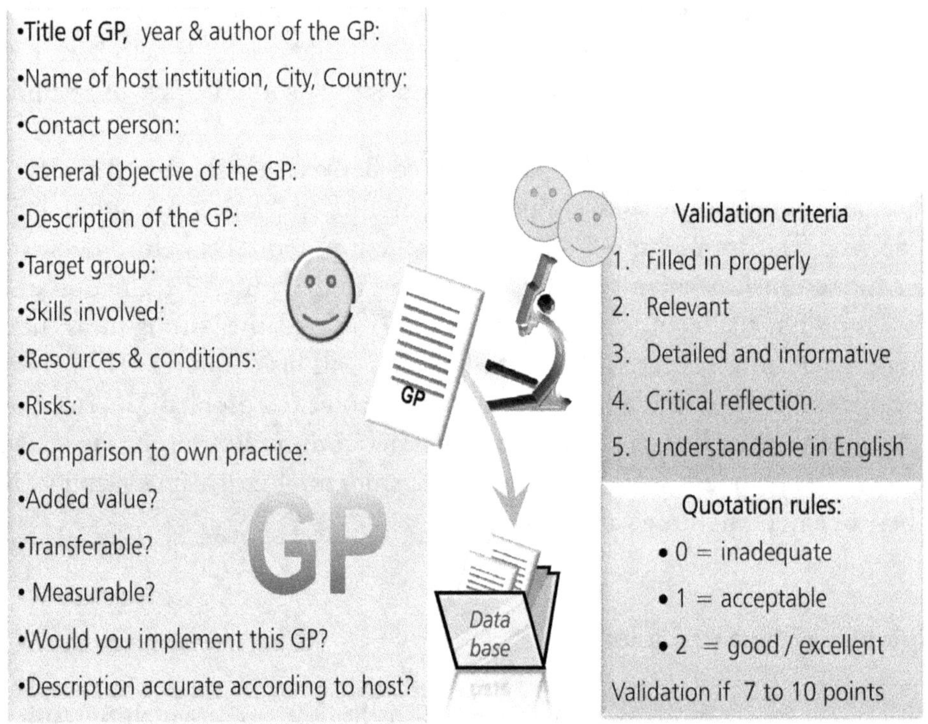

Figure 12. Validation of best practices (for B & C trainees).

tices (BPs): the title of the BP, year and author of the BP, the name of the host institution, contact person and the objective of the BP, its general description, target group, the skills required for this best practice, the resources required and the potential risks. The intern will issue a critical opinion on the added value of the BP, the possibility of measuring it, transferring it elsewhere, etc.

Best practices are subject to validation; the best practice is sent to the host to ensure there are no important errors in the writing of this best practice but also to another tutor of the ECEtt network who will provide ratings for different parameters: has the practice been completely filled in?, is it relevant to the professional sector in question?, is it detailed and informative?, is critical thinking satisfactory? is the writing correct? is it understandable in English? For each of these parameters, the tutors will give a score of 0 if it is "insufficient", 1 if it is acceptable and 2 if it is good. For a best practice to be valid and published in the referential, it must total between 7 and 10 points and cannot include any zero grades.

Referential of best practices

When best practices are validated by the tutors, they enter into a database of best practices. The referential of the ECEtt network includes different databases. Three of them are coordinated by Proyecto Hombre, Madrid. These are best practices in the sector of drug rehabilitation, those dealing with networking (with families or services), and best practices targeted at specific audiences. Other databases gather best practices in social work and in prevention and multi-area materials such as research and human resources.

"Ecett-Networks" and "Ecethos"

From 2003 to 2010, the ECETT network was the initiative of Trempoline NGO, which was legally responsible for ECEtt. The development of ECEtt was made possible thanks to private sponsors, European subsidies and co-financing partners in the ECETT projects: Trempoline, CeIS- Formazione, Proyecto Hombre, MONAR, Kethea, Coolmine House, Solidarnost, Aurore and CEID in France.

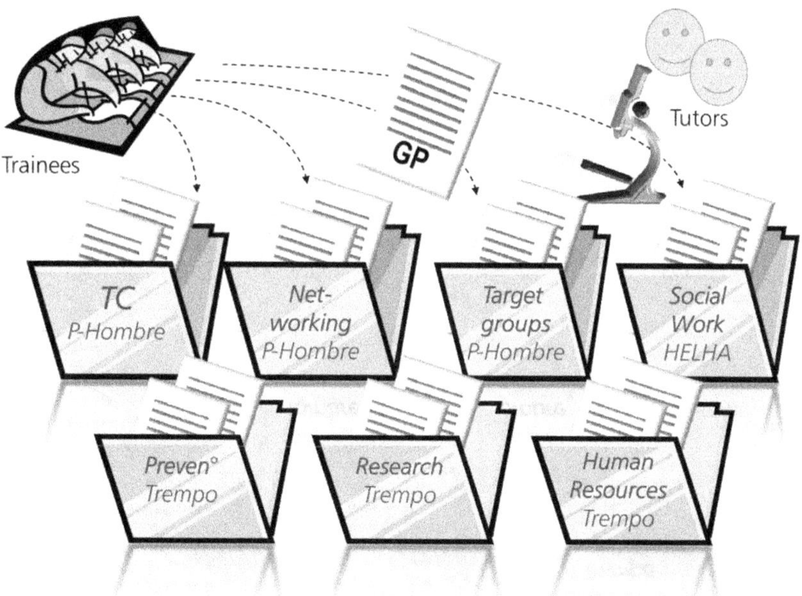

Figure 13. Database of "best practices".

The survival and development of the network ECETT requires the network to be legally and financially autonomous to enable survival beyond the periods subsidised by Europe. ECEtt's development plan of is based on three main points:

1. creating "Ecett-Networks" NGO, a non-profit organisation, including partners in human-based professions (addictions, social work, prevention, etc.).
2. selling MECETT (the learning method of ECEtt), which is transferable to many professional sectors and that is owned by Ecett-Networks NGO. MECETT is a common platform for various businesses.
3. creating Ecethos, a company that provides consultancy for the implementation of MECETT for private or public clients. Ecethos helps clients buying MECETT to structure their network of expertise and to structure the learning process for their staff. The profits generated by Ecethos are divided between Ecethos and Ecett-Networks NGO, in order to support the continued exchange of information within sectors of human-based professions.

12 The reasons for the rise and fall of the Bremberg empire

Vera Segraeus

National Board of Institutional Care
Uppsala University, Sweden

vera.segraeus@telia.com

Abstract

Sweden has played an important role in the TC history. The first TC World conference took place in Norrköping 1976 and the first European TC Conference took place in 1982 in Eskilstuna. The person behind this was Lars Bremberg, a visionary drugs activist who founded Vallmotorp 1973. My presentation will deal with the rise and fall of the Swedish TC movement.

The enthusiasm about the new methods of treatment that appeared at the beginning of the 1970s led to an uncritical acceptance of them by many researchers and society at large. The acceptance of TCs did not, to begin with, have much to do with their ability to produce favourable results, but rather with the fact that they were regarded as an alternative that was fit for human beings as opposed to the "inhumane" forms of treatment that characterised the old, custodial-oriented establishments. Treatment was advocated instead of detention. However in the 1980s, the wind of opinion had already changed direction; the uncritical belief in the TC concept was replaced by a critical questioning of both TC methods and results. But the Vallmotorp Foundation underwent a rapid and remarkable development during that period. On February 1991 Vallmotorp had 192 registered students and 9 geographically separate units. In addition, Vallmotorp and Lars Bremberg had started Daytop

Sweden and the Nordia Foundation, and the 3 organisations had a common head office in Katrineholm Uniswed for some time. In the mid 1980s Uniswed had a joint capacity of about 600 students. Inspired by Vallmotorp, a great number of other TCs were founded across the country at this time.

Three years later in 1994, Vallmotorp and many other Swedish TCs had diedd. What happened? This work discusses the various reasons that have been put forward for this development in Sweden.

Key words

Therapeutic Community; development; history method; culture.

Introduction

Sweden has played an important role in the TC history (Jones,1970; Segraeus, 1984). The first TC World conference took place in Norrköping 1976, and the first European TC Conference took place in 1982 in Eskilstuna (see EU-ROCON, Third generation of Therapeutic Communities. Proceedings of the First European Conference on Milieu Therapy, 1984). The person behind this was Lars Bremberg, a visionary drugs activist who founded Vallmotorp 1973 (Bremberg, 1978). This article will deal with the rise and fall of the Swedish TC movement.

Lars Bremberg had academic qualifications in law and the humanities, and had previously worked as teacher, journalist, lawyer and director of the Board of Temperance in Stockholm. Bremberg was inspired by Henderson Hospital and saw Vallmotorp as a Maxwell Jones-type Therapeutic Community. The enthusiasm about the new methods of treatment that appeared at the beginning of the 1970s led to an uncritical acceptance of them by many researchers and society at large. The acceptance of TCs did not, to begin with, have much to do with their ability to produce favourable results, but rather with the fact that they were regarded as an alternative that was fit for human beings as opposed to the "inhumane" forms of treatment that characterised the old, custodial-oriented establishments. Treatment was advocated instead of detention. However in the 1980s, the wind of opinion had already changed direction; the uncritical belief in the TC concept was replaced by a critical questioning of both TC methods and results.

The reasons for the rise and fall of the Bremberg empire

In addition to Vallmotorp, Lars Bremberg started Daytop Sweden and the Nordia Foundation, and the 3 organisations shared a head office for some time in Katrineholm Uniswed. In the mid 1980s Uniswed had a joint capacity of about 600 students. Inspired by Vallmotorp, a great number of other TCs were founded across the country at this time. The number of yearly treated drug-abusers and mixed substance abusers doubled between 1983 and 1991 (Jan Blomqvist 1996). One reason for this was the HIV/AIDS infection among abusers, which rose during the 80s and was considered a threat to society, requiring institutional treatment. The Vallmotorp Foundation underwent a rapid and remarkable development during that period. On February 1991 Vallmotorp had 192 registered students and 9 geographically separate units. Three years later in 1994, Vallmotorp and many other Swedish TCs were heavily threatened. What happened? In my presentation I will discuss the various reasons that have been put forward for this development in Sweden.

The economic reason

The first reason was economic. In Sweden the local governments of municipalities hold the greatest responsibility for large parts of the Swedish welfare system, e.g., for the treatment of alcohol and drug abuse. These services are mainly financed through local taxes, municipal fees and state subsidies. As a result of the weak economy during the late 1980s and early 1990s there had been substantial cuts in the state subsidy system to local governments and increases in local taxation were halted, restricting the municipalities' ability to take action. For the municipalities, this was a new economic situation. In general, during the 1980s, money was "no big problem" for them, when it came to carrying out their share of welfare tasks. But in 1994 the context was different. Lack of money became a big problem. Before 1986, subsidies were directly connected to the number of institutional beds, but from 1986, they were principally given as general, not earmarked, subsidies to the municipalities. This new system, together with the economic, crisis, was one of the main reasons for the reduction of residential treatment for substance abusers.

The political/ideological reason

The second reason was the political/ideological question. In 1980 Sweden got a new Social Service Act that stated that the two principles "standardisation" and "proximity" should be considered important in social work. It also indicated that treatment should take place in various forms of non-institutional care if possible. These principles are in contrast to earlier legislation that had a stronger moral and repressive perspective on alcohol treatment.

Organisation of alcohol and drug treatment in Sweden

From May to August 1993 a national survey was carried out by Bergmark and Oscarsson (NAT 1994) concerning the organisation of alcohol and drug treatment within the municipal social service organisations. Questions were asked about treatment policy, ideology, and motives, organisation, cost, resources and cooperation. 229 treatment institutions were identified, 157 were classified as alcohol units and 72 as drug units. There were 3307 beds in the alcohol category and 992 in the drug category. Drug institutions had fewer beds and were more expensive due to higher fees per day and a much longer recommended treatment period. The results from the data showed that the social service agencies gave clear priority to outpatient treatment. The data verifies a development during the beginning of the 1990s that probably led to a decrease in demand for institutional treatment. From the data one could see that the municipalities dominated the management of the outpatient departments, while private organisations played a substantial role in residential treatment.

The Minnesota model

Another ideological reason was the introduction of the Minnesota model in the middle of the 80s. Very soon AA and the Minnesota model totally dominated the alcohol residential treatment. It became important in Swedish alcohol treatment because it had all the characteristics that Swedish alcohol treatment lacked. It was commercial, professional and claimed that treatment could be completed in 28 days. The TCs had a one-year programme, mainly for drug addicts. They were mostly private and received no subsidies, which meant that the changed policy had quick and hard consequences for them.

The scientific reason

A third reason was the lack of support for the efficiency of the TC model (Segraeus 1984)… The fact that treatment research did not show a better outcome for institutional treatment compared to outpatient treatment was a sign for politicians not to put resources into long-term expensive residential treatment. In Sweden a dissertation by Lars Lindström (1986) had great importance. He had three main research questions. *1)* Is treatment more effective than no treatment? *2)* Are some types of treatment more effective than others? *3)* Do certain types of clients do better in certain types of treatment? He made a thorough investigation of controlled studies of the results of different types of alcohol treatment and found that the answer was no to all three questions. No type of treatment was better than any other in creating long-term results. This of course was a disaster for long-term institutional treatment.

Several large-scale projects have been conducted in the US aimed at creating an ongoing dialogue between treatment units and researchers within the care sector for substance abusers, such as DENS (Carise *et al.*, 2002; Rawson & Branch, 2002). This project has employed ASI as a foundation to identify change and trends with regard to the addicted population, and has created a framework for future studies and for comparisons between various client groups. Through the DENS project, a number of concrete and positive results have been generated:

Corresponding projects within the Swedish care sector for substance abuse are fairly few in number, and the SWEDATE project could possibly be the only one of its kind (Berglund, *et al.*, 1991).

The SWEDATE project

In SWEDATE, (a.a.1991, Segraeus 1987) the largest and most extensive investigation of substance abusers in Sweden. Interviews were conducted with drug addicts who were admitted to various treatment centres during the years 1982-83. A comprehensive question was posed: *"What type of treatment is the most effective for which type of patient?"*. Assisted by various types of questionnaires/ interview instruments, some 1,656 clients were studied as to their backgrounds, 31 treatment centres were reviewed as to their treatment and care organisations, and 387 individuals from the original client population were interviewed a year after their treatment had been concluded. The results did not give a full answer to that question. Of the clients in the study, 51% (198 of 387) reported no use of drugs one year after treatment termination but if you include the criteria of no or only little consumption of alcohol during that time, there were only 37% successful cases. If you also add the criteria of having no institutional care or criminal offences during the follow-up time, the number is reduced to 22%. If you add that the clients should also be socially integrated, which means having an income from work and sufficient housing, the success rate is reduced to 15%. The results depend on what you are asking for. These results of course did not make the politicians more optimistic.

Another objective of the SWEDATE project (ibid), in addition to the purely scientific aspects, was to develop, in conjunction with the units participating in the project, a self-evaluation instrument that could be used on an ongoing basis for status reports and in the development of methods. The conclusions from SWEDATE paved the way for the DOK project (Documentation within the care sector for substance abusers). DOK applied the experience of the Swedate project when it was developed both for Compulsory Care by the National Board of Institutional Care and for the Voluntary care system for substance abusers (Jenner & Segraeus 1997, 2005, 2009).

Vallmotorp did participate in the Swedate project and the results were average. There is also an academic dissertation about Vallmotorp by Thomas Ohlsson (2001), who was a close collaborator to Lars Bremberg and one of those who introduced transactional analysis (TA) at Vallmotorp in 1976. Thomas Ohlsson studied TA-therapy carried out at seven units of the "mature" large-scale Vallmotorp from 1990-92. At Vallmotorp, 2111 psychotherapy sessions were documented for 67 students over a time period of 20 months. The results from Vallmotorp were in short: Students who had more than 80 group therapy sessions improved more than those with less therapy, and better-qualified therapists had better results (Ohlsson 2001, 2009). These results came too late to be of any help to the Vallmotorp foundation.

The Delphi study

At the Department of Social Work in Stockholm, a research project was conducted in the early 1990s aimed at achieving, through dialogue between researchers and therapists, a description of accumulated knowledge and experience in the institutional care of substance abusers. I was the leader of the project (Vera Segraeus

1994, 1996). The main purpose of the study was to gain detailed knowledge about the respondents' point of view on a large number of subjects related to treatment. The project itself can be classified as caring model research. The study comprises an exploratory pilot study at nine institutions and what is termed a Delphi study – a written dialogue with 24 rehabilitation units. My main concern here will be to present some results from the Delphi study.

The sample of institutions was based on a total survey of "residential rehabilitation centres" designed mainly for substance abusers (Bergmark & Oscarsson 1988). The project only included adult rehabilitation units. Altogether, 28 units were invited to take part. Four dropped out. In three cases this was due to turbulence in the staff group or to a change of leader. Of the 24 remaining, 20 completed all the "rounds" of questioning. Eleven units dealt mainly with drug abusers, eight with alcoholics and five with substance abusers in general. 2 Vallmotorp units participated.

The people who took part in the Delphi rounds were experienced staff who, on average, had been working for 10.2 years in their rehabilitation units. Twelve of the participants were superintendents or heads of their various activities. Five had some kind of specialist position, such as senior treatment officer or methods developer.

The results show that the Delphi participants agreed that the ideological approach is important, but there is a clear difference between those working with drug treatment and those working with alcohol treatment. The preferred approach among drug treatment staff is to combine the psychological and the social treatment model. TC-oriented drug treatment participants stated that the social side of TC treatment has always been strong but it is now being surpassed by the psychological side. Participants working within alcohol treatment units instead stress first and foremost the possibility to choose recovery, to take responsibility for one's own recovery as it is presented in the Minnesota model.

One problem, according to the respondents in the Delphi study was to get social workers to be more humble and to admit that "no single treatment method is suitable for everybody, but also treatment staff need to be more humble and realise that no one method fits everyone". The lack of adequate cooperation between medical care, social welfare and correctional treatment was also mentioned as a problem. In Sweden, the responsibility for drug abuse treatment is shared between the municipality and the county council and they tend to firstly see to their own finances and try to pass the responsibility onto someone else.

Most of the respondents agreed about the criteria for good treatment. The competence of staff was emphasised. "The theoretical basis for treatment must be clear and the results must be documented and an adequate treatment model and well-educated staff is needed". The respondents did not doubt that there were good opportunities for the professionalisation of treatment, but here again a lot of problems were seen. Professionalisation has been described as "becoming aware of what you do and why you do it". Were education and training to lead to some form of accreditation, it would elevate the status of the entire caring sector. The most important change towards professionalisation is the growing interest in education.

There was also a question about the harder conditions and the fear for cuts in the economic resources of TCs. At the Vallmotorp Foundation, they pointed out that "the time in treatment tends to be shorter; social welfare does not pay for longer stays. The municipalities also try their own open ward alternatives". They also pointed out "the need to get people to stay in treatment, to decrease the dropout rate, which means modifying former rules and principles". They wanted more family treatment, smaller groups, less staff, shorter time in treatment, more education-training and cooperation with authorities. The private TC organisations did fight for their existence. In three years they were almost all shut down.

In the beginning of the 1990s the psychologist Rolf Karlsson at Vallmotorp found that the fundamental principles of the TC were hard to live up to. The democracy was gone. The power of the leader made the staff and clients more passive. The open communication was hard to maintain. The foundation had grown too much to have an open dialogue. The symptom-tolerance was less, especially in initial phases and at the end of treatment. Reality confrontations were less common. Group techniques were still in focus, but they were more structured and dedicated to specific tasks. It was obvious that Vallmotorp no longer worked according to the TC principles (Ohlsson, 2001).

The general resistance to research and the large gap between research and practice has been a main obstacle in times when there is more demand on evidence. Some of the reasons for the lack of an alliance between practitioners and researchers in Sweden are said to be rooted in fundamental historical differences in their respective working climates, levels of education, and their assignments. Other explanations mentioned are the differences in how much store is set by research findings compared to the importance of experience (Anderberg & Dahlberg, 2006).

In conclusion, I believe that basic documentation, conducted on an ongoing basis, concerning the clients and the interventions involved in the treatment of substance abusers is imperative in order to create a self-reflecting knowledge-based practice and research that attempts to identify effective treatment methods and convey their findings (Segraeus, 2009).

The professional/cultural reason

The fourth reason was professional. There was a great resistance towards the Daytop model in Sweden. The hard encounter meetings with humiliating elements were condemned. The hierarchical model also gave the leader possibilities that could be abused. Power abuse was considered to be rather common and the clients needed support. The leaders were often former drug addicts and did not always behave professionally or as good role models. The alcohol question did not have high priority in the Swedish TCs for drug addicts. For example, Swedish clients and staff members got a bad reputation at international conferences for drinking too much alcohol. The needs for special treatment for women and families were hard to handle within the TC structure (Segraeus, 2000; 2005). Power abuse, deficiencies in treatment and high economic costs and a great deal of money spent on representation gave the TCs a bad reputation.

Conclusions

The Vallmotorp/ Daytop concern was strongly affected. It had grown very fast. Bremberg was an inspiring leader and therapist but his way of dealing with money was questioned. He wanted to expand his activities abroad, so he started a Treatment centre in Thailand, Bremberg House, but that was too much for the Swedish authorities. The National Board of Health and Welfare reacted to the plans and the Stockholm Municipality withdrew their economic support to Vallmotorp and so did a lot of other municipalities, which led to an economic crisis for Vallmotorp. It was hard to handle the situation, so Lars moved abroad and the Vallmotorp, Daytop Sweden and Nordia Foundations were closed. Thereby much good competence was lost. During the few years of existence, the so-called Uniswed had established chains of treatment including halfway houses and an outpatient care and support systems that was highly effective and well built up. We still do not have anything like it in Sweden even though the need is obvious.

Today the clients in residential care have become a negatively selected group with bad prognoses and a great need for care and social and often psychiatric help. The TC treatment institutions' high ambitions led to a high drop-out rate that indicated that their treatment approach did not match the needs and conditions of the clients. In later years those clients have mainly got compulsory treatment. In 1994, the National Board of Institutional Care took over compulsory treatment from the county councils. Today they have 15 institutions for alcohol- and drug addicts. The yearly intake is about 500. In coming years, if compulsory treatment will no longer be an alternative, I am afraid that clients will be on the streets or in shelters.

When we consider the internal reasons for the fall of the TCs in Sweden, we have learnt that the role of management in the organisation is very important. The lack of structure can lead to chaos and in other instances to a transition to an authoritarian control in the hands of a charismatic leader, often with disastrous results. The internal and external boundaries of the organisation must be clarified. This development is a step towards the professionalisation of institutional care and treatment of substance abusers.

We can conclude that the idea of the TC has provided a foundation for the development of the institutional treatment of drug abusers in Sweden for two decades. Lars Bremberg was unique in starting both a democratic and a so-called hierarchic American-style TC. The fall of the TCs had both external and internal causes. It is a tragedy because the TCs were in a transitional phase when they had to close down. Sweden was in the forefront and could have given some important contributions to drug treatment development.

According to the historical and developmental perspective outlined by Gunderson (1978), treatment has progressed from care and support to involvement and structure. Gunderson calls the last step validation, that is to say, feedback is received from the environment. This kind of feedback or confrontation, which involves interpreting one's own behaviour as it is perceived by others, is the very basis of change. The importance of the other components in the TC lies in their creating conditions for this process to take place.

If you see drug abuse as a lifestyle problem you realise that a change of lifestyle cannot be done easily or by taking a pill. The TC is an effective tool, if you use it right. From the two decades of Swedish TC experience you can learn that the capacity to change and grow might be significant, but you have to be aware of the risk of power misuse within the organisations. You should document what you are doing and base your development on research-based knowledge as much as you can. But the even higher demands for evidence-based knowledge make it harder for social and psychological interventions. In Sweden a national investigation is going to propose that treatment for substance abuse will be transferred to the medical field and only care and social needs will be handled by the social authorities. The chances for further development of voluntary institutional TC-type treatment is thus getting even smaller.

References

Anderberg, M & Dahlberg, M (2006). *Strukturerade intervjuer inom missbrukarvården -som en grund för kunskapsutveckling.* Academic Dissertation, Växjö University Press.

Berglund, G *et al.* (1991). The SWEDATE project: Interaction Between Treatment, Client -Background, and Outcome in a One-year follow Up. *Journal of Substance Abuse Treatment.* Vol.8.161-169.

Bergmark, A & Oscarsson, L (1988). Projekt: Behandlingskultur och alkoholmissbruk, DSF (DSF (D88/2012:1-2013:1).

Bergmark, A & Oscarsson, L (1994). Swedish alcohol treatment in transition? Facts and fiction. *Nordisk Alkoholtidsskrift* vol 11, 1994, English Supplement.

Blomqvist, J (1996). *Från ideologi till ekonomi. Institutionsförlagd missbrukarvård under tre decennier.* FoU rapport nr 1996:2 Socialtjänsten.

Bremberg, L (1978). *Vallmotorp.* Aldus.

Carice, D *et al.* (2002). A successful researcher-practitioner collaboration in substance abuse treatment. *Journal of Substance Abuse Treatment, 17* 1-2, 67-77.

EUROCON, Third generation of Therapeutic Communities. *Proceedings of the First European Conference on Milieu Therapy 1984).*

Gundersson, JG (1978). Defining the Therapeutic Processes in Psychiatric Milieus. *Psychiatry,* vol 41.

Jenner, H & Segraeus, V (1997). Documentation as a useful tool in the care and treatment of drug abusers. A presentation of the DOC-project. *ITACA Magazine* 1997; 2: 15-40.

Jenner, H & Segraeus, V (2005). The Swedish DOC system- An attempt to combine Documentation and Self-evaluation. *European Addiction Research* nr 4/05, vol 11, 186-192.

Jenner, H & Segraeus,V (Eds.) (2009*). Evidence and Practical Knowledge in Substance Abuse Treatment- A basis for discussion,* Växjö University Press, Växjö University.

Jones, M (1970). *Det terapeutiska samhället.* Stockholm.

Lindström, L (1986). *Val av behandling för alkoholism.* Liber förlag.

Ohlsson, T (2001). *TA i missbruksarbete. Transaktionsanalytisk psykoterapi som behandlingsmetod för drogmissbrukare I miljöterapeutisk vård.* Academic Dissertation Lund University, Psychology department.

Ohlsson, T (2009). Vallmotorp, pioneer school for life. Paper presented at *the 12th International EWODOR Symposium,* University of Sterling Scotland Oct 19.

Rawson, RA & Branch, C (2002). Connecting Substance Abuse Treatment and Research: Let's make a Deal. *Journal of Drug Issues* 32 (3) 769-782.

Segraeus, V (1984). Research on the treatment of Alcoholics and Drug Addicts during the 1970th in Sweden. In proceedings from *the First European Conference on Milieu Therapy. Third generation of Therapeutic Communities. Eurocon 1982.*

Segraeus, V (1987). *Institutionell narkomanvård. Organisation och innehåll. Metodproblem vlid utvärdering av social behandling av missbrukare.* Akad. avh. Sociologiska institutionen Uppsala Universitet.

Segraeus, V (1994). Var står vi? *Accumulerad kunskap och erfarenhet inom institutionell missbrukarvård, utifrån en dialog forskare praktiker.* Forskningsrapport från Statens Institutionsstyrelse, (SiS) nr1 1994.

Segraeus, V (1996). Accumulated knowledge and experience in the treatment of substance abuse. *Scand J Soc Welfare,* 1996:5:268-277.

Segraeus, V (2000). Terapeutiskt samhälle i förändring. In: Hagqvist, A & Widdinghoff, B (Eds). *Miljöterapi igår idag I morgon.* Studentlitteratur.

Segraeus, V (2005). Terapeutiskt samhälle - kvinnobehandling på männens villkor. In: Hilte, M (Ed.). *Kön behandling och kunskap- om olika vägar ut ur missbruk och social marginalisering.* Studentlitteratur.

Segraeus, V (2009). Documentation as a bridge between practice and research. In: Jenner, H & Segraeus, V (Eds.). *Evidence and Practical Knowledge in Substance Abuse Treatment- A basis for discussion.* Växjö university press.

Social and politic factors

13 The United Nations and drug demand reduction policies

Xavier Fernández-Pons

Department of International Law and Economics
Faculty of Law
University of Barcelona, Spain
xavierfernandez@ub.edu

Abstract

The term "drug demand reduction" is usually used to describe policies or programmes directed towards reducing the consumer demand for narcotic drugs and psychotropic substances covered by international drug control conventions.

Drug demand reduction was traditionally a "secondary" issue in the international drug control conventions (see article 38 of the Single Convention on Narcotic Drugs of 1961 as amended by the 1972 Protocol, article 20 of the Convention on Psychotropic Substances of 1971 and article 14 of the United Nations Convention against Illicit Traffic in Narcotic Drugs and Psychotropic Substances of 1988).

In order to intensify drug demand reduction policies in all countries, the General Assembly of the United Nations adopted, in 1998, the "Declaration on the Guiding Principles of Drug Demand Reduction", whose application is periodically monitored and evaluated. Two Plans of Action (1999 and 2009) have tried to detail this Declaration.

This presentation examines the possibilities to "standardise" drug demand reduction methods using international legal instruments. There continue to be considerable differences between the drug demand reduction policies applied throughout the world. Demand reduction strategies should be carefully designed, based on scientific evidence and taking into account differences in gender, education, local conditions and intercultural diversity.

Key words

United Nations; international drug control conventions; drug demand reduction; pharmacological treatment; psychosocial treatment; scientific evidence.

Introduction:
The work of the United Nations Organization in international drug control

According to the terminology used by the United Nations Organization, the term "drug demand reduction" is used to describe policies or programmes directed towards reducing the consumer demand for narcotic drugs and psychotropic substances covered by international drug control conventions (United Nations Office for Drug Control and Crime Prevention, 2000). These policies and programmes include a wide variety of interventions concerning: prevention of initial consumption, treatment and rehabilitation, social reintegration, harm reduction and measures in the criminal justice systems (assistance to drug users in prison, alternatives to prison, etc.).

"Drug demand reduction" is one of the three pillars of international drug control, together with the control of supply and the persecution of illicit drug trafficking. The United Nations Organization has played a key role in the development of international drug control instruments (Bettati, 1995; Fernández-Pons, 1998) and has bodies dedicated to this issue, among them: the Commission on Narcotic Drugs, the International Narcotics Control Board and the United Nations Office on Drugs and Crime.

The Commission on Narcotic Drugs (CND) was established by the United Nations Economic and Social Council as one of its functional commissions on 16 February 1946 (resolution 9(I)). The Commission assists the Council in supervising the application of international drug control conventions. It also advises the Council on all matters pertaining to the control of narcotic drugs, psychotropic substances and their precursors. The Commission reviews and analyses the global drug control situation, considering the interrelated issues of the prevention of drug abuse, the rehabilitation of drug users and supply and trafficking of illicit drugs. It takes action through resolutions and decisions. The Commission on Narcotic Drugs has important normative functions under the international drug control conventions. It is *inter alia* authorised to consider all matters pertaining to the aims of these conventions and see to their implementation.

The International Narcotics Control Board (INCB) is the independent and quasi-judicial monitoring body for the implementation of the international drug control conventions. It was established in 1968. It had predecessors under the former drug control treaties of the League of Nations. The International Narcotics Control Board is responsible for reviewing whether measures taken in a country are in line with the international drug control conventions.

The United Nations Office on Drugs and Crime (UNODC) was established in 1997, as part of the United Nations Secretariat and integrating various previously existing funds and programmes. The UNODC has approximately 500 staff members. Its headquarters are in Vienna and it operates 20 field offices as well as a liaison office in New York and has permanent presence in Brussels. It relies on voluntary contributions, mainly from governments, for 90 per cent of its budget. It has released a new Menu of Services published in October 2010, which provides a detailed overview of how clients can access targeted assistance and the range of publications and online tools that are available. The UNODC can help in very different areas, including "drug abuse prevention and health". Through educational campaigns and by basing its approach on scientific findings, the UNODC tries to convince young people not to use illicit drugs, drug-dependent people to seek treatment and Governments to see drug use as a health problem, not a crime (United Nations Office on Drugs and Crime, 2010a).

The United Nations Organization has promoted the three main international conventions for the control of drugs: the Single Convention on Narcotic Drugs of 1961; the Convention on Psychotropic Substances of 1971 and the United Nations Convention against Illicit Traffic in Narcotic Drugs and Psychotropic Substances of 1988. These are three legally binding instruments and are ratified by a large number of States.

The Conventions of 1961 and 1971 are primarily devoted to: providing the lists of narcotic drugs and psychotropic substances under international control, which may be updated by the Commission on Narcotic Drugs; stating the general principle that controlled drugs should only be produced and used for medical and scientific purposes; establishing a number of obligations for States to control the "licit supply" of controlled drugs (for specified medical and scientific purposes) trying to prevent their possible diversion to other uses; and providing for the criminalisation of illicit drug trafficking.

The Convention of 1988 is essentially concerned with: detailing the obligations of States in the criminalisation and persecution of illicit drug trafficking, the crime of money laundering in relation to the profits of drug trafficking; strengthening international cooperation (police and judicial) against drug trafficking, and providing controls for the drug "precursors" (chemicals used in illicit manufacture of narcotic drugs and psychotropic substances) (Roucherau, 1988).

Together, the three international drug control conventions give considerable weight to the regulation of the licit supply (for medical and scientific purposes) and the prosecution of illicit drug trafficking, but they pay less attention to drug demand reduction policies.

Provisions on drug demand reduction in the international drug control conventions

The international drug control conventions provide for "drug demand reduction" in some precepts. The 1961 Convention dedicates Article 38 to this issue, entitled "Measures against the abuse of drugs", which states: "The Parties shall give special attention to and take all practicable measures for the prevention of abuse of drugs and for the early identification, treatment, education, after-care, rehabilitation and social reintegration of the persons involved and shall co-ordinate their efforts to these ends [...]".

Article 20 of the 1971 Convention , entitled "Measures against the abuse of psychotropic", states that: "The Parties shall take all practicable measures for the prevention of abuse of psychotropic substances and for the early identification, treatment, education, after-care, rehabilitation and social reintegration of the persons involved, and shall co-ordinate their efforts to these ends [...]".

Article 14, paragraph 4, of the 1988 Convention states that: "The Parties shall adopt appropriate measures aimed at eliminating or reducing illicit demand for narcotic drugs and psychotropic substances, with a view to reducing human suffering and eliminating financial incentives for illicit traffic. These measures may be based, *inter alia,* on the recommendations of the United Nations, specialized agencies of the United Nations such as the World Health Organization, and other competent international organizations [...]". It also specifically refers to "[...] governmental and non-governmental agencies and private efforts in the fields of prevention, treatment and rehabilitation".

In any case, these articles from the three international drug control conventions on "demand reduction" are terse and their wording is very generic. This explains why, especially since the late eighties, there is a need to broaden and strengthen international instruments on drug demand reduction, trying to give a more "balanced" approach.

Promotion of other international instruments on "drug demand reduction"

The importance of drug demand reduction was confirmed by the International Conference on Drug Abuse and Illicit Trafficking, held at Vienna from 17 to 26 June 1987, which adopted the Comprehensive Multidisciplinary Outline of Future Activities in Drug Abuse Control. The Comprehensive Multidisciplinary Outline sets out fourteen targets in the field of demand reduction, as well as the types of activities needed to achieve them at the national, regional and international levels. The United Nations General Assembly, the Economic and Social Council and the Commission on Narcotic Drugs have all adopted resolutions endorsing the Comprehensive Multidisciplinary Outline and emphasising the need to pay increasing attention to demand reduction.

Moreover, at its seventeenth special session, on international cooperation against illicit production, supply, demand, trafficking and distribution of narcotic drugs and psychotropic substances, the General Assembly, by its resolution S-17/2 of 23 February 1990, adopted the Political Declaration and Global Programme of Action. The Global Programme of Action, in paragraphs 9 to 37, addresses issues related to the prevention and reduction of drug abuse with a view to elimination of the illicit demand for narcotic drugs and psychotropic substances and to the treatment, rehabilitation and social reintegration of drug abusers. Further attention was directed to demand reduction by the World Ministerial Summit to Reduce the Demand for Drugs and to Combat the Cocaine Threat, held in London from 9 to 11 April 1990.

In any case, the United Nations considered that it was necessary to adopt a legal instrument that deals specifically with the drug demand reduction, to show that the reduction of drug abuse must be a priority. This instrument, which will be presented below, was finally adopted in 1998.

The 1998 Declaration on the Guiding Principles of Drug Demand Reduction

From 8 to 10 June 1998, the General Assembly of the United Nations celebrated its twentieth special session, which was known as the World Drug Summit. One of the relevant resolutions of the Summit was the adoption of the Declaration on the Guiding Principles of Drug Demand Reduction (resolution S-20/3). This Declaration is not a legally binding instrument, but it is very important, being the first United Nations instrument specifically devoted to drug demand reduction. It has been considered as a "crucial aspect of the new strategy of the international community against drugs" (Udovenko, 1998).

This Declaration is a political commitment and shall "guide" the formulation of the demand reduction component of national and international drug control strategies. The Declaration provides a set of standards for policies on drug prevention, drug treatment, rehabilitation and social reintegration. According to the "guiding principles" of the Declaration, the drug demand reduction programmes should, *inter alia:* be based on a regular assessment of the nature and magnitude of drug use and abuse and drug-related problems in the population; cover all areas of prevention, from discouraging initial use to reducing the negative health and social consequences of drug abuse; embrace information, education, public awareness, early intervention, counselling, treatment, rehabilitation, relapse prevention, aftercare and social reintegration; encourage collaboration among Governments, non-governmental organisations, parents, teachers, health professionals, youth and community organisations, employers' and workers' organisations and the private sector; be designed to address the needs of the population in general, as well as those of specific population groups, paying special attention to youth; consider providing, either as an alternative to conviction or punishment, or in addition to punishment, that abusers of drugs should undergo treatment, education, aftercare, rehabilitation and social reintegration, in order to promote the social reintegration of drug-abusing offenders, wherever appropriate and consistent with the national laws and policies of Member States.

The 1999 Action Plan for the Implementation of the Declaration on the Guiding Principles of Drug Demand Reduction

The 1998 Declaration was still, in any case, a very generic text. With the aim of giving more specific patterns to the States, the General Assembly of the United

Nations adopted, with the resolution 54/132 of 17 December 1999, the Action Plan for the Implementation of the Declaration on the Guiding Principles of Drug Demand Reduction. The 1999 Action Plan is contained in the annex of the resolution, is not legally binding and is offered as guidance to Member States in implementing the 1998 Declaration. The 1999 Action Plan lists 16 objectives focusing, among others, on: the participation of relevant sectors of society in tackling drugs; and the development of appropriate tools and measures to assess and communicate the causes and consequences of substance misuse. It also stresses the need to address the different health, social and cultural contexts and recognises a wide flexibility for States to design and develop their own drug demand reduction policies.

This flexibility of the 1999 Action Plan shows the difficulties in trying to standardise drug demand reduction polices by international legal instruments. Indeed, there continue to be considerable differences between drug demand reduction policies applied throughout the world. The flexibility of the 1999 Action Plan may have its pros and cons. On the one hand, this flexibility allows a broad discretion to design drug demand reduction policies. On the other hand, it limits the ability to generalise the best policies. Regarding substance abuse treatment, the 1999 Action Plan emphasises the idea that programmes for reducing illicit drug demand, especially in terms of their relevance to population groups, must take into account their cultural diversity and specific needs, such as gender, age and socially, culturally and geographically marginalised groups.

The 2009 Political Declaration and Plan of Action on International Cooperation towards an Integrated and Balanced Strategy to Counter the World Drug Problem

After ten years from the aforementioned World Drug Summit of 1998, the Commission on Narcotic Drugs of the United Nations convened a high-level meeting on 11 and 12 March 2009 (attended by Heads of State and Ministers) to review progress in drug control in the last decade and agree on further steps to reduce the threat posed by drugs to health and security. The result of that meeting was the adoption of the 2009 Political Declaration and Plan of Action on International Cooperation towards an Integrated and Balanced Strategy to Counter the World Drug Problem. With both instruments, which are not legally binding, the United Nations Organization confirms the basis of the current international drug control regime, but it also makes self-criticism and stresses that "health" should be the main axis of the drug policies (Jelsma, 2011).

The Political Declaration recognises that countries have a shared responsibility for solving the world drugs problem, that a "balanced and comprehensive approach" is called for and that human rights need to be recognised in drug policies and treatments.

The 2009 Plan of Action proposes thirty remedies to problems in six areas of concern, namely: reducing drug abuse and dependence; reducing the illicit supply of drugs; control of precursors and of amphetamine-type stimulants; international cooperation to eradicate the illicit cultivation of crops and to provide alternative development; countering money-laundering; judicial cooperation.

The 2009 Plan of Action devotes considerable space to the issue of "Reducing drug abuse and dependence through a comprehensive approach". It identifies the main problems in this area and details the measures that Member States of the United Nations Organization should try to address them. Such problems and possible solutions are grouped into ten major areas and we will see them below.

a) Enhancing international cooperation

The 2009 Plan of Action notes that the commitments made by Member States in 1998 to attain significant and measurable results in the area of drug demand reduction have been attained only to a limited extent, largely owing to the lack of a balanced and comprehensive approach.

To address this problem, Member States should, among other actions: pursue a balanced and mutually reinforcing approach to supply and demand reduction, devoting more efforts to the realisation of demand reduction with a view to achieving proportionality of effort, resources and international cooperation in addressing drug abuse as a health and social issue, while upholding the law and its enforcement; and scale up international assistance in addressing drug demand reduction in order to achieve a significant impact; to that end, long-term political and financial commitments from Governments and the international community need to be ensured, including the strengthening of the United Nations Office on Drugs and Crime and other relevant international agencies.

b) Comprehensive approach to drug demand reduction

Some countries have implemented effective drug demand reduction policies. However, drug demand reduction measures are often limited in the range of interventions they offer. Measures are frequently planned and carried out in isolation and address only part of the health and socio-economic problems associated with drug use and dependence.

In order to overcome this situation, Member States should, inter alia: deliver comprehensive policies and programmes using a multi-agency approach, including health-care, social-care, criminal justice, employment and education agencies, non-governmental organisations and civil society, which should take full advantage of the activities of non-governmental and civil society organisations; and consider developing a comprehensive treatment system offering a wide range of integrated pharmacological (such as detoxification and opioid agonist and antagonist maintenance) and psychosocial (such as counselling, cognitive behavioural therapy and social support) interventions based on scientific evidence and focused on the process of rehabilitation, recovery and social reintegration.

c) Human rights, dignity and fundamental freedoms in the context of drug demand reduction

In many countries there is an insufficient emphasis on human rights and dignity in the context of drug demand reduction efforts, in particular regarding access to the highest attainable standard of health services. There is also a need for an improved understanding of addiction and the growing recognition of it as a chronic but treatable multifactorial health disorder.

The United Nations Office on Drugs and Crime has stressed that where systems of supposed drug "treatment" and "rehabilitation" force people into treatment as a matter of course and en masse, such systems violate international human rights standards. According to the United Nations Office on Drugs and Crime "with respect to drug treatment, in line with the right to informed consent to medical treatment (and its "logical corollary", the right to refuse treatment), drug dependence treatment should not be forced on patients. Only in exceptional crisis situations of high risk to self or others can compulsory treatment be ordered for specific conditions and for short periods that are no longer than strictly clinically necessary. Such treatment must be specified by law and subject to judicial review. Under no circumstances should anyone subject to compulsory treatment be given experimental forms of treatment, or punitive interventions under the guise of drug-dependence treatment" (United Nations Office on Drugs and Crime, 2010c).

To address this problem, all Member States, without exception, should ensure that drug demand reduction measures respect human rights and the inherent dignity of all individuals and facilitate access for all drug users to prevention services and healthcare and social services, with a view to social reintegration.

d) *Measures based on scientific evidence*

In many cases, drug use and dependence interventions aimed at prevention and care have been developed spontaneously by well-intentioned institutions responding to the urgency of a rapidly developing drug problem. Too often, however, those interventions were not based entirely on scientific evidence and a multidisciplinary approach.

To overcome this problem, Member States should: invest adequate resources in measures based on scientific evidence, building on the significant scientific progress achieved in that area; support and widely disseminate, in collaboration with the international community, further research to develop measures based on scientific evidence that are relevant to different socio-cultural environments and social groups; encourage innovative measures and incorporate evaluation in order to respond to present and future challenges; and take into account the possibilities given by new media and technologies, including the Internet, with a view to developing the scientific evidence base.

e) *Availability of and accessibility to drug demand reduction services*

Globally, the United Nations Office on Drugs and Crime estimates that between 149 and 272 million people, or, 3.3% to 6.1% of the population aged 15-64 used illicit substances at least once in the previous year, 2010. Considering only the problem drug users, estimates range from 15 to 39 million people, equivalent to 0.3%- 0.9% of the population aged 15-64 (United Nations Office on Drugs and Crime, 2011). It can be estimated that in 2008, globally, between 12% and 30% of problem drug users had received treatment, which means that between 11 and 33.5 million problem drug users did not receive treatment that year (United Nations Office on Drugs and Crime, 2010b).

A range of barriers to specific drug demand reduction services makes it difficult for those in need to access those services. Member States should ensure that access to drug treatment that is affordable, culturally appropriate and based on scientific evidence is available and that drug dependence care services are included in healthcare systems, whether public or private, with the involvement of primary and, where appropriate, specialised healthcare services, in accordance with national legislation; and ensure, where appropriate, the sufficient availability of substances for medication-assisted therapy, including those within the scope of control under the international drug control conventions, as part of a comprehensive package of services for the treatment of drug dependence.

f) *Mainstreaming community involvement and participation*

In many cases, interventions tend to be supported through isolated and short term initiatives and are not mainstreamed in the regular provision by Governments of public health, education and social services. Moreover, they do not involve all stakeholders at the community level in the planning, delivery, monitoring and evaluation of drug demand reduction measures, and they do not take full advantage of the activities of non-governmental organisations and civil society.

To overcome these problems, Member States should: ensure, as far as possible, that measures are mainstreamed in the provision of public and private health, education and social services (such as family, housing and employment services); involve all stakeholders at the community level (including the target populations, their families, community members, employers and local organisations) in the planning, delivery, monitoring and evaluation of drug demand reduction measures; and promote collaboration between governmental and non-governmental organisations and other members of civil society in the establishment of drug demand reduction measures at the local level.

g) *Targeting vulnerable groups and conditions*

Drug demand reduction interventions too often target the general population at large with a single standard approach and do not provide specialized programmes tailored to vulnerable groups with specific needs. Those groups include, among others, children, adolescents, vulnerable youth, women, including pregnant women, people with medical and psychiatric co-morbidities, ethnic minorities and socially marginalised individuals.

Member States should ensure that a broad range of drug demand reduction services, including those in the areas of prevention, treatment, rehabilitation and related support services, provide approaches that serve the needs of vulnerable groups and are differentiated on the basis of scientific evidence so that they respond best to the needs of those groups, taking into account gender considerations and cultural background.

h) Drug use and dependence care in the criminal justice system
In many countries there are limited alternatives to prosecution and imprisonment for drug-using offenders, and treatment services within the criminal justice system are frequently inadequate. Moreover, issues such as corruption, overcrowding and access to drugs and their adverse effects, including the frequency of transmission of infectious diseases within prisons, need to be addressed. Finally, increased emphasis should be placed on the transition between incarceration and release, re-entry and social reintegration. Member States should be working within their legal frameworks and in compliance with applicable international law and consider allowing the full implementation of drug dependence treatment and care options for offenders, in particular and wherever appropriate, providing treatment as an alternative to incarceration. This idea is developed in a "discussion paper" published by the United Nations Office on Drugs and Crime in 2009 and entitled "From coercion to cohesion: Treating drug dependence through health care, not punishment" (UNODC, 2009).

i) Quality standards and training of staff
Sometimes, inadequately trained personnel and a lack of certification and quality standards hinder the effective implementation of demand reduction measures based on scientific evidence. All Member States should: support the development and adoption of appropriate healthcare standards, as well as ongoing training on drug demand reduction measures; ensure that services are staffed, as far as possible and appropriate, with multidisciplinary teams, including physicians/psychiatrists, nurses, psychologists, social workers, educators and other professionals; and ensure, wherever appropriate, that the educational curricula for relevant service providers, including the curricula of universities, medical schools and other relevant professions, include training on the prevention of drug use and dependence and related care.

j) Data collection, monitoring and evaluation
The lack of data, particularly on the rapidly changing nature and the extent of drug use, and the lack of systematic monitoring and evaluation by

Governments of the coverage and quality of drug demand reduction measures are matters of great concern. Intensified international cooperation and support is necessary, including improved and coordinated data collection, monitoring and the evaluation of demand reduction programmes to inform demand reduction services and policy.

Therefore, Member States should, amongst other actions, increase their efforts in collecting data on the nature and extent of drug use and dependence, including the characteristics of the population in need, strengthening information and monitoring systems and employing methodologies and instruments based on scientific evidence; and develop and improve methods of objective national assessment by Governments to understand the negative impact of drug abuse on society, health and economies in a systematic and holistic manner.

Conclusions

Traditionally, the work of the United Nations Organization on international drug control paid less attention to drug demand reduction policies than to supply control and suppression of illicit traffic policies. The World Drug Summit, held in 1998, partially corrected this imbalance by adopting the Declaration on the Guiding Principles of Drug Demand Reduction. The 1999 Action Plan for the Implementation of this Declaration and the new Plan of Action of 2009 have tried to detail the principles to be followed by States in developing drug demand reduction policies.

The 2009 Plan of Action specifies a series of guidelines that should inspire these polices. Among them, the Plan of Action emphasises that Member States: should take, comprehensive measures, rather than isolated and partial measures, including health and socioeconomic aspects; should link measures to mitigate the adverse consequences of drug abuse (usually called "harm reduction") to prevention and treatment; and should ensure that drug treatment, including pharmacological and psychosocial treatment, is affordable, culturally appropriate and based on scientific evidence.

The repeated references in the 2009 Plan of Action to measures based on scientific evidence can be considered as the main element to try to improve and "standardise", where appropriate, policies to reduce drug abuse. This approach has been explicitly used in some recent reports by the Commission on Narcotic Drugs, such as the 2010 report entitled "New Challenges, Strategies and Programmes in demand reduction" (Commission on Narcotic Drugs, 2010).

This report reflects diverse experiences from many different countries, some promoted by the World Health Organization (WHO), on prevention, pharmacological treatment and psychosocial treatment. This report assesses, using a scientific basis, whether these experiences can be generalised. For example, with regard to pharmacological treatment, the report highlights that treatment with long-acting opioid agonists (LAOA), especially methadone, is an evidence-based treatment for opioid dependence, which is successfully implemented in many countries. Recent studies prove that methadone treatment is also effective in low-resource countries and that drug dependence treatment is an effective method for HIV prevention amongst injecting drug users. There was a significant reduction in heroin use in all countries and excellent retention in treatment in all countries, demonstrating that maintenance treatment can be successfully conducted in a range of developing and emerging economies with results that are similar or better than those in developed countries (Commission on Narcotic Drugs, 2010; World Health Organization, 2009).

Regarding psychosocial treatment, the report notes that the past three decades have been marked by tremendous progress in behavioural therapies for drug abuse and dependence, as well as advances in the conceptualisation of approaches to the development of behavioural therapies. Cognitive behaviour therapy, contingency management, couples and family therapy, and a variety of other types of behavioural treatment have been shown to be effective interventions for several forms of drug addiction, and scientific progress has also been greatly facilitated by the articulation of a systematic approach to the development, evaluation, and dissemination of behavioural therapies. The research findings on behavioural treatments have been positive, but there is still a great deal more to be done. Even the most powerful behavioural therapies are not universally effective, nor do all individuals who benefit from these treatments improve as quickly or as completely as desired. Basic neuroscience and basic research on behavioural, cognitive, affective, and social factors offer rich and relatively untapped sources of information on behaviour and behavioural change (Commission on Narcotic Drugs, 2010).

The current work of the Commission on Narcotic Drugs tends to confirm, therefore, that there are pharmacological treatments that can clearly be universalised, since its implementation in many different countries, both developed and developing countries, has been successful. Instead, psychosocial treatments often give very different results from one country to another or from one social group to another, showing that in such cases specific designs are needed.

Returning to the title of this book on "Substance Abuse Treatment: generalities and specificities", the current philosophy of the United Nations Organization on substance abuse treatment tends to seek a combination of pharmacological treatment, which (without prejudice to its adaptation to each patient) can be generalised, with psychosocial treatment, which must be specifically designed, taking into consideration not only the individuals concerned, but also socio-economic contexts and intercultural diversity.

References

Bettati, M (1995). *L'ONU et la drogue*, Editions A. Pédone, Paris.

Commission on Narcotic Drugs (2010). "New challenges, strategies and programmes in demand reduction", Document E/CN.7/2010/CRP.3.

Fernández-Pons, X (1998). "Las Naciones Unidas y la fiscalización internacional de las drogas", *Agenda ONU*, n. 1, 1998, 85-146.

Jelsma, M (2011). *The Development of International Drug Control: Lessons Learned and Strategic Challenges for the Future*, Global Commission on Drug Policies, Geneva, http://www.globalcommissionondrugs.org/Arquivos/Global_Com_Martin_Jelsma.pdf

Roucherau, F (1988). "La Convention des Nations Unies contre le trafic illicite de stupéfiants et de substances psychotropes", *Annuaire Français de Droit International*, XXXIV, 601-617.

Udovenko, H (1998). UN Press Release, Document GA/SM/45.

United Nations Office for Drug Control and Crime Prevention (2000). *Demand Reduction: A Glossary of Terms*, United Nations, New York.

United Nations Office on Drugs and Crime (2009). "From coercion to cohesion: Treating drug dependence through health care, not punishment", Discussion paper based on a scientific workshop, Vienna, October 28-30, 2009, http://www.unodc.org/docs/treatment/Coercion_Ebook.pdf

United Nations Office on Drugs and Crime (2010a). *UNODC Services and Tools. Practical solutions to global threats to justice, security and health*, UNODC, Vienna, http://www.unodc.org/documents/frontpage/MoS_book11_LORES.pdf

United Nations Office on Drugs and Crime (2010b). *World Drug Report 2010*, UNODC, Vienna.

United Nations Office on Drugs and Crime (2010c). "Drug control, Crime Prevention, and Criminal Justice: A Human Rights Perspective", Doc. E/CN.7/2010/CRP.6-E/CN.15/2010/CRP.1.

United Nations Office on Drugs and Crime (2011). *World Drug Report 2011*, UNODC, Vienna.

World Health Organization (2009). *Guidelines for the Psychosocially Assisted Pharmacological Treatment of Opioid Dependence*, WHO Press, Geneva.

14 Factors for effective long-term recovery: risk and challenges during the economic crisis in Greece

CHARALAMPOS POULOPOULOS

KETHEA
Athens, Greece

babis@kethea.gr

Abstract

During recent years, many significant changes have occurred at the economic, social and political level. These changes have affected the drug addiction field and the array of services provided within it. The financial crisis affects drug abusers and their families and it also affects their motivation for treatment, the retention of treatment programmes and the effectiveness of treatment itself by creating environments that are characterised by instability, lack of safety and depression. Furthermore, the economic crisis affects therapists and therapeutic organisations that feel the pressures of cutbacks in funding, together with the promotion of low budget methods and policies. Over the past year, Greece has started experiencing the full impact of the economic recession. The field of drug treatment and rehabilitation is no exception, given the fact that recession significantly affects both the recipients and the providers of treatment services.

The more the recession continues, the more likely it is that rates of drug abuse, alcoholism, addiction to gambling and prescription drugs, and mental health problems are going to rise. Recession could impact negatively on the mental and physical health problems of drug addicts, aggravate their addiction and accentuate their social exclusion. A bleak outlook for the post-treatment stage is more than likely to discourage drug users to approach treatment and rehabilitation services. High unemployment rates are going to make the vocational and social rehabilitation of former drug users even more difficult and they are more likely to increase the risks of relapse.

In this difficult period, social welfare organisations are being called upon to respond to the increasing new needs, while facing budget and personnel cuts that often force them to limit staff training and supervision. KETHEA's strategy focuses on finding and recording new needs that are relevant to the current socio-economic changes, on improving the accessibility, quality and cost-effectiveness of its programmes and on advocating policies that promote social justice and social care for vulnerable groups.

Key words

Economic crisis; unemployment; addiction; drug treatment; therapeutic communities; recovery; strategy.

The consequences of economic crisis

International crisis has several consequences for many countries in the world. Its effects on unemployment are going to affect population health. Eurostat (2011) estimates that unemployment rates in the Europe area in December 2010 reached 10%. In the European Union of 27, the same rate was 9.6%. These are the highest rates for the last ten years. The highest unemployment rates in EU member states were recorded in Spain, Lithuania and Latvia. The highest increases were registered in Lithuania (from 14.3% to 18.3%) and Greece (from 9.7% to 12.5%) between the third quarters of 2009 and 2010. In December 2010 the youth unemployment rate (for those under 25 years old) was 20.4% in the Euro area and 21% in the EU27. The highest rates in this age group were observed in Greece and Spain. The economic crisis leads millions of people into unemployment. In addition, Eurostat estimates that 23.179 million men and women in the EU27 were unemployed in December 2010. At the same time in EU16, 15.775 million men and women were unemployed. The European Commission (2009) estimates the current economic downturn as comparable to the

1930s recession. When people lose their jobs, they also lose their homes, their savings and their pensions. They can also lose their self-respect and they may "escape" into substance abuse and addiction.

Many scientists have expressed concern that the present economic downturn will affect public health as a result of job loss. Job loss contributes to mental health and addiction problems and to the adoption of less healthy lifestyles, followed by the increased consumption of cheap food with low nutritional value and by increased smoking and drinking as a response to stress. Poor disease management results from overburdened healthcare services or from long waiting lists in healthcare services that can no longer respond to the increased needs due to additional costs. The World Health Organization (2009) however has warned policymakers and the general public that *"it should not come as a surprise that we continue to see more stresses, suicides and mental disorders"*. The poor and vulnerable are going to be amongst the first groups that are going to suffer.

EMCDDA (2010) has also noted that more unemployed teenagers may start selling drugs as a way of increasing their income and thereby they may increase the availability and use of cannabis amongst their peers. The crisis also increases violence and criminal behaviour, deteriorates family relationships, increases early drop out from schooling, suicidal attempts, leads to social exclusion and reinforces environmental problems.

Two of the major consequences of economic crisis are the increase in unemployment rates and the consequent decrease in income resources. Unemployment, amongst other things, is linked to mental health problems. Paul and Moser (2009) presented a meta-analysis of mental health consequences on unemployed populations. They analysed 237 cross-sectional and 87 longitudinal studies. The results of their meta-analysis suggested that unemployed populations more often experience distress, depression, anxiety and psychosomatic symptoms when compared with working populations. It is worth noting that 34% of the unemployed reported psychological problems. On the contrary, only 16% of employed populations experience similar types of problems. Unemployment rates are also related with increased suicide rates and higher mortality rates.

Some people may also use substances as a form of self-treatment and in order to cope with negative feelings, frustration and emotional exhaustion. Stuckler and his colleagues (2009) tried to understand the relationship between mortality rates and economic changes in Europe over the last 30 years. Their study concluded that for the under 65s, every 1% rise in unemployment rates was associated with a 0.79% rise in suicide rates and a similar rise in homicides. When unemployment rates were increased by more than 3% the effects on suicide and death rates from alcohol abuse also increased at ages below 65.

However, it is important to note that mortality rates from drug dependence and toxicomania decreased. This phenomenon could be attributed to the reduction of drugs for recreational use or to the increase of mortality rates for other reasons in the general population. Nevertheless, the population of drug addicts is in a worse condition than the general population. Multiple problems are associated with drug use: financial, medical, mental health problems, vocational, educational, legal problems, family and housing problems.

Drug Addicts and Drug Treatment

According to the report and special issue of EMCDDA (2010; 2009) most drug addicts are unemployed, under-nourished and they experience more mental and physical health problems than the general population. They are also at higher risk in terms of mortality rates with their chances being 10-20 times higher than the general population. They also report 14 times more suicide attempts than the general population. Most drug addicts are multi-drug and alcohol users, they dropped out of school earlier than the general population, they are involved in criminal activities and they have experienced imprisonment as well as social racism and exclusion. They also experience more housing problems.

Long-term drug use and addiction are likely to result in impaired health, poor quality of life, a chaotic lifestyle and broken relationships, increased risks of unemployment, legal and medical problems and prolonged imprisonment. In Greece, one out of three drug users attending KETHEA programmes faces chronic or acute health problems, such as hepatitis, injection site ulcers, dental problems and accidental injuries due to falls. One out of two report pending legal issues, six out of ten report unemployment and two out of ten report temporary employment (KETHEA, 2011).

The economic recession may contribute further to the negative consequences of already existing drug-related problems. Recession is expected to accentuate the social exclusion of vulnerable populations such as drug addicts. The health condition, the legal status and the poor quality of life of drug users are expected to worsen when accessibility and availability of medical and social services decrease, due to budget cutbacks on service providers. Furthermore, the recent trends of increased inhalant use of heroin among Greek drug users may go back to drug injection, as drug users may seek more cost-effective but also more risky routes of drug administration.

Consequently, effective drug treatment programmes need to cover the multiple needs of drug users and not just help them stop their drug use. Effective treatment organisations need to address the individuals' drug abuse problem and any associated medical, psychological, social, educational, vocational and legal problems they may face. Treatment programmes need to address drug abusers' efforts for their rehabilitation and reduce social exclusion.

It is obvious that the effective treatment of drug addiction and social rehabilitation requires full support for coping with the above problems. This type of treatment support is not a luxury. It is a necessity, especially at times of economic crisis when the effects of drug addiction concern society as a whole. The prolonged period of drug use has several consequences for society in general. These include:

- Increased use of health services and other social benefits and social care institutions, which result in increased costs for the health and social welfare system.
- Increased delinquency, which results in increased costs for the criminal justice system.
- Increased rates of family violence and child neglect and abuse.
- Increased risks of Sexually Transmitted and other Diseases.
- Increase risks for expansion of drug use.
- Increase of social problems, such us public safety, social exclusion, etc.
- Reduction of productivity, which results in less public income from taxes.

In contrast to the above, drug treatment and social integration are followed by reduction in the above indicators and by resource savings.

French, *et al.* (2002) compared the economic costs and benefits of a modified therapeutic community (TC) in the USA for the treatment of homeless mentally ill substance abusers with "treatment as usual". The study considered employment, criminal activity, and the use of healthcare services as outcome measures and found that the economic cost of the average TC episode was $20,361 while the average economic benefit of such an episode was $305,273.

Ettner, *et al.* (2006) carried out a study based on the analysis of data from 43 substance abuse treatment providers in California with the help of the Drug Abuse Programme Cost Analysis Instrument. The researchers concluded that "on average, substance abuse treatment costs $1,583 and is associated with a monetary benefit to society of $11,487, representing a greater than 7:1 ratio of benefits to costs–or $7 in benefits for every $1 spent on treatment". The study interpreted these findings as a result of the reduced costs of crime and increased employment earnings. The researchers concluded the study claiming that "even without considering the direct value to clients of improved health and quality of life, allocating taxpayer dollars to substance abuse treatment may be a wise investment".

It is obvious that treatment is cost beneficial, because it costs less and has better results for the society. The resources that are saved even by reducing just delinquency due to offering treatment are much more than the resources needed for drug treatment programmes to properly function.

However, during an economic crisis, drug treatment organisations come across several contradictions that jeopardise the goals of treatment. The social and economic environment is changing rapidly, creating new problems and reinforcing the already existing problems of drug addicts and drug treatment organisations that are under fiscal pressure and staff shortages.

In addition, long-term effective client recovery is affected due to changes in the psycho-social characteristics and patterns of use that include increased unemployment rates and increased drug use and engagement in criminal behaviour. Furthermore, other changes that affect effective long-term recovery are observed and include family involvement and social networks, the therapist's background, engagement and empathy, the range of available treatment methods and those that are socially friendly towards drug use and pharmacotherapy environment.

In Greece, long term recovery at KETHEA is marked by three different phases: *a)* the induction phase; *b)* the intensive phase, and *c)* the rehabilitation phase. Each of these phases corresponds to different therapeutic programme units with their specific goals: *a)* Counselling Centre at the induction phase; *b)* Therapeutic Community at the intensive phase, and *c)* Re-entry Centre at rehabilitation phase. Finally, Family Support Programmes function at a parallel level offering services to the relatives and close family members of the addicted individuals. Some of the therapeutic programmes also offer special services in order to respond to specific characteristics and needs e.g. of the imprisoned addicts, of addicted parents, of employed addicts etc.

Treatment starts at the Counselling Centres. This initial stage of the treatment programme lasts for between approximately 8-10 weeks and involves a needs assessment, motivation and treatment planning. Counselling Centres prepare drug addicts in a safe environment to be admitted into a therapeutic community by providing information on the therapeutic community's goals and mode of operation, by strengthening drug addicts' motivation for treatment and by supporting them to stop using drugs. Counselling Centres refer drug addicts to the local medical services for HIV, HCV and other medical tests, they provide free coffee and lunch and they offer recreational activities. In addition, Counselling Centres are the first link that drug addicts' families and friends have with the treatment programmes.

The second phase of the programme takes place within the therapeutic community and lasts approximately 12 months. The TC goals are both social and psychological. This is the central phase of treatment. KETHEA runs therapeutic communities with live-in facilities and non-residential communities. Substance abuse is usually the symptom of deeper psychological, personal and/or social problems. Addicts use drugs in order to feel better or to feel "normal". Drug addicts crave for drugs and drugs become the central focus of their lives and define their activity and behaviour. Therapeutic communities were developed in order to lead members to an understanding of the underlying reasons for their drug addiction and towards a complete change in their behaviour and overall lifestyle. The therapeutic community helps former drug users to develop self-confidence and trust in others, help them to deal with stress and difficulties in a constructive way and to realise that asking for help does not imply a sign of weakness on their part. By discovering their abilities but also the limits of their capabilities, they learn new ways to deal with their problems. In order to achieve their goals, therapeutic communities apply self-help principles: each community member learns how to help himself/herself with the support of others. Therapeutic communities can thus be identified as an environment in which individuals co-exist and connect thanks to their common goal: recovery from drug abuse and reintegration into society.

Treatment programme attendance is on a voluntary basis but a prerequisite for the programme's success is the individual's active participation in the common daily programme. The basic rules forbid the use of alcohol, the use of psychotropic substances or their substitutes, verbal and physical violence and sexual relationships between community members. Daily living and maintenance chores in the community are based on community members and staff and the principles of self-management are applied: that is members' personal contribution, organised in groups with specific responsibilities (cooking, cleaning, paperwork, public relations, administration etc.) under the supervision of therapeutic staff.

Therapeutic communities also offer a systematic training programme that has multiple objectives: to help participants fill basic educational gaps (reading, writing, maths, etc.), to help them reconnect with schooling, to develop a career, to receive vocational training and support and to develop their personal interests. Additionally, medical and legal problems that members may have are dealt with in a systematic way.

When completing the therapeutic community programme, members proceed to the phase of social reintegration that takes place at the Re-entry Centres. Re-entry centres have guesthouses available to host members with no permanent residence up to the time when they will be able to find their own employment and accommodation. The goal, during this phase, is to teach individuals to function as equal members of the society on the basis of the new identity they have acquired during their stay in the therapeutic community. Special emphasis is placed on vocational training and rehabilitation, since these are prerequisites for complete social integration and essential relapse prevention factors. The phase of social reintegration or social activation usually lasts for approximately 10 to 12 months.

Effectiveness of treatment

Studies on treatment outcome have been carried out mainly in USA and the UK and have significantly contributed towards gaining a better understanding of treatment effectiveness. Most treatment effectiveness studies focus on measures of employment, on ex-users' participation in criminal activities, on improving family relationships and on finding a new home and a new way of life.

The Drug Abuse Treatment Outcome Study (Simpson *et al.*, 1997) demonstrates that better follow-up outcomes are present when clients stay in treatment for at least three months. The study also claims that the more time spent in treatment, the better the outcomes and it supports the need for a more careful study of the treatment process (Simpson *et al.*, 1997).

The National Treatment Outcome Research Study in the UK (Gossop *et al.*, 1997) argues that significant improvements in a range of drug use problems were present at the six month follow-up for clients that followed any type of treatment. Another study (Ouimette, Finney & Moos, 1997) demonstrates that even patients who were ordered to undergo treatment showed improvement, regardless of the type of treatment received at the one year follow-up. Gossop *et al.* (1999) suggest that there is little information available about the effectiveness of treatment delivered in special settings or in primary healthcare in the UK. The National Treatment Outcome Research Study was the largest in the UK on treatment outcome and showed positive effects for drug addicts receiving community-based methadone treatment at the six month follow-up.

In accordance with international practice, research was carried out in Greece by the National School of Public Health between 1999 and 2002 on the effectiveness of KETHEA's Therapeutic Communities. A five year follow-up study was carried out to research the status of the drug addicts admitted to a therapeutic community even for one day. The sample comprised of 388 clients from 4 residential and 2 non-residential therapeutic communities (1 for adolescents).

Measures were taken of illicit drug use, injection, psychological health, physical health, crime and employment. To validate self-reports, additional data from alternative sources (parents, spouses, peers and staff) in relation to drug behaviour was taken. The study was based on a retrospective design with randomly selected samples. Both semi-structured (EuropAsi) and open-ended face-to-face interviews were used to collect data at 5-6 years after initial intake. In addition, an analysis was carried out of the client's records taken at the initial intake for treatment.

The follow-up study focused on the measures of drug abstinence, illegal behaviour, family relationships, social networking, physical and psychological health and employment status. The results of this study were positive in linking treatment effectiveness with time in treatment. The longer a drug addict remained in treatment, the less likely he/she was to relapse. Positive outcomes are higher for those who completed 12 months of treatment in a therapeutic community. According to the study, 67.7% of those who remained in therapeutic communities for one year had had no relapse episodes five years later; 72.7% of the same group had had no further involvement with the criminal justice system (arrests, lawsuits, imprisonment, etc.) and 83.7% managed to find and sustain a job.

The research also revealed that therapeutic experience accounts for many positive changes in every area under study, even when treatment experience is short in duration. Therefore, even drug addicts who stayed for less than a year but a minimum of 90 days in a therapeutic community, experienced many benefits from their participation in the treatment process.

The benefits they received include overall improvement in their health status, HIV/AIDS and Hepatitis C prevention, less participation in illegal activities and better social and personal relationships. This improvement, according to the relevant research, is directly linked to the fact that a large number of individuals who stopped their treatment too soon managed to return to the same or a similar type of therapeutic programme within five years.

Therefore, approaching drug treatment services, even when the first attempt does not guarantee full recovery, is proved to be beneficial and reinforces motivation for treatment. However, the economic crisis is expected to change the patterns of use, the motivation for treatment and the rehabilitation processes.

The effects of crisis and the need for a new strategy

During the economic crisis, the expectation is that the patterns of problematic drug use are going to worsen. Drug injection, together with violence and criminal activities may increase due to poor finances. At the induction phase, drug abusers may be less motivated towards treatment and they may be more likely to question the effectiveness of treatment due to lesser opportunities for work and rehabilitation. In this depressive period drug abusers may tend to prefer substitution programmes that are more widely available (for financial reasons) and have low requirements of attendance and low pressure for changing drug habits.

In TCs or intensive-phase treatments, drop-out rates and acting out behaviours are expected to increase, especially during the personal crisis period due to the above reasons. On the other hand, in this time of economic crisis, family involvement and participation at the treatment process is expected to decrease, contributing to the problems of drop-outs. The uncertainty that drug addicts experience in relation to re-entry options and problems is also expected to contribute towards a development of a pathetic attitude and for some treatment members it is going to increase dependence due to the treatment setting and institutionalisation.

Finally, at the re-entry phase, it is going to become harder to find jobs. In addition the risk of losing jobs is also high. Most former drug addicts at re-entry phase experience worsened working conditions, they experience that their income is being reduced and they experience poor living standards and an increase in stereotypes and prejudices. These all lead to increased stress levels and as a result of this to an increase in drop-out and relapse rates.

Drug treatment organisations are also under the pressure of the economic crisis since their annual budget is reduced together with their staff reduction. These result in reduced accessibility and quality of services, in more competitiveness and conflicts, in bureaucracy and introversion. At times when support systems become less and less available, pathology is expected to occur in the treatment settings.

What can we do to confront this situation? What are the strategies in an environment of uncertainty and change?

Drug Treatment organisations need to adopt a new strategy that involves all interested parties in open communication, clarity and democracy in decision-making. They have to be flexible and have alternative options open when confronting crisis. They have to focus on vocational training and on developing social networks in order to support clients in the rehabilitation phase. New relationships, financial stability, employment retention and keeping away from drugs and criminal behaviour are the best cues for relapse prevention (Marlatt & Gordon, 1985) and long-term recovery.

Re-organisation is often necessary, together with innovation and the use of new technologies for better response to new needs. Networking at the national and international level are important variables in this process. Emphasis on research, evaluation and evidence-based practices are also highly significant with regard to resisting crisis. Finally, fighting for human rights and free access to public health and social justice are necessary to fight social and economic crisis.

The case of KETHEA

KETHEA, an NGO with Special Consultative Status at ECOSOC (Economic and Social Council) United Nations is a nationwide network of drug treatment, rehabilitation and social re-integration services in Greece. Its resources stem from state grants, donations and self-financing activities. KETHEA supports drug users and their families since the foundation of ITHAKI, the first Greek therapeutic community in Greece founded in 1983.

KETHEA offers its services within community, prison and residential settings and has the capacity to respond to clients with diverse needs, including adults, adolescents, parents, immigrants, refugees, prison inmates, alcoholics, gamblers and pathological Internet users, at every stage of their recovery. KETHEA programmes are drug-free and offer a comprehensive continuum of services, aiming at full recovery and social integration as an equal member of the society. All KETHEA services are provided free of charge. KETHEA also runs school- and community-based prevention and early intervention programmes and it is active in training and research in the field of drug and alcohol addiction.

Due to the financial crisis in Greece, KETHEA went through very hard times during which the organisation not only had to survive but also continue to offer high quality services to drug abusers and their families. The strategy the organisation adopted includes the following:

Re-organising services: more and better services with existing resources

At this time of economic and social crisis, KETHEA proceeded to re-organise its services. The main task was to restrain costs by making better use of its staff and infrastructure, improving the quality of services and facilitating accessibility by opening new gateways to treatment. This re-organisation is based on the conclusions drawn from the qualitative and quantitative evaluation of the services provided .

Increasing gateways to the KETHEA network of services in cooperation with local authorities

In order to facilitate better access for drug addicts and their families and to increase the number of admissions, KETHEA set up new priorities by establishing new Counselling and Intake Centres in areas with the greatest needs. While KETHEA was already running 24 Counselling Centres in different cities within the first half of 2010, three new Counselling Centres were established in collaboration with local authorities. In recent years, more than 15 local authority boards from various areas of Greece requested KETHEA to develop new services in their area. In response to that, KETHEA further developed its cooperation with the local authorities, which they are asked to provide the premises for the new units and to cover the initial running costs. KETHEA provides the personnel and offers full clinical and administrative supervision of the services.

Expanding prison programmes – promoting the principle of "treatment not punishment"

About half of the 11,364 inmates in the Greek prison system are serving sentences for drug-related offences (Hellenic Ministry of Justice, 2010). Within the Greek Criminal Justice System, KETHEA runs 21 Counselling Support Programmes for Prisoners and it operates three Therapeutic Communities and two Reception and Re-entry Centres upon release in Athens and Thessaloniki, respectively. KETHEA has striven to facilitate access to treatment for all inmates by launching new services and submitting proposals based on the "treatment, not punishment" principle for the amendment of drug-related legislation. KETHEA's goal is to increase the number of referrals to therapeutic communities and social integration centres and, in parallel, apply pressure to change the law in order to give drug abusers the option to seek treatment as an alternative to imprisonment for offences related to their drug addiction.

Innovative programmes for special and newly arising needs

KETHEA strives to meet the diverse and evolving needs of addicted persons with new services. In Athens, KETHEA has set up an intercultural support programme for immigrants and refugees, a programme for "legal" addictions (alcohol, gambling), as well as an Internet addiction support programme for adolescents and young adults. In Thessaloniki, KETHEA runs a special programme for addicted parents, which includes day-care and welfare services for their children. With funds from the National Lottery Organisation (OPAP), KETHEA started to operate a helpline for people addicted to gambling and their families. In addition to funds donated by a private entity (Stavros Niarchos Foundation) KETHEA is going to operate a new drug-free harm reduction centre in the heart of Athens using psychosocial methods. This approach includes street work programmes, medical and psychological support services, social welfare systems and referral services.

Focusing on social re-integration

As the economic crisis continues, former drug users face increasing difficulties to find full-time jobs and to ensure decent working conditions. KETHEA offers education and vocational training to its members throughout the stages of their treatment. To this end, KETHEA set up 22 re-entry houses for people who complete the therapeutic community programme. To support rehabilitation, KETHEA established four transitional schools and four Specialised Social and Vocational Integration Centres in northern and central Greece, Athens and Crete. It also runs production units offering training in graphic arts, carpentry, pottery, organic farming and multimedia applications. KETHEA has also developed local networks with employers and companies to facilitate the integration of its members into the labour market. However, the situation is still difficult given the fact that unemployment rates in Greece continue to increase, especially amongst young people and it has now reached 12%-14% (Eurostat, 2011).

Legal aid for programme members below the poverty line

Three out of four drug users seeking help at KETHEA report legal problems. Settling any type of legal problems with the criminal justice system is a prerequisite for recovery and for building a new life. To help its members who are below the poverty line to deal with the law, KETHEA offers counselling and legal aid and runs two offices in Athens and Thessaloniki in collaboration with the respective Bar Associations. During the financial crisis, many people cannot pay for legal services, therefore running the risk of imprisonment and relapse.

Networking with healthcare and social services

The organisation has developed a cooperation network with public entities and NGOs that are active in the field of healthcare, social welfare and education, with a view to better address the multi-faceted needs of substance abusers and their families. Furthermore, KETHEA has proposed concrete measures for co-operation between healthcare and social welfare organisations working in the field of addiction treatment (drug-free programmes, substitution programmes, hospitals, social services). The aim is to cater for a large number of substance abusers and to also save resources through networking. These measures are intended to tackle the problem of the "revolving door" and to provide a more direct response to users' needs.

Prevention and community development

In the field of prevention, KETHEA is increasingly focusing on intervention programmes for high-risk groups. Recently, KETHEA developed a new Community Intervention Centre in Athens that is close to one of the city's well known drug scene areas, in an attempt to respond to the new arising needs resulting from the socio-economic crisis and the expansion of drug use amongst young people in Attica. The Centre addresses the needs of adolescents and young adults facing personal, interpersonal and social problems together with drug use experimentation. The centre cooperates with schools and social services in the greater Athens area and offers a meeting place to youngsters together with psycho education, motivation and counselling services, crisis intervention, referrals and parent support groups.

Maintaining a dynamic relationship with society

In order to maintain open communication with broader society and to have social support, KETHEA has a multi-dimensional strategy. Firstly, every two years KETHEA elects an Executive Council that supervises the organisation. The council is elected by members of the past Executive Councils of the organisation, by staff members, family members and re-entry phase members. The candidates are prominent members of Greek society who are well known for their social activism and their professional life. Members represent different professional areas including the academic world, the justice system, businesses, the area of journalism etc. Secondly, KETHEA is supported by twelve active Family and Friends Associations working for KETHEA on a volunteer basis. These associations operate as a pressure group at the policy-making level. Thirdly, the organisation increases its resources through donations and runs media-sponsored awareness campaigns. Finally, it cooperates with NGOs and active citizens in social, environmental and cultural actions with the active participation of its programme members.

Promoting an international dialogue on recession

KETHEA actively participates in international organisations and forums aiming to promote international dialogue on the repercussions of the financial crisis on substance users and recovery services. The focus of the organisation is on the development of an effective policy on the above issues in the present conditions of economic crisis and the promotion of a drug policy for high quality services and to support human rights.

Documenting and improving quality and outcome Research

Research is the key instrument for meeting KETHEA's goals and objectives, such as the promotion of evidence-based practices, the constant improvement of the services provided and the adoption of an effective developmental strategy. To this end, KETHEA's methodology is based on internal and external evaluation systems that include the Management Information System, the Continuous Quality Improvement Evaluation System, the effectiveness of Therapeutic Communities and client and staff satisfaction studies. During the economic crisis it is necessary to provide evidence about the effectiveness of drug-free treatment programmes in order to be able to document our intervention, to inform policy through better monitoring, analysis and research and use the results to improve services.

Staff support and the continuous training of professionals

Staff members are the driving force behind KETHEA. In recognising this, the organisation systematically supports the development of its employee's professional knowledge and skills. KETHEA employs 542 people, 481 of whom work on a full-time and 61 on a part-time basis. The majority of them are treatment staff who offer direct services to drug addicts and their families and 20% of the staff members are programme graduates.

The recession has negatively impacted on staff morale due to cut backs on salaries, together with an increase in the work load and decrease in other resources. KETHEA offers its staff members systematic training and supervision, hoping to overcome the negative consequences of the recession by providing feedback to employees, by preventing staff burn-out and maintaining the high quality of services provided.

KETHEA focuses on creating a friendly, safe and efficient working environment by establishing open communication and decision-making, by ensuring equal rights and equal opportunities for all, by promoting transparency in administrative procedures and job selection criteria, by promoting professional ethics and by providing maternity/paternity legal rights.

KETHEA's initiatives for the promotion of scientific discussion, the exchange of knowhow and the diffusion of best practices between drug treatment and prevention professionals include training seminars, conferences and open days. KETHEA training programmes offer theory, practice and experiential workshops in the field of drug addiction treatment and prevention. These programmes are offered to KETHEA staff. Staff from methadone maintenance and other types of drug treatment services, are also invited to attend. KETHEA also offers professional certification programmes and internships to its services network. KETHEA also published the scientific journal "Exartiseis" and it has established the only specialised library on drug addiction in Greece. More than 250 places in KETHEA short-term and long-term training programmes are available for this purpose to its staff members. In addition, KETHEA together with the International Certification and Reciprocity Consortium in Greece managed to certify 168 substance-abuse counsellors and prevention specialists.

Decreasing expenses, increasing self-funding

Addiction treatment in Greece is provided free of charge since the Greek Ministry of Health funds directly funds the relevant agencies on an annual basis. A substantial part of KETHEA's expenditure is covered by state funding, which allows the organisation to provide its services to substance users and their families free of charge and without contributions from social insurance funds. However, the recession has already led to a significant reduction in funds allocated for the treatment of addictions. KETHEA tried to reduce its expenditure and increase the resources through self-financing activities involving businesses, grants, European programmes and private donations.

Educating the public and policy makers

KETHEA places emphasis on "educating the public and policymakers" on the consequences of the recession on mental health, drug abuse and social exclusion. For this purpose, KETHEA is organising nationwide awareness campaigns on a systematic basis using electronic and printed media. KETHEA has kept its awareness campaigns up and running throughout the year by means of open events, leaflets and publications, TV and radio adverts, web pages and social media ads and broadcasts on KETHEA Web radio. In addition, KETHEA increases public awareness using websites, facebook and twitter and sends research results, annual reports and other publications and leaflets to policymakers, government officials, other organisations etc. During the economic crisis, in order to educate the public and policymakers about the relationship between crisis and drug abuse, it is necessary to clarify that unless drug treatment organisations are reinforced, the effects of drug abuse are going to worsen. On the contrary, social and economic cost will decrease as a result of the decrease in drug use, delinquency, unemployment and improvement of health conditions.

Critique on the causes of crisis and Promoting Human Rights and Human Dignity

During the economic crisis it is necessary to defend the social welfare and health system and to promote peoples' right to receive high quality services based on human rights and social justice. While trying to respond in a creative and flexible way to the negative consequences of the recession, KETHEA systematically exercises political pressure with a view to defend the basic conquests of the Greek social welfare state. The Greek State should continue to allocate sufficient resources to public and free-of-charge drug treatment programmes. KETHEA urges the Greek Government to take into account the cost effectiveness of existing programmes in the long run, before making further cuts to public expenditure in the drug field. In this way KETHEA is trying to ensure the right of drug users and their families to access quality counselling and treatment services for free.

Conclusions

The crisis is going to have significant consequences in the coming years by reinforcing drug abuse problems, delinquency and social exclusion. It is necessary to constantly observe this phenomenon and new arising needs as much as the organisations' adjustment to the new needs. The need for a new strategy that is going to include innovative programmes, research and documentation, networking, the use of new technologies, continued training and staff education is vital. The case of KETHEA offers an example on how to survive an unstable environment. In drug treatment organisations it is necessary to respect personal needs and promote personal dignity and social justice. Drug treatment organisations should be able to defend the physical, psychological, social and spiritual integrity and well-being of all people in treatment and continue to promote change both at the personal and social level.

References

Edwards, G (2004). *Matters of Substance-Drugs: Is Legalization the Right Answer or the Wrong Question?* UK: Penguin Books.

EMCDDA (2009). *Annual report 2009, the state of the drugs problem in Europe*, Publications Office of the European Union, Luxembourg.

EMCDDA (2009). *Polydrug use: patterns and responses,* EMCDDA Selected issue, Publications Office of the European Union, Luxembourg.

EMCDDA (2010). *Annual report 2009, the state of the drugs problem in Europe*, Publications Office of the European Union, Luxembourg.

Ettner, SL, Huang, D, Evans, E *et al.* (2006). Benefit-cost in the California treatment outcome project: does substance abuse treatment "pay for itself"? Health Service Research, 41(1): 192-213.

European Commission (2009). *Economic Crisis in Europe:causes, consequences and responses,* European Economy, 7/2009, Publications Office of the European Union, Luxembourg.

Eurostat (2011). Available at: http://ec.europa.eu/eurostat/euroindicators

French, MT, McCollister, KE, Sacks, S, McKendrick, K & De Leon, G (2002). Benefit cost analysis of a modified therapeutic community for mentally ill chemical abusers. Evaluation and Program Planning, 25: 137-148. DOI: 10.1016/S0149-7189(02)00006-X.

Gossop, M, Marsden, D, Stewart, D, Lehmann, P & Strang, J (1999), Methadone Treatment practices and outcomes for opiate addicts treated in drug clinics and in general practice: results from the National Treatment Outcome Study. *British Journal of General Practice*, 49 (438), 31-34.

Gossop, M, Marsden, J, Stewart, D, Edwards, C, Lehmann, P, Wilson, A & Segar, G (1997). The National Treatment Outcome Research Study in the United Kingdom: six-month follow-up outcomes. *Psychology of Addictive Behaviours*, 11 (4), 324-337.

Guth RA & Thurow R (2008). A different banking crisis in need of fresh capital. *Wall Street Journal.* November 20, 2008, A16.

KETHEA (2011). Annual report of KETHEA services during 2010 available at: http://www.kethea.gr.

Levy, BS & Sidel, VW (2006). The Nature of Social Injustice and Its Impact on Public Health. In Levy, BS & Sidel, VW (eds.). *Social Injustice and Public Health.* New York: Oxford University Press (published in cooperation with the American Public Health Association), 6.

Levy, BS & Sidel, VW (2009). The Economic Crisis and Public Health. *Social Medicine,* Volume 4, Number 2.

Ouimette, PC, Finney, JW & Moos, RH (1997). Twelve-step and cognitive behavioural treatment for substance abuse: a comparison of treatment effectiveness. *Journal of Consulting and clinical psychology*, 65 (2), 230-240.

Schultz, KB (2008). *Divorce during recession*, available at: http://www.forbes.com.

Schumacher, HC (1934). The Depression and its effect on the mental health of the child. *American Journal of Public Health and The Nation's Health.* 24: 367-371.

Simpson, DD, Joe, GW, Broome, KM, Hiller, ML, Knight, K & Rowan-Szal, GA (1997). *Psychology of Addictive Behaviours*, 11 (4), 279-293.

Solantaus, T, Leinonen, J & Punamaki, RL (2004). Children's mental health in times of economic recession: replication and extension of the family economic stress model in Finland. *Developmental Psychology.* 40: 412-429.

Stuckler, D, Basu, S, Suhrcke, M, Coutts, A & McKee, M (2009). The public health effect of economic crises and alternative policy responses in Europe: an empirical analysis. *The Lancet.* Vol 374 July 25, 323.

Tapia-Granados, J (2008). Macroeconomic fluctuations and mortality in post-war Japan. *Demography.* 45: 323-43.

World Health Organization (2009). *The Financial Crisis and Global Health: Report of a High-Level Consultation, Geneva:* World Health Organization

15 Getting regular, early and brief alcohol interventions into primary care in rural New South Wales: the origins of the Murdi Paaki Drug and Alcohol Network

Rod MacQueen

Lyndon Withdrawal Unit
Bloomfield Hospital, Australia

rmacqueen@lyndoncommunity.org.au

Abstract

The Murdi Paaki Drug and Alcohol Network (MPDAN) has been working to improve clinical services for people with drug and alcohol related problems in rural New South Wales, Australia, for about 18 months. Its development builds upon several years of work and reflection upon practice outcomes by a variety of clinicians and managers. The model of service provision is put forward as a pragmatic response to a complex health problem, drawing upon a diversity of evidence and literature, which seeks to bring about major changes in the way such problems are conceptualised and addressed. The Network seeks to improve clinical services, community health, worker morale, engagement and wellbeing and in time to demonstrate a community development approach to health service development. It suggests a need to understand and better address the current ineffective way of managing alcohol-related problems, and to implement the evidence from a wealth of literature for a less bureaucratic, community development approach. This could bring about major health improvements effectively and efficiently.

Key words

Alcohol; screening; intervention; Aboriginal health; service development.

Introduction

Whilst it would be tempting to describe origins of the Murdi Paaki Drug and Alcohol Network (MPDAN) as an example of the implementation of current best practice, or as a logical developmental process where careful planning and documentation preceded each step, this is not at all how things happened. So when I was asked to expand upon the presentation given in Barcelona, I was troubled; this was a scientific conference, and it would be normal to explain how things happen in the traditional manner, starting with a hypothesis, arguing how we would seek to test this hypothesis, all written up as a meticulously planned process, each step logically following, until we came to the proof and conclusions. And in the third person, of course. But the presentation given at the conference described a personal journey, the slow evolution of an idea, a process and eventually a clinical service, because that is what happened. Happily, the editor agreed that the same approach could be followed in this chapter, for which I am most grateful, because describing our service evolution in a linear, connected way would be to support an untruth. In fact, the process described in this chapter may be how most change takes place in clinical services, if not in most research projects including those in the hard sciences (Kuhn, 1959).

Robert Merton describes and illustrates this "Shandean" progress of the discovery process (after Sterne's 1760s book, The Life and Opinions of Tristram Shandy, Gentleman) in his lovely book "On the Shoulders of Giants" (Merton, 1993), the reading of which led to much relief as I realised that our often shuffling, pragmatic, backwards and forwards progress was probably very common. This is not to say that we acted without an evidence base, and there are years of experience, reading, discussion and reflection amongst the staff involved in the project to draw upon. It is merely that the need to act preceded the rigorous documentation of every element of the process, which may be a necessity in complex, evolving situations (Fraser & Greenhalgh, 2001). This then will be a personal account of how I believe we came to our current position, and others may, if asked, tell the story slightly differently. Many people were involved in the evolution of this programme – some will be mentioned by name, with their approval, and as ever, any errors, points of dispute or problems remain purely mine.

It is important to note from the outset that nothing discussed in this chapter should be used to diminish the fact that the determinants of an individual's or community's health frequently lie well outside of that person or community. The social and structural determinants of health are very important throughout rural New South Wales and more so amongst Aboriginal communities (Gray, 2005; Marmot, 2011). There is a large and growing body of literature discussing these determinants (Marmot, 2000; Marmot & Wilkinson 2001). At the same time there is a growing tendency to focus upon the individual's choices to the exclusion of any discussion, let alone redressing, of the bigger determinants of health – I do not wish to support such a view even by implication. In this article I describe merely the evolution of a clinical service: we believe it will lead to a community better able to advocate for changes to these more complex determinants (Syme, 1997, 2003; Baum, 2007), as well as to the expected improvements in individual and family health, but this remains to be seen. Our starting point was this: inasmuch as a recurrently funded clinical service operates in our area, and accepting that we do not currently have much capacity to effect the other determinants of health but we do know something about clinical services, can we provide and support a good and improving drug and alcohol (D&A) service, and do better at helping improve our communities' health?

Improving drug and alcohol services

My first involvement in the delivery of clinical D&A services outside of my own city began in about 2003, with visits to Broken Hill to support the methadone programme, as part of my Area Health Service job. This initially involved visiting two days per fortnight, later reduced to two days per month. On these visits, I worked with people from Maari Ma Aboriginal Health Corporation and on one occasion, I was asked by Kate Gooden, then a Community Development worker, to be part of a programme to develop a workbook for better informing primary care and other frontline workers how they could work with people who experience D&A problems. Maari Ma was then in the unusual, perhaps unique, situation where, as an Aboriginal health service, it was providing or supervising all population health services through an agreement with the (state government funded) Area Health Service. The workbook (Laycock, 2004) was developed over some months, after which we introduced the finished product to workers who had contributed to the discussion and its development. Kate and I visited a number of worksites and towns that I had not previously visited, and became acquainted with many health workers as well as those working in other support programmes, such as community housing and telephone counselling services.

The feedback from these visits indicated clearly that most of these workers would greatly value training in the area of engagement and problem sensing, discussing change, and other pragmatic aspects of caring for people with drug and alcohol problems. Interestingly, the Stages of Change model (Prochaska *et al.*, 1992), consistently proved to be a mind expanding concept leading to productive discussion amongst most primary care workers. Consequently, an extra day was added to each area visit after the methadone clinic, without there being too much time or expense incurred (as flying to Broken Hill is the only practical way to maximise work time, but costs over $A500). It was about this time that Kate and I, supported by the management, decided we should gently push for more screening and brief intervention (SBI) with regard to alcohol use. Most workers believed they saw many people with problems caused or exacerbated by alcohol use, but few felt willing or able to raise the issue. We began to explain that this was not specialist or indeed difficult work. My first exposure to the WHO research on SBI for alcohol occurred in about 1985, and it now appeared that the time had come to actively promote this approach (Babor, 2007; Heather, 2011).

At this time I met with an Aboriginal health worker who was to have a considerable effect on my life, Justin Files. Justin is a Barkinje ("people of the river") man, from Menindee, who now works as the team leader of primary care in Maari Ma. But at this time he was a clinical worker responsible for much of the organising and arranging of clinics, staff training and support, and liaison with others such as visiting doctors. His attention to detail in making sure people attended clinics and felt safe and comfortable was remarkable; he taught us all about getting better results by paying attention to the details and respecting people's understanding of our service, something I was to read about only much later (Gawande, 2007). I also learned a good deal about Aboriginal history, personal, local and in general, and though Justin feels I have not learned nearly enough to be culturally competent, having not been mentored in that area, he feels I have some respect for and understanding of other people's experience that has changed the way I view clinical services.

Much of this learning took place whilst driving in the car, as we would spend up to 2-3 hours travelling to do a clinic or a teaching session. In turn, Justin learned about the logic behind screening and brief intervention (SBI) and how it could be applied in our area, as well as about the spirit of motivational interviewing (MI) and other clinical issues. Kate and I travelled a good deal as well, and on those trips we would discuss service development right down to the details of how to work with individual managers or workers who we felt may understand and advance our cause.

We began working with any individual or group with an interest in improving D&A services. In some towns this was the Aboriginal health service, in others the Area Health Service, and it soon became clear that even in small towns, there could be 2 or 3 health service providers who rarely spoke together. Although all sites agreed that better D&A services were a high priority, we could on occasions run a well publicised community discussion group and nobody from one or other service attended because we were in the wrong meeting room. This silo approach has not entirely disappeared, even though we made it clear, and continue to do so, that we would work with anybody who was interested in working in this field. We (perhaps naively) believed that good, evidence-based services were desired by all people, or would be once they saw what we had to offer, but I am now not so sure that is always the case.

Initially the plan was to promote the use of AUDIT (the WHO developed Alcohol Use Disorders Identification Test), then we considered using an abbreviated version, AUDIT C. Finally, beginning with a well person health check in one site, we settled on a simple question asked by the primary care workers, namely, "Are you worried about your alcohol use or someone else's use? Would you like to talk to somebody about this?" We considered that there was a limited capacity at that stage for workers to do any follow up, even a brief intervention, so a formal screening followed immediately by a brief intervention (SBI, see Babor, 2007) was not possible. On the other hand, these two questions did not take much time or skill, and gathered some data whilst exposing workers to, at least, the beginnings of SBI. At the first run in one site, 12 people answered in the affirmative and made appointments to see me on the next visit. Ten of these attended, even though the visit was some two months later, and six wished to talk about their own alcohol consumption whilst four wished to speak about the consumption of a person about whom they were concerned. It was tempting to introduce a screener for alcohol use at that stage, and we could have attempted this in a policy-driven, top down manner. But there would be little point doing this unless there could also be a brief intervention linking it to a health issues worrying the patient at that moment. That is the motivating moment, whereas if it is not done with some degree of skill, it is unlikely to do any good and may even do harm (Rollnick *et al.,* 1992). Consequently, we identified early (in 2004) the need to work on developing the infrastructure, including the workers and their willingness and capacity to do this work, and the managers who identify and support this approach. This has proven to be harder and slower than we first thought.

It became clear that we needed to consider whether the current views and practice concerning SBI within health services, workers and the community exists because this is what many people find most comfortable. The assumption we made is that most people would rather be healthier, and if we could effectively link alcohol use to poor health outcomes, or to other problems, they would be inclined to seek change. But this may not be true. One of my concerns remain, that many people may like to keep health problems clearly externalised, as issues that visit them, as it were, in moments of weakness but that definitely reside out of their own person. In this approach, problems can be excised (or even exorcised – Cohen, 2000) by an outside agent, an expert, whereas what a population level health promotional approach seeks is that people live longer and healthier lives by living in healthier communities and by better understanding the health risks and benefits of certain activities and behaviours. Around the world, we are not seeing much implementation of SBI in primary care settings (Heather, 2011), despite workers and communities stating very clearly that alcohol and other drug problems are both prevalent and important. We have tried to learn what concerns workers about SBI, but so far there is no clear picture. Perhaps an additional problem is that both workers and patients have internalised a socially learned moral weakness or deficit model of alcohol and drug problems (Treloar, 2006; Trucco, 2007), a situation perpetuated by an abstinence-is-best approach modelled in TV shows and by several high profile actors and singers, hardly tempered by a tradition of boom and bust drinking in many rural communities (Hunter, 1993). Some discussions with emergency accommodation workers, for example, revealed that despite their view that alcohol use played a major part in the presentation of most clients, many of whom stayed several weeks, they did not discuss alcohol. When we suggested gentle intervention was preferable to ignoring the issue, they replied that their client would most likely not accept a referral to detox and long term rehabilitation! Clearly, the logic of brief motivational interventions, and of harm reduction, was not yet understood.

We also had to better improve our understanding of why people did not keep appointments with the D&A team, a fairly common occurrence. One insight is that even when D&A workers are not judgmental in their approach, many of our patients have met so many others in the community who are judgmental about alcohol use, and they themselves may have accepted the deficit model, that they believe we will exhibit similar behaviours. So they stay away. This implies that health services and workers have done net harm and reduced the likelihood that people will present, at least until they are quite sick. In many consultations, when people do actually present, workers have reported spending the first 15 minutes defusing the patient's anger about how they were treated recently by another health worker – this militates against early presentation of alcohol problems per se, and suggests an even greater need to engage in screening and brief interventions on all possible occasions when people present to any arm of the health service. Our challenge was not about better clinical services alone, but was also to change the community's conception of alcohol use and subsequent problems.

The Clinical Leadership Programme

About this time, I moved from work at the Area Health Service to working with a non-government organisation, The Lyndon Community, based in Orange. Whilst, in theory, this would severely curtail the capacity to expand services, it had become clear that in practice, the Area Health Service was bound up in a process ensuring that change, let alone rapidly grasping local opportunities as they presented, was virtually impossible. Several opportunities, some with funding attached, including training of junior medical officers and teaching medical students in D&A medicine, passed by because the bureaucratic climate ensured those responsible for the decisions felt unable or unwilling to respond. At about this time, the Area D&A and mental health services were being amalgamated as a result of State Health policy, a process currently being reversed. These processes absorb much energy, but do not address clinical services, and it became far easier to bring these ideas to fruition in a non-government organisation despite an ongoing shortage of funding and staff. There has been no cause to reconsider this decision after some seven years. The Lyndon Community and MPDAN now train a junior doctor on regular rotation, teach students from 3 medical schools, and support Aboriginal Health trainees, for example. The management recognised the opportunity to further expand our range of services and sought funding from the Commonwealth (Australian) Government under the Proceeds of Crime Act, to promote a programme that later became known as the Clinical Leadership Programme (CLP). This enabled the organisation to move towards funding my position full-time, and we were thus able to continue work with Maari Ma. Initially I flew to various sites with the Royal Flying Doctor Service (RFDS), which operates a regular shuttle service for health staff, whilst later we funded these trips from our budget.

Commonwealth funding was also used for some trips through the Medical Specialists Outreach Assistance Programme (MSOAP) which, though set up principally to provide conventional one to one clinical services, did have the capacity to pay for some staff training and development. Quite simply, there had been no effective D&A service in many towns for so long that no assessment, triage and referral system was possible, even if we had intended to operate a more typical clinical service. Over this period, we also developed increasing links with community-controlled Aboriginal health services in a number of towns, at least in part because, as they were flexible NGOs, they were willing and able to work in new ways with new people – and they wanted a better D&A service.

An experienced colleague, a Wiradjuri descendant, Lynette Bullen, was employed to help run the CLP, and we were able to work together for three years looking at a new model of clinical service development and delivery. We had noted the failure of the usual top down, bureaucratically heavy service, which often resulted in a succession of 5-year plans, manuals and guidelines along with an inability to deliver relevant services that respect and support local staff and conditions. A service could begin differently by supporting and enhancing the existing clinical services, poor though they may be, and working with non-D&A primary care and other workers who are most enthusiastic about evolving the services with our support. We were keen to promote and teach the spirit of MI, and realised that this was best demonstrated by working in a respectful way with co-workers and management, as well as with our patients. We were asking workers to change their behaviour (e.g., practice SBI in primary care, rather than ignoring alcohol use) and there was no reason to believe that workers change behaviour by means any different to our patients (Miller & Rollnick, 2002, Chapter 14). We realised this was evolving into a discrete model, a bold new approach we thought. As we better defined its characteristics and consulted the literature in a more targeted way, we discovered that this approach has, at least in part, already evolved in a number of places. This was both encouraging and disappointing – encouraging because it implied we might be on the right track, treading a path someone else has felt worth exploring and disappointing because we wanted to be bold pioneers! Entities variously called practice-based research networks and primary care practice-based research networks have been documented in the literature for over 20 years (Mold, 2005), and they seem to have evolved to address some of the same needs.

The CLP thus consisted of two workers from Orange, spending about half their time visiting outlying towns, usually flying with the RFDS shuttle service, with support especially from Kate Gooden, Justin Files and other staff at Maari Ma. On these trips, our brief was that we would do whatever was most likely to improve both clinical services and the capacity of the individual or organisation to maintain and expand on any gains made. In practice, we believed several interconnected strategies were needed. The traditional reason for visiting outlying communities would remain – firstly we would provide specialist drug and alcohol clinics, also addressing comorbid mental health and other issues. This was acceptable to and desired by patients, managers and funding bodies, though we realised the trap here – the better we did our job, the more likely it would be that other workers would see all D&A problems as belonging to someone else (ideally far away, in another town!). Secondly, we would provide education, training and support, through set educational pieces but more often working with individual workers, with their own readiness to change and their understanding of how and why they address D&A problems, in the spirit of MI. Management would also be challenged, encouraged and supported to help their workers change, and later to merge the boundaries between good practice, quality improvement and research so that practice change could become locally informed and owned. In the third step we would use new funding to employ a researcher who would stand back a little, overview what we all do, collect appropriate qualitative and quantitative data, and most importantly guide us to become more effective, efficient and evidence based. This has now led to the first MERI (Monitor, Evaluate, Review and Implement) review, which will be discussed shortly.

The fourth step would be to engage with local communities, and key individuals, in defining research priorities, implementing relevant local research, and helping change the health delivery system to be more relevant, responsive and efficient, a community-based participatory research process. Over 15 years ago, Sanson-Fisher, drawing upon several years work by many people, noted that most research in the D&A field was descriptive, and very little was based around intervention (Sanson-Fisher, 1994). Earlier, in Alice Springs in 1986, a group of 200 researchers noted that Aboriginal control over relevant research was highly desirable but usually lacking, and that participatory research may be a good model (Humphery, 2001). In most regards progress is not being made in implementation research, noted again by Sanson-Fisher (2008) whilst others have noted that Indigenous participation in the research process is still unusual (Kowal, 2005).

An example of a failed trial of SBI giving insight into this area was published in 2002. An attempt was made to conduct a primary care-based alcohol early intervention at an urban Aboriginal health service. The data supporting the intervention was solid, but it proved impossible to recruit sufficient people to run the trial and it was abandoned (Sibthorpe, 2002). Whilst there are many difficulties in running a randomised controlled trial (RCT) in a primary care setting, my learning from the trial's failure is not to put the cart before the horse in expecting workers and patients to support externally-directed research before their own capacity to define the role of evidence and the need for good research is supported and developed. A community development approach may avoid this problem by beginning with locally defined problems and locally developed research (Minkler, 2003; Mold, 2005), with an RCT, as part of a collaborative research network, not impossible but some years down the path. It may be both more effective and more efficient than the current top down approach, when one considers the current evidence-practice gap (Shakeshaft *et al.*, 1997; Green, 2005). However, this approach devolves power, money and control away from big city funding and research bodies, towards smaller community groups, and contrasts markedly with current approaches such as NICE in the UK, the NIH in the US and the Clinical Excellence Commission in Australia. For example, a recent review of "translational research", getting new evidence into routine healthcare, notes that less than 2% of the US NIH's funding is directed towards this practice development process, and of that very little goes to practice-based research (Woolf, 2008).

The Murdi Paaki Drug and Alcohol Network model

As it transpired, the CLP was rather ambitious and these steps took several years more to implement, but are now part of the MPDAN model. A combination of qualitative and quantitative, process and outcome data is required to document this change process, but we are confident this work represents the best possible way to redress the complex inter connected problems currently inhibiting the development of better D&A services, such as staff recruitment and retention, lack of a clear model including resistance to SBI, poor status of D&A workers and lack of promotional and career opportunities, poor training and support for GPs, and many more.

And so MPDAN began this way: the Commonwealth had a desire to improve clinical drug and alcohol services in western NSW particularly amongst Aboriginal people. They had engaged in discussion with a number of Aboriginal health services and other organisations and employed the services of a colleague, Dr Kris Battye, and her team to engage in a community consultation process. All of the Aboriginal organisations consulted were keen on The Lyndon Community continuing its engagement with their organisation or community and despite concerns by the Area Health Service, it was this model that was eventually funded. The Lyndon Community became the major fund holder and in a genuine partnership, the Area Health Service undertook to match the services to a large extent, such that they are now making a valuable contribution to this process.

What became clear is that although there was considerable planning involved in the initial development (Battye, 2008), the success of the CLP in engaging rural communities and the capacity of The Lyndon Community to be flexible was fundamental. We needed to respect the clearly expressed desire to improve D&A services without being welded firmly to one method of service delivery. During the course of the CLP, for example, we realised that using the insights provided by the MI literature and the spirit of MI in dealing not just with clients but also fellow workers and even management, was far more likely to change practice than using any other means. We also believe firmly that enhancing the capacity of primary care to both start the discussion about alcohol and other drug use and begin (if not complete) the management of such problems was the most evidence-based, effective and efficient way of using our resources. We were aware of the considerable body of literature concerning SBI for alcohol problems in primary care. I was also aware, however, both from experience in working with general practitioners and other primary care providers, and from reading the literature, that getting SBI into primary care had proven to be a difficult nut to crack over most of the planet.

A recent review by Heather makes this point clearly (Heather, 2011); he feels optimistic that the change can occur, and I agree, but I do not think it will come from a top down approach. This seems to have failed over the last 30 years, confirmed by the literature on the slow diffusion of evidence into practice across many fields (Shakeshaft *et al.*, 1997). We decided to help develop and support, rather than direct, the community where the community includes those affected, their families, community care workers, managers, general practitioners and members of the board. We do not adopt a Rogerian non-directive approach, and take it as given that people prefer good health to poor health, and inclusion to exclusion. We wish to help others discover the rationale supporting an SBI approach, as opposed to the more common late (or non-) intervention approach. This has lead to heated discussion on whether we were engaged in true community development or not, since we have our own agenda. I do not know the answer to that, and in time we may be compelled to learn some humility and engage in more fundamental community development, as Syme suggests (Syme, 1997), but we continue.

Physically the MPDAN organisation looks like this. There is a central hub in Orange, in which are located the office staff and management, which functions as a central point for outreach workers to recharge their enthusiasm, develop ideas and programmes, and reduce isolation and burnout. As well as supervising the Network, the manager seeks funding and support for expansion, such as employing and supporting Aboriginal health trainees and workers, and the hub now employs four Aboriginal workers. The hub also functions as a resource centre for any workers seeking information on projects or problems that they are addressing at the moment. Each group of towns also has a local site worker, whose job it is to use local knowledge to coordinate activities throughout their town or towns. Initially there was some debate about whether these people should perform a little, a good deal, or no clinical work, focusing upon coordinating clinics by outreach staff, education and training, liaising and advocacy, etc. There was concern about the propensity of D&A workers to slip back into the old model, where all (late detected, high threshold, and definitely not early brief interventions) drug and alcohol work was passed to the D&A worker. Thus the more conscientious and hard-working the worker, the more self-defeating this approach became as their own burnout became guaranteed, whilst at the same time, primary care services would develop no interest in, or capacity to deliver, SBI. After some debate, it was agreed that the site worker would engage in some clinical work so as to keep up their clinical skills, and so as to be aware of the problems and issues confronted in each town. It may give them some credibility with other workers and enable the demonstration of a different style of practice (specifically, an MI approach and SBI when appropriate). But the major part of their job would remain supporting other workers and facilitating the evolution of better practice within each outlying site. Getting hold of workers who share this view, and getting outlying areas to see that this is a good model for service development, or at least one worth trying properly, remains a difficult issue, not least because so many D&A workers have been raised in a different model, to which many still cling despite the growing evidence of a need to change (Miller, 1995). This is a generic problem Kuhn identified many years ago (Kuhn, 1970), and in this case it is one in which the revolution has not yet occurred.

The third arm of the MPDAN model is the outreach worker, each responsible for a few outlying sites, preferably in close geographical proximity to limit travel times and distances. This worker would also engage in a mix of service development, site worker support, supervision and mentorship, and clinical work for much the same reasons as the site worker. They would also bring back to the hub issues, problems and difficulties they had encountered that would be discussed and addressed at the hub – resources could then be found or developed to address these needs including personal visits, video teleconference support, or increased visits by the outreach worker as well as screening tools, position statements and so on to support practice and co worker evolution. The fourth component is the addiction medicine physician who would visit outlying sites and the hub as required, as determined by the outreach and site worker. They would triage patients to be seen and, just as importantly, identify issues to be addressed with staff, through formal and informal training, mentorship, and supervision. The physician would also engage in problem-defining and lobbying at a higher level than may be possible with each individual worker. In addition, the physician would engage with local general practitioners, who in many towns are the sole primary care workers and in many cases have worked in the town for considerable years. Regrettably, poor medical practice such as inappropriate prescribing of benzodiazepines and opioids as well as poor advice and referral has been well documented as an ongoing problem (Martyres *et al.,* 2004; Maxwell, 2011). Reducing problems from poor prescribing would lead to considerable improvements in health in some areas, let alone the gains that could be made if and when general practitioners were truly involved in SBI. Resolving this issue involves a whole of service approach, offering and modelling real local alternatives in rural areas, such as increased opioid substitution, detox facilities and, in the end, a commitment to more SBI having grasped the importance of a population approach to D&A (Rose, 1992). Our local and hub outreach workers use every opportunity to work with general practitioners and their Division, and we regularly have evening meals with GPs in some sites, have brief case discussions by phone or face to face, send relevant journal articles (Gourlay, 2009) and we are working towards a trial 6-8 hour structured teaching and discussion programme in one site now.

The geographical challenge in addressing clinical needs across our area should not be underestimated. Western NSW covers about 444,000 square kilometres, slightly less than the area of Spain as a whole at 504,000 square km. But the population density (and thus the infrastructure) is clearly a good deal less with 154,000 overall in our area, amongst them 9,000 Aboriginal people, compared to 46,000,000 people throughout Spain. This currently leads to a considerable amount of driving and flying, which is within the capacity of the budget at present but is not sustainable either financially or personally in the long run. Most sites now have videoconferencing facilities, many purchased through MPDAN, and the next phase is to encourage staff to use this equipment more frequently for a broad variety of purposes. We have already engaged in 1:1 clinical consultations, mentorship, clinical case discussions with small groups and didactic lectures to bigger groups, as well as for management meetings. Again, this often involves modelling and leading from the front – each site worker and each outreach worker should ideally use the equipment at the slightest provocation if only to demonstrate to others that it is an easy process resulting in useful support. Far too often, the equipment does not work as well as it should and we end up demonstrating that despite our wishes, the technology is not yet foolproof. This may be addressed in time when the National Broadband Network leads to better line speeds for most rural towns, but that may well take some years. In addition, equipment managed by one group does not always talk well with equipment managed by another, though when the equipment works well, the process is quite dramatically effective. For example, patients have been interviewed by video conference, having never met the interviewer face to face, and good clinical outcomes occur even given the constraints of the medium. The Area mental health service has for 5 years operated MHEC-RAP (Mental Health Emergency Care Rural Access Programme) which involves giving referral site workers from outlying hospitals and community health clinics, access to a psychiatrist (on this site, actually sitting under the Murdi Paaki hub site) 24 hours per day for assessments of and consultations with patients felt to be mentally ill or disordered. The results from this programme have been uniformly positive, and we can learn from their strengths, weaknesses and problems how to better advance our process in this regard.

We seek to evolve and demonstrate a new model involving early recognition of alcohol and other drug related problems, a focus on brief interventions where appropriate, and a careful triage approach before people move into more intensive treatments. In addition, putting effort into supporting the learning of other primary care workers, talking with them about what they currently do and why they continue to do it, using an MI approach with our co-workers as well as with our patients, is essential for this process. This entailed us learning a good deal more about adult learning principles, and about what does not work when it comes to bringing about change in both individual workers and in the workforce in these community areas. What evidence do we have so far that we are on the right track? This comes from two sources. First, we have avoided the most common pitfalls, such as an expert model with short term focus, which has lead to so much squandering of resources and opportunity in the past. The recently released Commonwealth report on programmes addressing Aboriginal health and wellbeing (Commonwealth, 2010) suggests most programmes have not done as well as they should have and represent at least a "dismally poor" return on investment, if not a national disgrace. It suggests effective approaches must involve partnerships, longer term non-piecemeal funding, respect for local conditions, working across many dimensions, and many other factors we believe are part of our model. We have learned from our failures over the years (MacQueen, 2007), and though this is not enough in itself, it fits with an iterative, self-correcting approach that should move us closer to the best possible model. Secondly, we have just undergone our first formal review, which has enabled us to learn, for example, that the cultural awareness and competence amongst hub and outreach staff is in serious need of attention – we shall address this very shortly, by working more closely with our local workers and other Aboriginal staff to more clearly define our training needs. Once the second and subsequent reviews are done, we will be able to determine whether we are moving towards our defined goals. Improvements in health outcomes, for which we are striving, will probably not be measurable for some years, but other factors such as staff retention, recruitment of Aboriginal workers, and community satisfaction can and are being monitored.

Present and future of the project

There are criticisms about this project; that it bites off more than it can chew; attempts to do too much; is untargeted because it doesn't have a single unifying hypothesis that it's exploring, and that it may be better to focus services on one town rather than trying to do too much and diluting our resources. These concerns have some validity. But the brief answer is this: given that clinical services are going to continue being provided in this area, can they be done more efficiently and more effectively so as to lead, in time, to measurable health improvements in the population? Of course the answer is yes, services can always be better (Gawande, 2007), but the issue then becomes one of how to most effectively use limited resources and how to monitor whether we are moving in the right direction. In this respect there has been considerable debate within MPDAN itself as well as in our partner organisations. To some extent, each organisation pursues its own philosophies explicitly or implicitly, and has a different set of factors effecting workforce activity. There is not much we can do about this in the short term, though we can learn more from each organisation by respecting that the way things are is quite possibly the best they can be given the constraints that operate in that town at this time. This is consistent with our evolutionary model, rather than a revolutionary approach to healthcare "reform" often admired by politicians.

Quite simply, there is no way we can (or perhaps need to) have all the answers before we proceed with our model – but how can we tell whether this intervention or any subsequent change in focus is appropriate and should even be commenced? What is the difference between a plan, created with a great deal of enthusiasm but that eventually turns out to be on the wrong path, as opposed to a plan that turns out to work well? Can we know from the beginning how things are likely to go in complex, non-deterministic systems? The answer is no. Does this then leave us free to head off in any direction we think is appropriate or can there be more guidance than just political expediency, hunch or intuition? My short response is that having taken on board as much of the available literature across a broad number of fields, as it is possible for a few people to absorb, and having had some tentative runs at using certain principles when engaging with individuals and communities, such as a respectful MI based approach, a non-expert model, avoiding the shortcomings of fly-in fly-out models and so forth, we can build on these insights incorporating the best available evidence, use the resources that we have (such as they are) and move forward with confidence. The major source of confidence is that this has become an iterative, self reflecting process whereby nobody is thoroughly welded to a particular approach, model or style (though we had to start with a model), which monitors the impact of interventions to date to modify subsequent interventions. Many individuals and organisations are welded to firm beliefs that limit their capacity to change, especially in D&A services, where almost everybody has firm views on why people end up with problems, and what kind of responses are needed (Peele, 1990).

In general, our belief is that the general understanding of these issues is poor (Peele, 2001), and responses are too often political or bureaucratic rather than evidence based and respecting of local conditions. Fortunately the local response to relevant information, education and training is gratifyingly positive, sufficient to encourage us to continue. We are aware of these problems, and accept that some people will cling to the old deficit model and late intervention approach, but we remain optimistic that a significant number of people will slowly but steadily move towards a different way of addressing these problems in their community.

And in the end, I need to ask, have we managed to implement SBI in primary care? Sadly, but not surprisingly, the answer is no – but we believe we are close, and that this multi-faceted, community development, evolutionary approach is the most likely to succeed of all the approaches we have seen.

References

Babor, TF, McRee, BG, Kassebaum, PA *et al.* (2007). Screening, Brief Intervention, and Referral to Treatment (SBIRT): Towards a Public Health Approach to the Management of Substance Abuse. *Substance Abuse, 28,* 7-30.

Battye, K (2008). Framework for the delivery of Social and Emotional Wellbeing services to the Murdi Paaki Region. *Report to the Commonwealth Dept of Health and Ageing.*

Baum, F (2007). Cracking the nut of health equity: top down and bottom up pressure for action on the social determinants of health. *Promotion and Education, 14,* 90-95.

Cohen, P (2000). Is the addiction doctor the voodoo priest of modern man? *Addiction Research, 8,* 589-598.

Commonwealth Department of Finance (2010). Strategic Review of Indigenous Expenditure. Accessed at: http://finance.gov.au/foi/disclosure-log/2011/docs/foi_10-27_strategic_review_indigenous_expenditure.pdf.

Fraser, SW, Greenhalgh, T, Plesk, P, Wilson, T & Holt, T (2001). Coping with complexity: educating for capability. *British Medical Journal, 323,* 799-803.

Gawande, A (2007). *Better: A surgeon's notes on performance.* NY, Metropolitan.

Gourlay, DL & Heit, HA (2009). Universal Precautions Revisited: Managing the Inherited Pain Patient. *Pain Medicine, 6,* S115-S123.

Gray, D (2005). *Preventing substance misuse among indigenous people: a comparative review.* 8th National Rural Health Conference, Alice Springs, March 2005.

Green, LA & Seifert, CM (2005). Translation of research into practice: why we can't "just do it". *Journal of the American Board of Family Medicine, 18,* 541-545.

Heather, N (2011). Developing, evaluating and implementing alcohol brief interventions in Europe. *Drug and Alcohol Review, 30,* 138-147.

Humphery, K (2001). Dirty questions: Indigenous health and "Western research". *Australian and New Zealand Journal of Public Health, 25,* 197-202.

Hunter, E (1993). *Aboriginal health and history: Power and prejudice in remote Australia.* Melbourne, Cambridge Uni Press.

Kowal, E, Anderson, I & Bailie, R (2005). Moving beyond good intentions: Indigenous participation in Aboriginal and Torres Strait Islander research. *Australian and New Zealand Journal of Public Health, 29,* 468-470.

Kuhn, T (1959). The essential tension: tradition and innovation in scientific research. Proceedings from *The third University of Utah Research Conference on the identification of scientific talent.* Chapter 2: 21-31.

Kuhn, T (1970). *The structure of scientific revolutions.* Chicago, University of Chicago Press.

Laycock, A (2004). Alcohol handbook for frontline workers. Available online at http://catalogue.nla.gov.au/Record/3304055.

MacQueen, R (2007). Learnings from failures - what not to do in a rural D&A service. Conference proceedings from the *Transcultural Psychiatry Section Conference,* Cairns.

Marmot, M (2000). Social determinants of health: from observation to policy. *Medical Journal of Australia, 172,* 379-382.

Marmot, M (2011). Social determinants and the health of Indigenous Australians. *Medical Journal of Australia, 194,* 512-513.

Marmot, M & Wilkinson, RG (2001). Psychosocial and material pathways in the relation between income and health: a response to Lynch *et al. British Medical Journal, 322,* 1233-1236.

Martyres, R, Clode, D & Burns, JM (2004). Seeking drugs or seeking help? Escalating "doctor shopping" by young heroin users before fatal overdose. *Medical Journal of Australia, 180,* 211-214.

Maxwell, J (2011). The prescription drug epidemic in the United States: A perfect storm. *Drug and Alcohol Review, 30,* 264-270.

Merton, R K (1993). On the Shoulders of Giants. A Shandean Postscript. Chicago, Free Press.

Miller, WR, Brown, JM, Simpson, TL *et al.* (1995). *What works? A methodological analysis of the alcohol treatment outcome literature.* Needham Heights, Allyn and Bacon.

Miller, WR & Rollnick, S (2002). *Motivational Interviewing; preparing people for change.* New York, Guilford.

Minkler, M, Glover Blackwell, A, Thompson, M & Tamir, H (2003). Community based participatory research: implications for public health funding. *American Journal of Public Health, 93,* 1210-1213.

Mold, JW & Peterson, KA (2005). Primary care practice-based networks: working at the interface between research and quality improvement. *Annals of Family Medicine, 3(Sup 1),* 512-520.

Peele, S (1990). Addiction as a Cultural Concept. *Annals of the New York Academy of Sciences, 602,* 205-220.

Peele, S (2001). What Addiction is and is not. *Addiction Research, 8,* 599-607.

Prochaska, JO, DiClemente, CC & Norcross, JC (1992). In search of how people change. Applications to addictive behaviors. *American Psychology, 47,* 1102-1114.

Rollnick, S, Heather, N & Bell, A (1992). Negotiating behaviour change in medical settings: The development of brief motivational interviewing. *Journal of Mental Health, 1,* 25-37.

Rose, G (1992). *The Strategy of Preventive Medicine.* Oxford, Oxford University Press.

Sanson-Fisher, R (1994). Allocation of research funds in the drug and alcohol field: report of the consensus workshop. *Drug and Alcohol Review, 13,* 79-86.

Sanson-Fisher, RW, Campbell, EM, Htun, AT, Bailey, LJ & Millar, CJ (2008). We are what we do: Research outputs of public health. *American Journal of Preventive Medicine, 35,* 380-385.

Shakeshaft, AP, Bowman, JA & Sanson-Fisher, RW (1997). Behavioural alcohol research: new directions or more of the same? *Addiction, 92,* 1411-1422.

Sibthorpe, B, Bailie, R, Brady, M, Ball, S, Sumner-Dodds, P & Hall, W (2002). The demise of a planned randomised controlled trial in an urban Aboriginal medical service. *Medical Journal of Australia, 176,* 273-276.

Syme, SL (1997). Individual vs Community Interventions in Public Health Practice: Some Thoughts About a New Approach. *Health Promotion Matters, 2,* 2-9.

Syme, SL (2003). *Social determinants of health: the community as an empowered partner.* Address to Communities in Control conference, Melbourne, April 2003.

Treloar, C & Holt, M (2006). Deficit models and divergent philosophies: Service providers' perspectives on barriers and incentives to drug treatment. *Drugs: Education, Prevention and Policy, 13,* 367-382.

Trucco, EM, Connery, HS, Griffin, ML (2007). The relationship of self-esteem and self-efficacy to treatment outcomes in alcohol dependent men and women. *The American Journal on Addictions, 16,* 85-92.

Woolf, S (2008). The meaning of translational research and why it matters. *JAMA, 299,* 211-213.

16 Social exclusion and immigration: new patterns of drug use among young marginal migrants

NÚRIA EMPEZ

Department of Theory and History of Education
University of Barcelona, Spain

nempez@ub.edu

Abstract

With the arrival of irregular non-European immigrants, we found an increase of immigrants in a social exclusion situation. The paper will focus on the new patterns of drug or substance consumption for the purpose of mood elevation ('getting high'), among a specific group of socially marginal immigrants. I will emphasise the new patterns of drug abuse that were eradicated in Spain, such as "inhalants" (volatile solvents, gases, aerosols and nitrites) using a case study: unaccompanied minors.

I will start by explaining who these new migrants are, I will continue with different drug uses among this group and end with some of the difficulties in drug treatment among social excluded immigrants and some proposals in order to begin to think about how to solve the problem.

Key words

Drug use; social exclusion; immigration; unaccompanied minors.

Introduction

The arrival of non-European immigrants in Spain during the last decade has produced social, economic and cultural changes. We can group migrants by ethnic group of origin, age and gender; but we can also do so according toadministrative status and social standing. There is a minority group (within the total migrant group), that crosses borders with an irregular administrative status, which we commonly call 'illegal'. A small part of this group is children who migrate alone are known as unaccompanied minors (UAMs).

The use of dangerous substances among certain groups seems to have appeared among young Maghrebi immigrants who came unaccompanied to Spain: These problems are noted in official speeches and reports in the press. The problem of drug use appears to be greater among those who are still "illegal" (in an irregular administrative situation).

If we take a look at the data on immigrant drug abuse in Catalonia (from the Xarxa d'Atenció A les Drogodependències a Catalunya / Drug Attention Network (XAD)), we can see that from 1995 to 2002, the number of immigrants initiating treatment for drug abuse nearly doubled: from 469 to 877 (4.4% to 6.9%). This number may have risen simply because there were more immigrants in Spain and not necessarily because more of them had drug problems). We also have to take into consideration that many immigrants do not have a national health card (possibly due to a lack of 'empadronamiento' or civil registry), which means that they do not have access to public health services.

I will explain the new patterns of drug abuse that were eradicated in Spain, such as "inhalants" (volatile solvents, gases, aerosols and nitrites) using a case study: unaccompanied minors.

I will start by explaining who these new migrants are and follow with the different drug uses among this group. I will conclude with some of the difficulties in drug treatment among socially excluded immigrants and some proposals in order to begin to think about how to solve the problem.

The aim of this article is to understand a little better what we mean when we refer to UAMs in a situation of social exclusion. Most of them, being drug consumers, it is important to understand their situation, their expectations. It is also important to acquire knowledge that can be useful to better understand the phenomenon. This is important to be able to design policies that are more appropriate for this group, which can be implemented in projects and programmes that take into account their characteristics and needs in order to protect and care for these children and adolescents. Moreover, it is also necessary to disclose the current immigration policies and child protection policies (with a longitudinal perspective of the last 10 years) and the possible relationship of these individual processes with children.

Background of the present study

My previous work examined the lives of unaccompanied minors in Catalonia, Spain, which is where many Moroccan children come (Empez, 2003). This work was based on my experiences in my job as a Social educator with young immigrants in the city hall of Manresa (Barcelona) since 2003, specialising in immigrant cases and dealing with Spanish policies that refer to the handling of unaccompanied children who migrate to Spain. I began in a participant observation in 2001 in Barcelona. My Master's thesis (Empez, 2003) on unaccompanied minors included four years of fieldwork in Barcelona, including visits to Tangier, Morocco, with some of the families of children I met in Spain. My longest most recent fieldwork in Morocco was based on family migration dynamics, funded by the Max Planck Institute for Demographic Research, which was part of my PhD dissertation for the Autonomous University of Barcelona. During the fieldwork in Tangier, from April to October 2006, I studied socialisation practices and reproductive strategies among families who send migrant children to Spain and the process of decision making in child migration. The findings then took me back to Catalonia, where I interviewed professionals in the minors' protection system dealing with unaccompanied minors; some of them in a marginal situation.

During the fieldwork, I mostly relied on qualitative methods: participant observation, open-ended interviews, group discussions, informal conversation, analyses of media, and so on. I had contact with many boys who were trying to cross to Spain from the port: some living on the street, some from rural areas, some in temporary street situations and some of whom came from the city of Tangier. My subjects included people from Tangier and rural people from the district of Beni Mellal; families of children (and children themselves) who Spain sent back as "minors" for family reunification; adults who wanted to migrate; families with children in Spain; ex-unaccompanied minors who were repatriated from Spain as adults; families with adult members living in Europe; young workers; students; older women; people living or working in the port; school teachers; NGO (non-governmental organisation) workers; and members of Moroccan authorities also with unaccompanied minors living on the street and unaccompanied minors in protection centres. The research also included secondary analyses of survey data (CERED, the Spanish Municipal Register, the Spanish Census, etc.).

Who are these children?

Children who migrate alone are defined by the European Union Council Resolution 97 / C 221/03 of June 26, 1997 as:

> Third-country nationals below the age of eighteen, who arrive on territory of the Member States unaccompanied by an adult responsible for them, whether by law or custom, and for as long as they are not effectively in the care of such a person.

They also have a special mention in the children's' rights convention , where it mentions that:

> 20.1. A child temporarily or permanently deprived of his or her family environment, or in whose own best interests cannot be allowed to remain in that environment, shall be entitled to special protection and assistance provided by the State.

The situation of unaccompanied minors (UAMs) began to surface in Spain in the late 90s, when the media uncovered the street situation in which some Moroccan children who had migrated alone, without any responsible adult were found. Many of them had migrated under a truck or a bus from their departure countries (Morocco and Algeria) to large cities like Barcelona and Madrid.
At the time different questions arose:

– Why did children migrate alone from Morocco to Europe?
– Why had children in streets situation in large cities appeared? Empez (2003, 2005)

These young migrants as Suarez (2006) noted, are a new migratory actor under Spanish Law. Undocumented minors from 16 to 18 who come without their parents have an opportunity to gain a residence permit before they turn 18. The years between 16 and 17 years of age are what I call a *"two year window of opportunity"* (Empez, 2005). It is a time of 'liminality,' during which they could either be repatriated or legalise their status.

This "liminal" situation generates a stress factor that, added to the complicated adolescence stage, could be a push factor to start consuming drugs

There have been various policies to address the situation of UAMs, but most indications show that these children are not welcome; which prioritises the irregular foreigner status over the minority fact.

Most of the children who migrate alone continue to migrate hidden under trucks and buses in the Tangier-Algeciras route. There has also been an increase in juvenile cases that migrate in small boats that use dangerous routes, not only in Moroccan cases but also in cases of south-Saharan children. In the Canary Islands we can also see the start of cases of girls who migrate alone, see Jiménez (2006, 2007), Trujillo & Morantes (2007), Empez (2007), CONRED (2005), UNICEF (2005).

Legal framework and action policies

In this case, the migration -because they are minors- has some contradictions, at the moment Spain has a strict and restrictive foreigners law that has been modified several times with extraordinary regularisations (one in 2001 and another in 2005, where a working contract and one year civil registration was required). On the other side, inside Spanish territory the law enforces the protection the unaccompanied minors, regardless of birthplace (Law 1/1986), simply because they are minors.

We can divide the legal framework of the migrant minors into three levels of action:

1. International level
2. State level
3. Regional Level

Articles 39 and 53.3 of the Spanish constitution place minor protection competency under the regulation of autonomous regions, but each autonomous region has its own rules.

Based on my professional experience as a Social Educator in immigration, we can create a standard itinerary of the migrant minors when they arrive in an Autonomous Region:

1. Detection of the minor, transferral to the minors section of the public prosecutor's office, and admission in an emergency protection centre. Here they will start the first institutional proceedings.
2. Diagnosis of the minors' age: if they don't have official documentation (passport, identity card, etc.) the bones will be measured based on arm radiography to detect the estimated age. A medical exam is also required. Afterwards, they will send these papers to the judge and the pathologist will determine if the person is over or younger than eighteen.
3. If it is confirmed that the person is a minor and the minor doesn't have any legal representation, the judge will send them to a protection centre, with the objective of complying with the protection measure. The Provincial Delegation of Social Affairs is in charge of fulfilling this action, and at the same time they will inform the Public Prosecutor's office of the minor's internship in the protection centre.
4. Documentation research about the situation of the minor in the country of origin is then initiated. They will submit the identification data provided by the minor to the Provincial Government Sub-delegation, , with the aim of starting the administrative procedure to resolve the identity and the personal and family circumstances of the minor in order to make a decision about whether to return the minor to the country of origin or not. In this process, they will also ask the Consulate of the origin country using the data given by the minor with the same aim mentioned above. At the same time this data is sent from the Consulate to the ministry of the interior of the country of origin, in the case of Morocco it is called the *mkadem* (District Governor) of the neighbourhood were the minor lives; this is done to also determine the age, name, surname, address, data of the parents and siblings and other information that may be considered to be of interest.

The Consulate will call the minor to an interview to compare the data. With the information collected directly for the Consulate they will request a new report from the *amaala's* office (Real Power Delegation) or the *wilaya's* office. Then, the police will make an investigation with the data provided by the *mkadem.*

After this study, if the *mkadem's* report coincides with the police's report, the latter will be handed to the police, who will give it to the *wilaya,* and the latter will send it onto the Consulate. Later, the consulate will make an appointment with the minor to inform him about the results obtained in the investigation. If all the data coincides, they will make the Moroccan passport for the minor.

At the same time, the protection centres management, after having been informed of the results of the study, will start arranging the residence permit pleading 'exceptional circumstances'.

In fact, the General Directorate of Childhood Care (DGAIA) is the organisation that has regional powers over the minors' protection system in Catalonia. Their recent policy has been to try to carry out familiar reunification, or to only take care of the child's guardianship and to avoid full custody duties. This means that if the minors are not sent back, they will offer them protection in a centre (food, lodging) as long as they are minors, but they will not provide them with a residence permit and when they turn eighteen, they will have to leave the protection system without having solved their administrative situation.

Talking with a few minors who were invited to leave the DGAIA's protection system because they had family in Spanish territory, they explained that their situation was not considered an emergency due to the fact that they had family in the country. For this reason they had been requested to 'voluntarily abandon' the protection system.

When speaking to these minors, they expressed the fact that not being legalised by the regional government would not dissuade them from migrating. Very few minors would accept family reunification. When a person decides to migrate, risking the loss of their own lif in the attempt, they will not come back without having accomplished their objective and it is this fact that makes us find more and more teenagers in a street situation, undocumented and without the possibility of working or earning their own living in legal terms. We must also take into account that most of the boys that are sent home will try to come back again.

Drug use

The relationship between migration, drug abuse and treatment is complex and not clear (See Casas, Collazos, Qureshi *et al.*).

Some of the possible factors in drug consumption among immigrants in social exclusion are the acculturative stress, the difficulties to access services because of ignorance or fear, different views on drug use and mental illness and the easy access to drugs.

One of the characteristics that contribute to the marginalisation of children on the street is their association with the collective image; and in the media to drug addiction. Drug abuse can lead to social exclusion processes, poor living conditions (skin diseases, infectious, STDs, sexually transmitted diseases, some liver diseases and bad nutrition).

It should be noted that drug use is in a minority compared to the entire group of unaccompanied minors. Consumption increases if children are at risk of social exclusion and living on the street.

Drug: the concept used in this article is Kramer, Cameron, quoted in Díaz, 1998:155: "drug means any substance or drug that introduced in the living organism may modify one or more of the functions. It is a broad concept internationally, as it covers not only medicines for the treatment of patients especially, but also other active substances from the point of view drug" (Kramer, Cameron, 1975:13).

It is also worth defining the terms of use and consumption, as they have to do with the relationship that makes some of the smaller objects of our study concerning substance abuse.

Consumer: "consumption is defined as the introduction of a substance in the body in any way or by any method that allows absorption. This definition does not exclude the symbolic aspects of the individual-substance" (Díaz, 1998:157).

Usage: "it is considered regarding the use of any substance that does not mean consumption" (Díaz, 1998:157).

As an example we have the case of minors who do not take drugs but sell them, small traffic…

In any case, this article will focus on the young people who use drugs. We can mention the consequences that the World Health Organization (WHO) marks:

> The early onset of drug use and its continuity appear closely associated to behaviors such as sexual precocity, delinquency and school failure. They are also linked to the following environmental factors: family breakdown, poverty, lack of accessible and useful recreational activities, lack of suitable accommodation when the child cannot remain at home, change of place, oppression and discrimination, availability of drugs and, in some cases, pressure from the dealers (WHO, 1994:7).

Non-integrated-UAMs are, as a group or community, youth at risk, because of their illegal status, stress and helplessness, because the lack of family references creates a personal situation of distress and uncertainty in the future, etc.

Among the factors that influence consumption, we can find: the easy access to drugs, the insecure neighbourhoods, stress from migration, uncertainty about their future, their will to forget part of the past and the present, alcohol consumption patterns among standard Spanish youth, lack of concerned adults, concern about (and loss of contact with) the family, stress from hours spent in the street in a marginal environment, frustration about the migratory project and reality.

We can also say that the more time these minors spent on the street, the greater the risk to abuse drugs, mainly due to the harshness of the environment and the accessibility of substances.

It is important to highlight the physical and social changes that the boys experience if they are using drugs or they are in a period of abstinence: both are marked by consumption (in this case, greed in acquiring certain consumer goods that are highly valued among young people such as branded sportswear, mobile phones, etc.). While consuming, they neglect their physical and health status and initiate an escalation of violence and robberies that usually ends up with contact with the youth justice system.

Principal consequences of use

- *Physical:* (Direct consequence of consumption): dizziness, vomiting, breathing problems, eye problems, mouth sores, colds, etc.
- *Psychological:* Anxiety, alexitimia, paranoia, depression, and hallucinations.
- *Legal:* Fines for consuming in public spaces, lawsuits for selling drugs, thefts and robberies carried out during consumption.
- *Social:* Bad behaviour, loss of non-consumer network, loss of education, work, and abandonment of protection centers, etc.

The main drug consumed by UAMs are inhalants. Some of them also consume other drugs such as cannabis, cocaine or medical drugs. Alcohol and tobacco can also be consumed.

Most Unaccompanied Minors are **not** drug consumers, but there are growing concerns about patterns of drug consumption among them because of their early starting, the amount of toxic drugs sometimes consumed in short periods of time and the resurgence of forms of consumption that were almost eradicated in Spain (e.g., inhalants).

Inhalants

Volatile chemicals that are legal to use (solvents, glue, etc.). The product is usually inhaled after impregnation with a cloth or a sock and is inhaled through the nose or mouth. Consumers tend to put small amounts in plastic bottles that are stored in their pocket.

Given its low price and that it easy to obtain, the product is consumed primarily by the youngest boys, from 12-15 years. With the arrival of adolescence, this drug is usually replaced with other illegal drugs.

Regarding Catalonia, the product is available in most supermarkets and/or chemists and is often stolen by the kids from large shopping centres. It must be added that the use of inhalants usually occurs within a group that shares the same product between several members of the gang, but we can also find kids consuming alone. These are usually in a worse situation.

The profile of an Unaccompanied Minor Inhalant consumer in Catalonia is male, usually from an urban area in Morocco, from 14 to 18 years old. They are usually kids, who alternate their life in the protection system with life on the streets, sometimes consuming other substances, and sometimes we can even find children who are mentally ill.

The UAM Inhalant users tend to distribute the same product in smaller doses in plastic bottles for individual use; they do it to share costs and in order to make it more manageable, because these bottles tend to fit in their pockets. Once the bottle is full, the solvent is impregnated in a cloth or a sock, in a piece of absorbent material and then inhaled through the nose or mouth. Afterwards, they seal the bottle again and keep the rest of the content for later.

Another practice method is to pour the content directly into a plastic bag and inhale it.

Inhalants can be categorised into: Glues and adhesives, gas ignition, solvents, propellants and fuels.

They are substances that have a depressant action, disturbing the central nervous system; their administration method makes them quickly absorbed as they pass directly through the blood to the lung alveoli and rapidly reach the brain.

We can say then that they have an immediate effect, which usually occurs within 5 minutes of consuming, and its duration is between 15 and 45 minutes, effects that can be enhanced if mixed with other substances such as alcohol or barbiturates.

The solvent effects are several, among them are:

- In the short term:

  – Dizziness, drunkenness and euphoria, then confusion, disorientation and difficulties in movement coordination. Hallucinations, euphoria, remarkable perception disorders, lack of the ability to reason, difficulties in speech. Loss of appetite, variation of the emotional feeling of wellness from sadness or negative feelings. Feeling similar to alcohol intoxication (floating sensation, dizziness, etc.) Acute poisoning:
  – Drunkenness, delusions, diplopia, respiratory depression, risk of death by suffocation.

- In the long term:

  – Liver, brain and kidney damage . High tolerance. Sudden withdrawal after chronic use produces some degree of lethargy, depression and irritability, but physical dependence has not been demonstrated. Psychic dependence. Personality deterioration.

According to the DSM-IV (Diagnostic and Statistical Manual of Mental Disorders.) (American Psychiatric Association) an abstinence syndrome in consumers between 24 to 48 hours of consumption can be produced with a duration of up to 5 days, with symptoms such as sleep disturbances, tremors, irritability, sweating, nausea, and fleeting illusions. This syndrome has not been well documented and seems to lack clinical reliance, as inhalant dependence does not include a physical abstinence síndrome.

According to witnesses cited in the literature, the effects described by a user are:

  – "I felt good, it was like I was turning into a crazy person, it was like having an engine in the brain, I liked walking in the street because these hallucinations make you feel as if you were walking on air, you feel as if you've got powers" (Empez, 2000).

– "Real cool, me, my head was this (uuuuummmmmm) like a small motor that works good, not afraid of anything, It made the hunger go away and it gave me courage to steal" (Empez, 2000).

The group under study uses inhalants casually, the exact reason is unknown, but according to Luchini consumption may be related to identification.

According to Luchini: "The drug is, thus, marginalising the element but is integrated into the daily lives of children". The reasons for the alternatives between individual consumption and consumption in the group are not well understood. We have presented the hypothesis on collective consumption of inhalants being understood as a challenge, trespassing from childhood to adulthood. Through this challenge, the child is claiming membership in a particular social group: the children of the street. Collective consumption of inhalants may be linked then to the issue of collective identity" (Luchini, 1999:237).

Although inhalant abuse is a practice that occurs in Morocco, most UAMs began to consume in Barcelona, the ones who consumed in Morocco are street children from a very marginal area, who usually do not have sufficient skills to migrate.

Unlike what happens with other substances, inhaling is closely tied to social exclusion and marginalisation, so the UAM who are in this situation already show a certain degree of self-neglect, as it is one of the most noticeable substances, they pass from neatness and body cult, from a concern for their appearance, to abandoning themselves.

Cocaine

A substance that comes from the coca plant and stimulates the central nervous system (Erythroxylon Coca). It mainly comes from South America and is later treated through a chemical process. Usually, we can find it in white powder form but it can also be seen as rock. The most common way of consumption is to snort it and/or to smoke it, although it can also be injected.

The effects of consumption tend to be: The 'high' (within minutes of consumption), dilated pupils and increase in heartbeat, breathing and body temperature. It usually causes euphoria, a sense of control and physical fatigue. It may reduce alertness, make you feel apparently better but it can also cause headaches, insomnia, irritability and it may impair concentration, memory and attention.

After an hour or two, the effect declines and tiredness comes. Symptoms of anxiety and depression can also appear. High doses can cause hallucinations, paranoia, violent behaviour, anxiety attacks, panic attacks and/or paranoid type reactions: a persecution complex.

This is a drug that causes a high psychological dependence characterised by a strong urge to continue consuming, but it also generates a high tolerance, this is, the need to increase the dose to achieve the same effects.

According to Gawin and Kleher (1984), the clearances of symptoms usually start nine hours after consuming and can take months. The classic symptom of physical discomfort may not appear likewise with opiates, but the psychological desire to consume it will. Its abstinence syndrome can often result to provoke aggressive behaviour and delirium. We must keep in mind that the cocaine consumer profile is diverse, and does not fit into a certain stereotype. "Derivatives of cocaine (cocaine hydrochloride and crack cocaine paste) including or not the coca leaf, are characterised by being multi-phased: there is an existence of a wide variety of itineraries, profiles, situations, types, methods of consumption and administration forms. In addition, it must be said that its consumption is irregularly spread in the various strata of the social structure, both in the standard and in marginalised population" (Díaz, 1998:288).

Amongst the UAMs I had contact with, the ones who had used cocaine were also linked to small-scale traffic, or had done "post" work; which is someone who does the 'middleman' job; between the dealer and wholesaler. In these cases the drug was usually used to pay their own consumption.

If we look at different patterns of consumption, although we are not able to make generalisations, we could say that the most common type of consumer among the UAM, is the one Díaz calls the *"Instrumental Consumer"*:

The instrumental consumers use drugs for specific purposes that are not necessarily related to the contexts of having social fun. The consumption of cocaine is intranasal; coca paste consumption can also been found. This consumer profile has similarities with the recreational type but some risk factors should be included in this case: higher levels of consumption (as consumption increases also increase the problems). Another reason that may lead to escalation is boredom; fighting it is a way to escape from problems, and it ends up to be an objective in itself and not a means to enhance fun. It is too, a causal association to job performance and career success (Díaz, 1998: 289-290).

Here, what we have talked about is consumption associated with sale and/ or traffic; to acquire sufficient courage for petty theft or robbery, etc. added to recreational use.

If we take into consideration that inhalants are cheap and easily available (stolen from supermarkets) but on the other hand cocaine means having considerable economic resources (the price is more or less established at €60 a gramme), we can almost link the consumption of cocaine to theft and sale.

The typologies of children who consume cocaine are often found in situations of social exclusion and marginalisation:

> When it comes to the previously marginalised population, consumption is an aggravating factor that deepens and consolidates particularly harsh living conditions. In these cases, consumption is a problem among others and often plays a key role to survive in a hostile environment or to escape it (Díaz, 1998:290).

Alcohol

Alcohol is a liquid substance obtained from the fermentation of certain fruits and grains; it is a central nervous system depressant. Even if in Muslim religion -practiced by most citizens of the Maghreb- it is prohibited to consume this substance that is considered "haram", alcohol is already consumed by some adults and youth "occasionally" in the Maghreb; in fact, it is relatively easy to obtain. Once the migration process has been completed, many of these young people start to consume alcohol, although not every day in a social way; it is more associated with a holiday or the marginal world.

We could say that they start drinking intermittently seeking the approval of their peers. For local adolescents, mixing alcohol with other psychoactive substances is a common practice (cannabis, cocaine, amphetamines), while for adults in their thirties, the mix with sedatives, tranquilisers, hypnotics and/or tobacco is more common; in the case of UAMs, their exclusion makes the drug use pattern not just as recreational, but also marginal. As it is more frequent to find alcohol consumption mixed with sedatives (varying quantities and frequencies of consumption, according to the child's personal situation).

In the case of the UAMs , who are the object of this study, the majority are not alcohol consumers (as it is considered "haram" within the Muslim religion). Only a small part consumes in celebrations, when they go to a disco, etc. (for social recreational use). The other small minor group with problematic consumption mixes alcohol with benzodiazepines (sedatives) with the purpose of escaping from reality or getting the courage to commit robbery or violent acts. We need to note that alcohol mixed with other drugs increases the psychoactive effects of both substances and the risk of overdose.

Psychoactive drugs

Psychoactive drugs are chemical drugs for therapeutic use. If they are used outside the therapeutic context they can lead to problematic use. We can classify the psychoactive drugs as: sedatives, hypnotics, anxiolytics (barbiturates, benzodiazepines) and psycho stimulants and amphetamines. Hypnotics and sedatives are often used to evade reality and are used in combination with other drugs such as alcohol, which enhances their effects.

Some of the UAMs mix pills with alcohol to enter into a semiconscious stage; these drugs are cheap and easily available. In the Raval, a district of Barcelona, especially in Calle Sant Pau, we can find a lot of people selling pills, the majority of whom are heroin users who have prescriptions for themselves or their families and they sell at the price of around 3 euros per pill.

In this context, I could report cases of kids , who exchanged psychoactive pills for cannabis, as is the case of a group of UAMs in Santa Coloma de Gramanet.

Cannabis

Cannabis is obtained from the Cannabis sativa plant and its most important and active ingredient is called delta-9-thetrahidrocannabinol (THC).

- Styles:

  - Marihuana-preparation: obtained from grinding the plant's previously dried up heart, leaves and branches.
  - Hashish-extract is obtained from the resin of the plants, which is dried and pressed into brown shaped tablets.
  - Hashish Oil: Obtained from filtering the resinous substance, the concentration of THC is much higher than in other styles.

Cannabis uninhibits the higher nerve centre. When cannabis is smoked, the physiological and psychological effects are more subjective in 20-30 minutes, reaching the most critical point after 45-60 minutes and fading away in two or three hours. However, when cannabis is ingested orally, the effects can take an hour to make an effect, and two to three hours to reach the peak; the effects disappear gradually.

We must keep in mind that most of the cannabis sold in Spain comes from Morocco; from areas where its consumption is more or less socially accepted and especially from areas where it is cultivated, such as Ketama and Chefchaouen in Rif. Here, hashish is as integrated as alcohol is in the Spanish cultural pattern; for this reason, many young people consume it without any problems, associated to sporadic consumption.

Most street children consume hashish and some devote themselves to selling it. Since the law is not as harsh with children, there have been cases where children are used for small trading duties or for mail by adults that are to a lesser or greater extent are dedicated to drug traffic. In this context it is important to mention the diversities in cultural connotation of hashish for a Moroccan or for a European, as there are differences, at least in terms of the moral implications of consumption.

Some difficulties in drug treatment among socially excluded immigrants (including unaccompanied minors)

This relatively new population of drug consumers represent a challenge when talking about assistance programmes to stop drug use. We must take into consideration the difficulties and the characteristics of this group, to start thinking about useful programmes; some of the characteristics we must face are:

- Lack of social networks or a family to encourage keeping up a treatment and remaining clean.
- The marginal environment where drugs are available and the socially excluded immigrants are located.
- Difficulties in paying some resources such as therapeutic communities, etc.
- Increase in use of emergency services, but decline in monitored treatment.
- Lack of information in their own languages (some of the marginal immigrants are also illiterate).

- For those without a residence permit: fear of being deported if they go to a health centre.
- Difficulties with immigrants that don't speak fluently; it is difficult to offer proper psychological support.
- Professionals that lack information about cultural specificities.
- Lack of specialist resources for young consumers.
- Entrances and exits in Justice Centres.
- High mobility, difficult tracking, mobile phones that do not work, addresses that expire, homelessness and squat houses, etc.

Conclusions and proposals

We can tell that different families' strategies to migrate are responsible on one hand, when it concerns their Government policies, but it is obvious they also take into account the policies of the destination country. If they send their children to a country it can be understood that they have an idea of the law and the chances of success in each country.

Having a child represents an opportunity of success in the future; more children, more opportunities to succeed in Europe to help the rest of the family, even the extended family.

The complexity of these issues depend on immigration laws. As some are under State jurisdiction and others such as minors' protection laws are subject to regional legislation, many children end up travelling from one autonomous region to another trying to legalise themselves. If they don't see progress in their administrative situation, they decide to move somewhere else. This places them in a 'liminal' position, given the two years they have to be repatriated or arrange their administrative situation. It should not be surprising that some get tired of waiting and having no trust in the protection system, they decide to live outside the boundaries of the Administration system; on their own. However, it is important to point out that: even though the general population expresses their contempt when they talk about the majority of young non-accompanied minors in a street situation in Catalonia; calling them "street children" without homes, manners, or discipline, many were members of stable families of modest means in their country and they became street kids when they arrived in Spain.

The kids who are sent to migrate are not just the ones who predict their families' success, but ones who have certain age characteristics and depend on Spain.

We should mention how this evolved and how young migration is producing changes in Moroccan families; changes in the roles within the family members, in the members' behaviour and changes in the expectations and pleasure that is put on each member of the family.

The laws for foreigners and the minors' protection laws are changing constantly, so we will have to see how this is going to affect the migration process and the vital events of the people who have emigrated or who are thinking of emigrating. These legal shifts affect not only the health and welfare of the children who come from North Africa but also the way society considers them.

We should remark that minors are subjects, subjects who move but are invisible. So as a result they are especially vulnerable and undefended. As a society we should act with responsibility when it comes to minors; we should think that they are subjects with rights and subjects who need protection.

Drug use among unaccompanied minors can be interpreted as a way to handle the stress of this "liminal" position; the weight felt by some of the children who migrate at a young age is unbearable and they don't feel capable of acting as adults. We can see others factors, such as the accessibility to drugs, acculturative stress etc. With heedless structural changes in laws, heedless north-south inequity, we have to start thinking how to attend the specificity of this new community of drug consumers.

Some of the proposals could be; coordinating transversal work among relevant social agencies (social services administrations, health affairs administrations, NGOs, etc.); using street educators as figures of proximity and trust; better prevention materials adapted to their living conditions; training professionals in cultural and ethnical specificities; attending emotional needs; reestablishing the social and family network, even if it is located in the origin country; creating alternative spaces with activities to occupy their time away from consumption and creating specific therapeutic communities for teenagers.

References

American Psychiatric Association (1995) DSM-IV. *Manual de diagnóstico y estadística de los trastornos mentales*. Barcelona, Masson.

Ararteko (2005). *Situación de los Menores Extranjeros No Acompañados en la CAPV*.

Arbex, C & Jiménez, A (2004). Menores inmigrantes y consumo de drogas: un estudio cualitativo. *Revista de la Asociación Proyecto Hombre*, 53. 2005.

Comas, M (coord.) (2001). *L'atenció als menors no acompanyats a Catalunya. Anàlisi de la realitat i propostes d'actuació*, Col·lecció Finestra Oberta n.º 19, Ed. Fundació Jaume Bofill, Barcelona.

Con RED (2005). Rutas de pequeños sueños: Los menores migrantes no acompañados en Europa. Barcelona: *Fundación Pere Tarrés.* http://www.peretarres.org/daphneconred/estudi/informe.html

Díaz, A (1998). Hoja, pasta, roca y polvo: el consumo de los derivados de la hoja de coca, Barcelona. Universidad Autónoma de Barcelona.

Díaz, A (2000). El estudio de las drogas en distintas sociedades. Problemas metodológicos. In the book. *Contextos, sujetos y drogas: un manual sobre drogodependencias.* 31-42 GRUP IGIA, Ajuntament de Barcelona-FAD, Barcelona.

Empez, N (2000). *"Prospección con menores inhalantes de cola en Managua"* (Nicaragua) Unpublished document.

Empez, N (2003). Menors No Acompanyats Estrangers Indocumentats: Una Aproximació al Fenomen. Barcelona: Universitat Autónoma de Barcelona. PhD Master Thesis.

Empez, N (2005). "Menores no acompañados en situación de exclusión social". En Fernández, Tomas, *et al.* (eds) *Multiculturalidad y Educación: Teorías, Ámbitos, Prácticas.* 314-333 Madrid: Alianza Editorial. Chapter in a book

Empez, N (2007). "Social construction of neglect: the case of unaccompanied minors from Morocco to Spain". Working paper MPIDR.

Empez, N (2008). "Menores no acompañados, breve aproximación". In the book. *Frontera Sur* 239-251. V V.AA. Barcelona. Virus ed.

Empez, N (2009). "The Fieldworker as social worker: dilemas in research with Moroccan unaccompanied minors" Chapter in a book Van Liempt, I & Bilger V (Ed) *The ethics of migration research methodology. Dealing with vulnerable immigrants.* 155-168. Sussex Academic Press. Brighton –Portland.

Empez, N (2010). The transnational affected: Spanish State Policies and The Life-Course Events of Families in North Africa. Chapter in the book *Everyday Ruptures, Children, Youth, and Migration in Global Perspective,* 174-189. Ed by Caty Coe [*et al.*], Vanderbilt University Press, Nashville.

Fundació Salut i Comunitat (2005). Manual para la prevención de drogas entre jóvenes y menores migrantes.

Jiménez-Álvarez, M (2003). Buscarse la vida: Análisis transnacional de los procesos migratorios de los menores marroquíes en Andalucía, Fundación Santa María.

Jiménez-Álvarez, M (2006). "Menores inmigrantes o los vulnerables de la globalización", En: Checa Olmos, F, Arjona, A & Checa Olmos, JC, *Menores tras la frontera,* 63-83. Icaria Antrazyt.

Jiménez-Álvarez, M (2007). "Donde quiebra la protección: las reagrupaciones familiares sin garantías". *Informe Anual de SOS RACISMO.*

Jiménez-Álvarez, M (2007b). "Una mirada transnacional: los menores migrantes como nuevos rebeldes de la globalización". International seminar *La migration des mineurs non accompagnés: les contextes d'origine, les routes migratoires, les systèmes d'accueil, Maison des Sciences de l'Hommes et de la Société,* Poitiers 10-11 octobre 2007.

Jiménez-Álvarez, M & Lorente, D (2004). Menores en las fronteras: de los retornos efectuados sin garantías a menores marroquíes y de los malos tratos sufridos. Report. *Federación SOS Racismo.*

Kramer, JF & Cameron, DC (1975). Manual sobre la dependencia de las drogas. *OMS.* Ginebra.

Laranga, M, Marcó, A & Buscallà, RM (1999). Menors immigrats: sols o desemparats? *Fundació Jaume Bofill* http://www.fbofill.cat/intra/fbofill/documents/publicacions/209.pdf

Lucchini, R (1996). *Niño de la calle. Identidad, Sociabilidad, Droga.* Barcelona: Los Libros de la Frontera.

Quiroga, V (2003). Els petits harraga. Menors irregulars no acompanyats d'origen marroquí a Catalunya. Phd Thesis. Universitat Rovira i Virgili, Tarragona.

Qureshi, A, Collazos, F, Antolín, M & Tómas-Sábado, J (2008). Estrés aculturativo y salud mental en la población inmigrante. *Papeles del Psicólogo.* Vol 29.

Qureshi, A, Revollo, H-W, Collazos, F, Visiers, C & El Harrak, J (2009). La mediación intercultural sociosanitaria: implicaciones y retos. *Revista Norte para la salud mental* nº 35. 56-66.

Senovilla, D (2007). Situación y Tratamiento de los Menores Extranjeros No Acompañados en

Europa. *Observatorio Internacional de Justicia Juvenil* (OIJJ).

Síndic de Greuges (2006). Informe i recomenacions. La situació dels menors immigrats sols. http://www.sindic.cat/ficheros/informes/37_Situaciomenorsimmigrats.pdf

Suárez Navaz, L (2006). "Un nuevo actor migratorio: Jóvenes, rutas y ritos juveniles transnacionales". In: Checa y Olmos F, Arjona A and Checa Olmos JC, *Menores tras la frontera. Otra migración que aguarda.* 17-51. Icaria Antrazyt.

Trujillo, MA & Morante, ML (2007). "Las niñas y adolescentes que emigran solas a España. Las influencias o determinaciones derivadas de su condición de mujeres". International workshop: *La migration des mineurs non accompagnés: les contextes d'origine, les routes migratoires, les systèmes d'accueil, Maison des Sciences de l'Hommes et de la Société,* Poitiers 10-11 octobre 2007.

Van Heijningrn, H & Van Der Winden, B (1999). ed. TESIS *"Los huelepegas, vivir en el callejón de la Muerte",* Tesis, Managua.

17 Politics and ethics for a journal editor

RICHARD PATES

Cardiff School of Health Sciences
Llandaff Campus
University of Wales Institute Cardiff
United Kingdom

dr_pates23@hotmail.com

Abstract

Scientific peer reviewed journals are the main conduit for the dissemination of scientific information, discovery and debate across all sciences. In the field of addiction there are more than 80 journals published in the English language and many others published in other languages across the world.

As editors, it is part of our role to act as gatekeepers, encouraging the publication of good and original work and filtering out the less interesting information, the poor science and the unoriginal work that is submitted. However, as the paper will discuss this is not always straightforward as we also depend on reviewers to impartially review papers for us and they do not always agree with each other. I also believe that we have a role in encouraging young and new talent to publish their work and also to encourage work from emerging countries, particularly those who are non-English speaking who are at a disadvantage in getting their work published.

To do this job efficiently and fairly we usually work with international colleagues as an editorial team and an international advisory board. We need to take account of the ethics of publication in terms of ensuring that work published is the author's own work, not plagiarised, work of all the named authors and ethical in terms of the subjects of the research. Emerging issues are often politically controversial within our field, for example the emergence of harm reduction 25 years ago and the current debate of the reawakening of the recovery movement.

Key words

Peer reviewed process; plagiarism; open access journal; international advisory board; ethics of publishing; politics of publishing; impact factor.

Introduction

This paper will discuss the role of the journal editor in publishing peer reviewed scientific papers. Most, if not all of the readers of this book will have published scientific papers based on their research, opinion pieces based on controversies in their fields, review articles based on a specialist corner of their field or even letters to learned journals. These publications remain very important for the individual, their reputation, the reflection of their abilities when applying for jobs, etc.

For the field, peer reviewed scientific papers are a crucial part of any academic subject. Lafollette (1992) defined a journal as "a periodical that an identifiable intellectual community regards as a primary channel of communication of knowledge in a field and as one of the arbiters of the authenticity or legitimacy of that knowledge". So a journal:

- Provides a forum for communication among scientists.
- Sets intellectual standards in a field.
- Sets the agenda of what to study.
- Provides an institutional memory of a field.
- Brings information to the public.
- Certifies that the author's work is authentic.
- Can advance the author's career.

It is therefore the lifeblood of our and all other scientific communities. But most of us will know the frustrations of being authors, trying to get papers published, being refused publication and trying to convince editors of the value of our work. There are more than 80 journals in existence just on the subject of addictions, drugs, alcohol, etc. Thousands of papers are published every year, but also of course thousands are also turned down. The difficulty of keeping updated in our field would be almost impossible were it not for modern search engines that have revolutionised scientific research in the past 30 years. Then, in order to search for papers on a particular subject one had to go to printed volumes of abstracts and search through these volumes and then for any journals not held in that library, requests had to be made to a central library for a copy of the needed paper.

This has been further complicated by the proliferation of journals over the past 45 years. Until the mid-1960s there were about 10 journals published internationally on the various subjects of addictions, in English and other languages. There are now more than 80 journals published across the world, meaning a huge number of papers being available to researchers which, without the use of electronic search engines, would make it almost impossible to identify and access papers needed for research.

The future of academic publishing is very much in a process of change because of the process of electronic publishing. Twenty years ago papers were submitted via the postal services, papers were sent out to reviewers by mail and all the consequent correspondence was undertaken in a similar way. Papers are now generally submitted electronically, forwarded to reviewers in the same way and all the corrections etc are similarly handled. This has led to a greater efficiency in handling manuscripts and should have led to a faster turnaround of decisions on accepting or rejecting of papers although the human factor of the efficiency of the reviewer is still probably the one factor that influences the speed of decision making.

In addition to this journals are published on line as well as in print copy and the on line version usually is published earlier than the print version. Some journals are now only published on line and may be available on subscription or as open access journals. Being published on line means that papers can be purchased on line buying just one paper rather than subscribing to a journal and selling papers in this way is a lucrative source of income for the publisher and gives a wider access to the potential reader. Journals usually publish the abstract of papers that can be accessed free of charge. There are some people who think that the future of publishing paper copies of journals has a limited life and that in future learned articles will only be published on line.

Peer reviewed journals generally do not charge authors for publication. The journal may be owned by the publisher, or by a scientific society on behalf of the members. The editor is often not paid, the advisory committee are not paid and the reviewers are not paid. This means a relatively cheap cost for the publishers who do not have to pay for copy or the work in handling manuscripts. The income is generated by subscriptions either to individuals or institutions (or in the case of scientific societies from membership fees) but also increasingly from articles sold individually on line.

Open Access Journals

Open access journals are published on line and do not charge subscriptions for the journal. This means that the articles in the journal are available to anyone free of charge. The "openness" also refers to the fact that provided the article is cited there is a freedom to re-use the material as long as it is not for commercial gain giving the user the right to download articles and re-use tables and figures without needing to obtain permission from the copyright holder (libre open access) (Sutton, 2010). The open access journals that are published by professional publishing houses or by independent publishers usually charge a publication/article processing charge to cover costs of publication. As Sutton points out that although they were regarded with scepticism initially, a number of high profile publishers have now launched open access journals, including Springer, The Oxford University Press, the BMJ group (British Medical Journal) and Nature. Open access journals are also achieving good results in terms of impact factors with five open access journal being first in their fields and many more ranked as second or third (Sutton, 2010).

Sutton describes three routes for the open access journal:

1. Authors can choose to submit their work in full open access journals and for this the author will expect to pay a fee.
2. To use one of the open choice programmes offered by most established publishers. In this case the author chooses to have their article libre open access, within a journal that otherwise are subject to license and subscription arrangements.
3. A third route, "the green route" is to publish the paper in an institutional or subject archive or repository. Librarians can help in depositing the paper in the appropriate archive.

Sutton (2010) mentions the scepticism that greeted some of the early open access journals but as she points out the quality of many has now been accepted and validated.

However, Davis (2009) tested the system by submitting a paper to Bentham Publishers who had spammed Davis with submission requests and invitations to join the editorial board. Using SCIgen, which is software that generates grammatically correct but "context free" content (ie nonsense), Davis produced a paper that was complete with figures, tables and references but was in fact entirely nonsensical. He submitted the paper to a journal *The Open Information Science Journal*, which is a journal that claims to peer review papers using two fictitious author names from a fictitious institution, The Center for Research in Applied Phrenology (CRAP). The paper was acknowledged and 4 months later it was accepted "after a peer reviewing process" and requesting the authors to submit a fee schedule and pay a fee of $800 to a PO box in the United Arab Emirates. Davis subsequently retracted the article claiming that some errors had been discovered. While it should be recognised that this is an unusual example of what would appear to be an organisation that claimed to be peer reviewing papers (which it clearly had not), it is a lesson for authors to be careful and to ensure that they investigate the journal's editorial board and policy. If a paper has been peer reviewed it will then supply the reviews, which in this case was not done. If an author is going to part with what is quite a large sum of money to get the paper published they need to be careful as to the integrity of the journal.

Role of journal editor

Editors are usually offered the job of editor either because they have played a more minor role in the journal previously or because the post has been advertised. Often the editor has had little or no training and therefore has to learn on the job. The editor is then in an important role for the prestige and future of the journal and at the same time has to act as a "gatekeeper" for the scientific role of the journal. Our role is to publish good and original work and to filter out the less interesting information, the poor science and the unoriginal work.

Papers come into the journal (most journals now only accept papers on line) and are entered onto the database, many journals now use a fully computerised system. The editor will look at the paper and make a decision as to whether it should go out to review (we do not wish to waste reviewers time with poor work) and will choose 2 or 3 reviewers whose experience and interests would reveal them to be suitable to review the paper.

The reviewers will review the paper, make comments on the paper and recommend acceptance, acceptance with minor amendments or major amendments or rejection. The editor will review these comments and then make a decision on whether to accept the paper and under what conditions. Papers are rarely accepted without some recommendation. It is hoped that reviewers will broadly agree on the outcome for the paper but on some occasions there is disagreement and in the most extreme cases the reviews will be diametrically opposed with one review being "accept" and the other review being "reject". On these occasions the editor must make a decision about the outcome for the paper and will usually request a third review. Reviewers give their services free and are usually conscientious and efficient. We choose reviewers who have knowledge of the subject of the paper but occasionally we receive reviews that are inadequate, which make a recommendation but with little or no comment. This is unfair to the author of the paper who needs adequate feedback in order to improve the paper. We also ask authors whether they have a preferred reviewer or a non-preferred reviewer. Where a reviewer is suggested this can be helpful but quite frequently the preferred reviewer declines. What is interesting is that reviewers recommended by the author do not seem to give any preferential review to the authors.

We also work with an International Advisory Board made up of experts from throughout the world who will represent the journal and also act as reviewers. This is an important role, especially if we wish to be seen as international and having representatives across the world gives us access to areas not easily covered. We also have Associate Editors for the regions, North America, Europe, Australasia and sub-Saharan Africa. Their role is to represent us in their region, encourage submissions and handle some of the papers from their region.

So this in theory is how the journal works and how your paper will be handled when submitted. But…

How do we work?

The problems with running a journal are that despite a smooth plan for the throughput of papers and a very efficient electronic system for handling the papers there are still problems. For example when you are sent a paper for which there are no precedents in terms of subject, you cannot rely on your database of reviewers. Sometimes you may make approximations and at other times you cannot find anyone to review the paper. Even with mainstream subjects you might find a string of people who decline to review the paper which means that by the time you have contacted them and they have declined, contacted further people who decline etc you may have had the paper for 2 months without finding a suitable reviewer. This is unfair on the author who clearly wants their work to be reviewed as soon as possible.

We then have the problem of uneven reviews. We hope to have two reviews that roughly agree on whether we should accept the paper or not and yet occasionally we may have one expert who says reject the paper and one who says accept, both of whom are experts and who have considered the paper carefully. You then have to send it out for further reviews or make the editorial decision to publish or not. Has one reviewer taken a dislike to the author, as has happened, and despite the fact that these papers are reviewed blind it is often possible to work out who the author is. Has one of the reviewers misunderstood the paper? As a submitting author I have felt this sometimes to be the situation and if this happens I think it is appropriate to ask the editor to reconsider after examining your arguments.

The reviewing of submitted papers is the crucial centre of the publishing of academic papers. This is where the quality of papers is tested and the integrity of both the author and the journal rest on the decision that is made. What is important to note is that despite the huge increase in the number of journals published there are still more papers submitted than there is space for them to be published. Journals that are the most difficult to get a paper published in might have a rejection rate of over 80%. The paper might be quite suitable for publication but because it is competing with other papers it might not be deemed to be of sufficient quality or interest to be included. This means that if the paper is rejected but is still sound in methodology etc., it is worth submitting it elsewhere where it may well be accepted.

Ethics of publishing

There are a number of ethical issues that must be considered in relation to papers received. Although we expect academics to behave in an honest and ethical way, this is not always the case. Babor and McGovern (2008) list what they call "The seven deadly sins of publishing", which are as follows:

- Carelessness, for example citation bias that will produce a paper weighted in a specific cause and not objective by taking into account all the evidence.

- Redundant publication where some tables or literature is reported without noting the prior source. This can lead to copyright infringement.
- Unfair authorship credit where authors who have done the work are not included in the authorship credits and some authors (e.g. supervisors, heads of department) are included even though they have contributed nothing to the paper. It is good practice to ask for a declaration of who has done what on the paper.
- Undeclared conflict of interest, for example, where sources of funding are not declared. This is particularly true of the alcohol, tobacco and pharmaceutical industries. It is also useful to note that conflict of interest can apply to reviewers as well as authors, for example, if they are in the same department or have already reviewed the paper for another journal.
- Human or animal subject violations, where ethical approval has not been sought. This is stricter now than previously and one can think of famous experiments in the past where ethical approval was not sought or anticipated.
- Plagiarism where work of others is reproduced as one's own without citation. This can be poor referencing at one end of the scale or wholesale copying of work at the other. In the vast amount of information now being reproduced this is often difficult to police especially when it may be foreign language work that is copied.
- Scientific fraud where results of work are fabricated, data is falsified or there is misappropriation of others' work or plans given in confidence.

The difficulty we have as editors is to identify any of the above. There is a reliance on the honesty and integrity of the academic community and in the vast majority of people this is the case. For those few, detection may be difficult and may rely on sharp-eyed editors, reviewers or readers. In some cases, such as a lack of proper citation, this may be the due to inexperience or sloppy work but in the case of scientific fraud or plagiarism this is usually deliberate. It is however important that we do try to root out these cases of misappropriate submission in order to maintain the integrity of our field.

Politics of publishing

The politics of journal publishing are curious. As editors we have editorial freedom to publish what we think is appropriate subject to libel laws! However, the journal is owned by a publisher or a learned society and we must be aware that if we publish material damaging to them or against their principles this may cause us problems. One of the interesting things that happens over time is the way in which different topics or methodologies become popular. A few years ago it was very difficult to get work based on qualitative methods published in the addiction field. Whether this was because reviewers and editors did not understand the methodology or because it was felt that "it was not proper science" with statistics etc., is hard to know. My view has always been that qualitative methodology is important to our field because it helps us to understand some of the finer details of our subject that may be missed in quantitative studies. For example, one of my fields of research is injecting and without detailed qualitative discussions with injectors we would never have understood some of the minutiae and beliefs about injecting. The publication of qualitative studies is much more common and acceptable in most journals.

In terms of topics these again become popular. When harm reduction became a practical intervention with drug users in the early 1980s it was initially probably too avant-garde for many journals. This is now mainstream and quite acceptable and we talk about harm reduction for alcohol and tobacco. One of the themes that is now becoming popular in the drug field is the issue of long-term methadone maintenance versus recovery and the regaining of abstinence. A few years ago this would have seemed to be contrary to the politics and policies of harm reduction but in the UK at least it is becoming an important issue in the field and attracts some interesting papers. This is likely to remain a controversial topic for a while but what we need to inform the debate is high quality papers on the subject.

Other issues that are more complicated are when an author has a particular view and has great animosity to any suggestions of criticism. Is this a question of an author being ahead of the field or being way out of touch with the rest of the field? It is the sort of issue editors sometimes need to consider and act carefully.

Impact Factors

Impact factors are a method that is used to measure the quality of the journal. This has become increasingly important as many academic institutions expect and demand that their academic staff publish in high quality journals with high impact factors. The organisation that assigns impact factors is Thompson Reuters via the Institute for Scientific Information (ISI). Journals have to apply to ISI to be included and acceptance is not automatic. Impact factors are published each year for all journals that are indexed in Thompson Reuters *Journal Citation Reports.*

The impact factors of a journal is calculated by an average number of citations received per paper published in that journal for the two preceding years. So for example, the impact factor for a journal for 2011would be calculated as follows:

1. The number of times articles that were published in 2009 and 2010 were cited in articles in indexed journals during 2011.
2. The total number of citable items (articles, reviews, proceedings and notes) published by the journal in 2009 and 2010.
3. The impact factor is then calculated by dividing the first figure by the second figure.

One of the duties of the editor is to try to improve the journal's impact factor and thus the desirability of being published in it. This is sometimes circular because people will want to publish in a high impact journal but in order to get a high impact factor there needs to be papers of high quality and high importance. There are other methods where a journal can improve its impact factor such as by publishing more review articles that tend to be cited more frequently than research papers. It is also important to ensure that all papers cited in an article are referenced, which sometimes is not the case.

Other methods have been used with less honest intent such as by encouraging authors to cite papers in your own journal, and by authors frequently self-citing their articles in the same journal. It is also true that pure science and medical journals tend to have higher impact factors; often because they have many more papers cited and often have many more authors, which tends to produce higher impact factors. So for example, a number of science and medical journals have an impact factor of above 30 whereas the journal with the highest impact factor in the addiction field has an impact factor of less than 5.

There are a number of critics of the system of impact factors that exclude journals not included in ISI and also journals not published in the English language and some suggestions that impact factor is not necessarily the same as the quality of the article. Because of the importance that academic departments place on impact factors this means that we cannot ignore them, we must try to improve our impact factors or prospective authors will not submit their paper to the journal.

Editorials

One of the privileges of being an editor is to write editorials. Whereas one needs to be objective and scrupulously fair in handling other people's papers one can use the editorial as an opportunity to air opinions, to test ideas and to be outspoken on certain issues. For example I have used the editorial as a platform to criticise the issue of human rights of drug users especially in the light of the Human Rights Act, the war on drug users in Thailand in the early 1990s and to draw attention to good work being done in developing countries. We have also published editorials by others criticising the use of the death penalty in other countries for possession of drugs, etc.

We have to remember when writing an editorial it is not the same as writing for a newspaper for which news needs to be current and because of the way they work news can be published the day after it happens. With journals there is a longer period of time between writing an editorial and the appearance of the printed version of maybe a few weeks so that it is pointless in writing about subjects that are very current and have a short shelf life.

Conclusions

The editor therefore has a role in maintaining fairness and trying to develop and produce a quality product in terms of the journal he/she is editing. We do act as gatekeepers for the scientific information that becomes available to the scientific community, a role which is important but for which there is very little reward other than the production of a successful journal.

One final role I consider we have is to encourage young researchers to publish their work especially when they are from a developing country where resources are few. Often very important work is coming from these countries without the opportunity to publish. In some parts of the developing world there is a lack of availability to the internet to research information or where electricity is intermittent and therefore authors are under a huge disadvantage in terms of producing quality articles. To this end I will offer advice to young researchers about the preparation of their manuscripts and help with language editing in order to bring the paper up to publishable standard.

References

Babor, TF & McGovern, T (2008). Dante's inferno: seven deadly sins in scientific publishing and how to avoid them, chapter 11 in Babor, TF, Stenius, K, Savva, S & O'Reilly, J (2008) *Publishing Addiction Science, A Guide for the Perplexed,* ISAJE, London.

Davis, P (2009). "Open Access Publisher Accepts Nonsense Manuscript for Dollars" *The Scholarly Kitchen* (10 June, 2009) http://scholarlykitchen.sspnet.org/2009/06/10/nonsense-for-dollars/ accessed on 7th. October 2011.

Lafollette, MC (1992*). Stealing into print: fraud, plagiarism and misconduct in scientific publishing,* University of California Press, Berkeley, CA. quoted in Babor, T and Stenius, K Chapter 1 A guide for the perplexed in Babor, TF, Stenius, K, Savva, S & O'Reilly, J (2008) *Publishing Addiction Science, A Guide for the Perplexed,* ISAJE, London.

Sutton, C (2010). The Rationale, Role and Working Methods of Open Access Publishing, *ISAJE newsletter,* July 2010.

Conclusions

Concluding remarks of 13th International Symposium on Substance Abuse Treatment

Conrad Vilanou

Department of Theory and History of Education
University of Barcelona, Spain

cvilanou@ub.edu

Right from the start, we need to recognise the distance that always exists between what we say and what is written, either before or afterwards. Words fly, as the classics said. Therefore, the following summary, as a closing essay or chronicle of the symposium, has been prepared based on the notes that were taken during the various sessions of the 13th International Symposium on Substance Abuse Treatment, in other words, thanks to the talks given by each of the speakers who, altogether and thanks to their enthusiasm, managed to convey the results of their research and reflections to the public. However, we have also taken into consideration the definitive texts that were prepared by the various speakers and that give meaning to this book, which is like a series of considerably improved and extended minutes of that event. So, we move between the spoken word and the written word, and we have tried to prepare a synthesis which, in as far as possible, captures the contents explained in this book through its different chapters. Not forgetting the passion that each of the speakers gave to their talk which, on most of the occasions, conveyed to us, together with the scientific considerations explained, a high sense of professional, intellectual and social commitment.

Nor should we forget that whilst the spoken word, in keeping with the poetic theory that defends the strength of the living word, transmits energy and passion, the logos of the scientific word, of the written word, are fairer and more precise. Therefore, in this summary, we have tried to capture both aspects, in other words, the nucleus of the spoken expression and the scientific coherence of the written texts. At the risk of being wrong, we believe that the tree of life cannot be separated from the tree of science, even more so when the object of the Symposium dealt with matters concerning one of today's most notable problems: the dependencies that human beings have on diverse substances, some of which are as old as alcohol and tobacco and others that have appeared more recently in human history, such as designer drugs. All of them are equally damaging for one's health, preventing people, as the academics of the 18th century intended, from attaining the adult age of the human being that requires, as a priority, not becoming dependent on any type of substance, or more particularly, drug dependency, whether or not there is tolerance towards the product in question (alcohol, tobacco, psychotropic drugs and drugs in general).

On the other hand, we believe that the so-called scientific asepsis is often a pure illusion as no author ever speaks without knowledge, but with the vision of his own personal career, his convictions, his scientific assumptions and, above all, with a stated desire to contribute towards solving the problems that affect the human being. This is why the modern dream (Cartesian and positivist) of any cold, abstract reason is a desire that will be difficult to achieve. So much so that the winds of Romanticism (with Goethe at the head of them) stated the existence of an overall conception of life, through a *nexus organicus* that linked the somatic, psychic and spiritual layers of the human being into an integral whole that possessed a great vital energy, which certain trends of thought –such as Bergson's philosophy– also made theirs. In recent times, on highlighting the emotional side of human life, we have tried to correct, as the Portuguese professor António Damasio stated some years ago, the "Descartes' error" which, in essence, was none other than that of dividing the human being in to reason and feeling, giving priority to reason, up to the point of identifying man as a *cogitans* being, avoiding the fact that he is also an *amans* being. Therefore, science and life, scientific precision and passion, methodological rigour and feelings, scientific data and personal emotions do not constitute, on most occasions, two isolated vessels but establish bridges of links and connections allowing us to state that they constitute a single reality in which things intermingle and relate to each other.

The emergent paradigms of complexity, whose origin can be found in systematic and cybernetic thoughts that depend on principles such as homeostasis, confirm the need to deal with questions and controversy through an overall vision that is removed from the unilateral temptation to offer simple answers, through the determinist logic of cause and effect. Beyond the laws that science discovers, we should not forget –when the subject of this study is mankind– the cultural and social aspects that a given historic-social frame always require. The data provided by science, above all experimental science, should be read and interpreted in the light of these historic-social links that determine human reality at all times and in all places. For example, it is well-known that Spain has been a country with high levels of alcohol consumption and that, in recent times, changes are taking place in the social uses of alcohol among young people. In fact, the traditional dichotomy between being a teetotaller or an alcoholic no longer serve to explain the social reality in which there are many occasional drinkers, particularly at the weekend. It has even been said that there are social drinkers who, if in the past were found in bars and taverns, now use collective festivals (for example, binge drinking in the streets) to get together in public places and drink large amounts of alcoholic beverages in a group. In the end, science, like life, cannot be divided into isolated, watertight compartments, but a joint vision is needed, which is even more convenient when trying to summarise, as we are doing here.

In addition, the philosophy of science reveals that today's scientists are aware that each of them speaks, and therefore researches, from a given scientific position, in other words from specific epistemological and methodological areas and, therefore, from a specific paradigm, as T. S. Kuhn stated. On the other hand, and independently of the theoretical framework and the paradigmatic option, a subject or matter is studied because there is a desire to solve a problem or, at least, to contribute to finding solutions that are not always easy. Without scorning interests of all kinds (political, economic, social, etc.) that are found behind any type of research, the fact is, as hermeneutics have confirmed, that the researcher's question presumes or advances a given response that will finally be corroborated or rejected.

In keeping with this argument of hermeneutic bias, we should be well aware that any interpretive attempt, and even more so if it is conclusive, is outlined from the vital situation position, or world view, that the author shares. Although the person writing is not directly related to the world of drug addiction, as Terencio said, nothing human is foreign to him. Therefore, this chronicler, with his pedagogical training and inscribed in the thought of spiritual sciences, tries to account in the following paragraphs what the *13th International Symposium on Substance Abuse Treatment* has meant, taking aspects and valuations even further than the particular content of each of the speeches that led to the book you are now holding. In fact, our intention does not stem so much from placing one's attention on the summary of each of the contributions, as from trying to scrutinise the categories that can be made out from the various chapters of which this book consists.

In this sense, and as a priority, it should be pointed out that most of the contributions come from Europe, although it is true that there are others –for example from Australia– while yet others give the symposium a western and perhaps Eurocentric slant on the matter. Unfortunately, the subject of drug dependency affects other countries and geographical areas, making up a global phenomenon in which the international organisations need to intervene, as stated by Xavier Fernández-Pons in his intervention. Therefore, the subject of drug addiction is reaching an increasingly planetary scale, even though the origin of the studies is limited to the countries that have achieved a certain level of welfare state, which have seen how their possibilities to act in view of the cutbacks derived from the latest economic crisis have cut off their possibilities. It should not be forgotten –and those of us who work in the world of education know this– that there is no better policy in the drug addiction area than prevention, above all if we take into account the early age at which many children begin in this world, starting with solvents, the use of which has proliferated among the most socially vulnerable populations. These children, as Núria Empez has shown, have emigrated alone, without their families and are found at risk of social exclusion, wandering the streets of the large cities in the hope that re-education associations take care of them.

From a professional point of view, the great diversity of the occupations of the various speakers should be pointed out: doctors, psychologists, pedagogues, therapists, lawyers, etc.). There is no doubt that this wealth of points of view enriched the meeting that thus took on an unmistakably interdisciplinary dimension, dealing with the treatment of drug addiction in a general, overall way. Each of the speeches can be seen as a particular point of view, a specific, determined part of this large puzzle under construction –always open to novelties– which is the regionalised attention given to drug addicts. This is a new phenomenon in the history of our culture as neither cigarettes nor alcohol were considered to be drugs until recently. In addition, the generalisation of the abuse of certain drugs, such as opium and morphine, did not become large scale until the end of the 19th century. Obviously, the two World Wars that took place during the first half of the 20th century made it easier for substances to circulate which, from a pharmacological point of view, aimed to attenuate the pain of the young people who were sometimes badly wounded, and who saw many of their companions die. Pain, as well as the wish to evade, was the trigger for many young people to enter the circuit of drug dependency which, after the Second World War, affected a generation of youths which, as correctly stated by Stefan Zweig, broke their links with yesterday's world.

Therefore, the history of Western culture during the second half of the 20th century facilitated the consumption of these substances, some of them, like tobacco and alcohol, because they were linked to the North American lifestyle which, through cinema and television, reached all young people. The winds that followed the youth freedom movements that took place in around 1968 did the rest, offering some of these substances as an opportunity for the freedom of young people tired of war and violence. The Vietnam War, which was a recent drama for North American soldiers and the culminating point in the midst of the Cold War, provided, if possible, an even greater proliferation of the use of these substances, which ended up reaching every corner of the world. Therefore, we are looking at an emergent phenomenon which, unfortunately, is spreading throughout the world, not only among mature people but also among younger people, generating the phenomenon of polyconsumption, which is a generalised reality today. In any case, considered as a whole, all the contributions dealt with the matter of health, looked at from different points of view, in such a way that the final horizon is always the same, the improvement of the psychophysical state of drug addicts.

Therefore, we are looking at a long-term concern in a history or narration that takes care of the health of human beings, something that has been inherent in humans since the origins of humanity and, most particularly, since the appearance of science. It should be added that this concern for the health of human beings covers all its aspects, not just the physical ones but also the psychic ones, because health constitutes a psycho-bio-social unit, as has been recognised by the most prestigious authors. Here, we should remember the doctor and psychologist Dr. Emilio Mira y López (1896-1964) who, in 1933, occupied the first Chair in Psychiatry at the University of Barcelona. If Juvenal coined the saying *mens sana in corpore sano* in his Satire 10, Baron Pierre de Coubertin, who brought back the Olympic Games in 1896, reformulated it with the expression *mens fervida in corpore lacertoso,* in other words a burning spirit in a muscular body. Emilio Mira insisted on the need to bring together in a single body the psyche and, also, society, establishing the formula of *mens sana in societate sana,* which affirms that the individual cannot be healthy in a sick society. Based on this premise, and in order to overcome any dualist temptation that limits human health to a psychophysical question, Emilio Mira, who can be found in all the manuals on the history of psychology, considered that somatic therapy (therapy of the body) should act in harmony with psychotherapy (therapy of the mind), without forgetting the social aspects in order to achieve health, as understood from a triple point of view: physical, psychic and social. Treating the body or the mind separately does not take us anywhere, as the human individual requires an integral, integrating treatment, through the overlapping of all the resources available, whether psychological methods, biochemical applications or social means. To do this, Dr. Mira insisted on the need to set up the bases of psychosomatic medicine, which he called integral or eubiatric medicine, (from the Greek *eu,* well-being and *bios,* life) This integral (eubiatric) medicine offers an overall, synthetic vision of the human being, which hopes to join and combine the Socratic and Hippocratic tradition, aims to move away from the dualisms that since Plato's times have not only split human knowledge but also the anthropology of man, something that the Cartesian philosopher emphasised by consecrating the separation between body and soul.

In fact, this historic genealogy, this archaeology in the terrain of rehabilitation has not been unnoticed by the speakers at the Symposium. Here we should mention the contribution by Rowdy Yates who presented, in great detail, the long path that has been developed to consolidate rehabilitation in a historic, far-reaching process. In fact, there is a long tradition in the rehabilitation area, the roots of which can be found in the 19th century, although the first tests date back to the 18th century, with the first associations for alcoholics. In an approach that brings to mind Dr. Emilio Mira's philosophy, Rowdy Yates opts for a bio-psycho-social model of intervention, therefore being in favour of an overall treatment that places a parenthesis on the use of methadone, though it is true that although it is momentarily successful, in his opinion, it does not solve the problem. Therefore we should tend towards a full recovery that is long-lasting and that takes into account the overall life of the person.

Despite the fact that most authors coincide in their desire to improve the situation of drug addicts, and that nobody denies the need to work in collaboration with the various agents involved, the fact is that one of the constant features that has arisen with greatest emphasis throughout the symposium has been the need to find evidence, with some people adding —and here we should quote Marica Ferri— the convenience that it should be "scientific". Therefore, one of the driving forces of this meeting is to find some scientific evidence that allows us to advance in the prevention and treatment of drug addiction. Naturally, this statement leads us to an exercise of interpretive hermeneutics and even epistemological reflection. What do we understand by evidence? This question is not trivial or gratuitous, even today, when we have attended, in the postmodern cultural context, an epistemological anarchism that has suspended the criteria of truth that have been valid since modernity, when an experimental protocol was required that reminded us that evidence should be clear and distinct (Descartes) or experimentally protocolised

(Claude Bernard). However, when dealing with human beings, evidence is never as exact as we would like it to be, as on occasions the informers –as often happens in the case of women– do not dare to state all their feelings, fears and troubles. The tree –the tree of life– cannot always be limited to the exact limits of the tree of science, with its protocols, laboratories and experiments, although it is no less true that the research group work directed by Ana Adan on chronobiology and addiction responds perfectly to these demands, typical of a piece of work carried out in a way that is precise and exact, from an objective point of view. In addition, we thus obtain experimentally verified data, concluding, for example, with regard to the circadian rhythms that abstinence improves sleep, while people who have an evening lifestyle are more given to consuming drugs.

With all this, and together with empirical proof, there were also some contributions that were notable due to their experiential scope, in other words, the experiences that they contribute and transmit. An experience is not the same as an experiment. An experience responds to qualitative criteria that concern the etymological sense of the word *sapere,* which is none other than to taste. While experiences are tasted and savoured, experiments respond to well-argued work schemes designed with hypotheses, experimental tests and, finally, relevant conclusions. Throughout these sessions, we have also seen contributions such as that of Georges Van Der Straten who, for thirty-five years, has travelled all over Europe getting to know different therapeutic communities. Here the trip, the contact with other people with similar concerns, contrast, comparison, loan and dialogue become a rich source of "evidence", although for some people they would not be strictly scientific, taking into account their personal and subjective nature. In this postmodern period, Georges has become a true nomad, crossing countries and borders in search of novelties and suggestions which, to him, are authentic evidence. Here, the lifeworld *(Lebenswelt)* is tinged with experiences and therefore evidence. This is not just a simple play on words but a genuinely tangible reality: the objectivity of scientific evidence cannot avoid the importance of subjective experience. It is also clear that scientific evidence –the true aspiration of any rigorous piece of work– depends on many variables that are, at times, personal and subjective. Drawing up questionnaires is not something gratuitous or fashionable, as we were told by Vera Segraeus, the results vary depending on the question asked. In *Sein und Zeit* (1927) Martin Heidegger insisted on this by pointing out that the question anticipates the answer, meaning that the success or failure of a programme or action may vary depending on the question marks that are established in a given question.

Perhaps we can identify the evidence in the sense that Marica Ferri indicated, which is none other than good practices, which involves the additional difficulty of having to immediately afterwards define what we understand by "best practice". It could be stated that good practices acquire this condition through the consensus of a determined scientific community, by positively valuing their successes and results. In the final instance, it is a line of demarcation of a practical, utilitarian nature that involves some provisional part to it, from the moment that this criterion of "best practice" can be reviewed, but which, meanwhile, offers the possibility of being transferred to other places. Here we should emphasise the importance of networking in order to communicate advances and deteriorations, with the aim of making everything that guarantees the success of a "best practice" available to interested parties. At the end of the day, the idea of "best practice" is defined according to its capacity to optimise a given reality, indicating the path to follow and imitate. Any evidence will be positive and accepted when it serves, as a best practice, to optimise resources and results in our actions. In fact more than evidence (facts), we have indications (signs) that show us where we should be going, gradually advancing and trying out new strategies in a prudent way.

Having analysed the various contributions from an overall point of view, the existence of some tensions has been detected –a kind of antinomy or opposition– that emerged more than once during the discussions of the Symposium, the presence of which was also detected when reading the various chapters that comprise this book. Being able to determine these tensions is important to be able to offer solutions that try to get away from the polarisation of the extremes that preside over these tensions. Therefore, while some contributions supplied data that was obtained objectively through well-designed protocols, other speeches recurred to the use of open interviews or to the use of observational methodologies. Therefore, we are moving between diverse tensions that, openly or latently, have presided over the explanations given, as well as the later discussions. While some people refer to patients, others talk about clients or users. While some people comment on the importance of pharmacology in treatment processes, others insist on the relevance of community work, in particular therapeutic communities, and of the benefits derived from mutual help in order to obtain best results. If some people appealed to the work of outpatients, others gave priority to collectives, whether families or communities, in particular, the therapeutic communities that are widespread in numerous countries, which encourages us to make a comparative reflection such as the one proposed by Ilse Goethals when contrasting European and American ones, showing that, in general terms, there are few variations.

Obviously, life in these communities is not free from danger, from the moment at which a long stay can generate the appearance of charismatic leaders. In addition, life in these communities can favour a lack of internal democracy, as well as some imperviousness to the relationship between action and research, not forgetting that they can take on the features of a more or less sectarian closed group. However, apart from these considerations, diverse speakers referred to this aspect, there is the danger that the current worldwide economic situation, not just at a standstill but going backwards in several countries, constitutes a serious danger for supporting actions in favour of the rehabilitation of drug addicts, a situation that affects the Mediterranean countries very seriously, as stated by Charalampos Poulopoulos when referring to Greece.

If some specialists are given to the use of drugs to look for immediate success, lengthening the time between relapses, others opt for long-term solutions in order to ensure the success of the treatment, avoiding relapses and, what is even more important, giving meaning to the life of the people who are following treatment. In the same way, there is some interest in finding definitive therapies while other people opt for a medical-based treatment that limits their objectives to improve quality of life. While some comment on the vulnerability of certain collectives, such as women who are more inclined to depression, other contributions stated the difficulty of the visibility of certain pathologies, particularly with regard to men. The gender variability therefore becomes an aspect to be taken into account in research, as Marta Torrens explained in her speech. At the end of the day, everything would seem to indicate that women are more given to depression than men and therefore, to the use of psychotropic drugs (tranquillisers, sleeping pills, etc.), making them more vulnerable to drug addiction, thus increasing the risk factor. Karen Briggs also took into account this gender variable on studying the treatment process of several mothers in diverse English therapeutic communities. Her conclusion seems to show that children have a positive influence on the recovery of mothers.

In the same way, we detected tension between those who opted for prevention and those who insist on the need for intervention. Some contributions were limited to specific geographical areas, responding to local logic, while others dealt with a more global context of a national character. In the same way, we could see that while some people opted for disseminating the advances and knowledge through portals on the Internet, there are others who emphasise limited circulation through specialist publications. In any case, we know that access to these specialist publications –classified by scientific organisations– is not easy, generating ethical questions that were analysed by Richard Pates as an editor. On the one hand, he stated the existence of a notorious inflation of the information in view of the high number of existing specialist magazines (80 alone in English). In fact, the scientific knowledge that is created around the matter we are dealing with is growing exponentially, although today we have search engines that help things. On the other hand, a series of relations are set up between the author, editor and reviewer that respond to logic that requires an ethical reflection, as the same filters are not always applied to all the articles that are reviewed. Whatever, the difficulties of access by authors to magazines with impact are serious, meaning that a deontology is imposed that regulates the activity of the editor who, at the same time, is overwhelmed by the large number of originals he receives and a reduced number of specialists who can carry out this anonymous, rigorous arbitration free of charge, aside from wheeling and dealing and string-pulling.

It is not easy to find a happy medium that is more or less balanced, which offers responses to these tensions that preside over the work of people interested in the study and treatment of drug addicts, meaning that we can conclude that there are no magical or universal solutions, but that therapeutic treatments are not mutually exclusive but complimentary. In any case, the great tension that exists in the treatment of drug addicts and that also occurs in other therapeutic areas is the result of a position of a philosophical nature, of an attitude that is somewhat a priori that determines the action to be taken. In keeping with this, we detected two main ways or paths that, in one way or another, are found in most of the contributions included in this book. For didactic purposes, we will give these two positions two names, which are phonetically similar but that are clearly different in their meaning. Specifically, we are referring to the terms "methadone" and "metanoia". Those who are in favour of the first, look at the subject of treating drug addicts with a medical approach, not stating notable restrictions in the use of methadone, which they compare to dialysis or insulin. This is a medical attitude that wishes to mitigate pain and lengthen the life of drug addicts, who are thus considered to be chronically ill. On the other hand, those who are committed to "metanoia", as the etymology of the word suggests, are looking for a radical change of life, looking at the life of the drug addict in an overall way, in other words, not only the biological aspects but also the psychic and social ones.

Those who opt for the "methadone" method are aware that drug addictions, aetiologies apart, are diseases that must be treated with drugs that alleviate the life of the people affected, based on the fact that they should supply analgesics to attenuate the effects derived from the diseases that, over time, have become chronic. The second group, on the other hand, are interested in the meaning of life, giving their therapy is a kind of salvation pedagogy, the aim of achieving a conversion or metanoia in the lives of the individuals affected. If the first group is found in the parameters of pharmacology and therefore, in a medical line that seeks to cope with the drug addiction, the second group recur to a pedagogical method (orthopedagogical in the words of our Belgian colleagues headed by Eric Broekaert, which is rooted in therapeutic pedagogy or *Heilpädagogik*) in order to achieve a qualitative leap which, along the lines of Víctor Frankl, shows that man is a being in search of meaning. Therefore there are two therapeutic horizons that cannot be presented as opposed and antagonistic, despite the existing tension, but as complementary, although we know that their respective starting points, their "a priori" and assumptions are diametrically opposed.

It is obvious that our position, which is rather eclectic and conciliatory, wishes to go beyond reductionist dualisms that have done so much damage in the history of science and thought, seeking a third area that wishes to put an end to the antinomic, dialectic games that so often impoverish work and scientific reflection. It is true that we detected tensions. It is true that we have observed the existence of great tension between those who opt for a medical solution and those who recur to a more holistic treatment (or pedagogic, if you like) of a therapeutic nature. The first are driven by emergencies and the second by ideals. The first apply a practical and even pragmatic sense while the second follow and look for the meaning of life. Therefore, we find two world views that, although are opposing, cannot be considered to be exclusive.

In fact, these two focuses, paradigms or world views, which at the same time generate two very clear forms of action, can be reconciled through a point of balance, a medium term, if we act prudently, in the way proposed by Aristotelian philosophy. For this, we think that we should recur to the use of common sense, which is so traditional in Scottish philosophy, for example. In short, it is a question of claiming the use of some degree of tact, as was claimed by Herbart at the beginning of the 19th century in the pedagogical area, which should be able to guide the therapist's action at any time. In this Symposium we have seen that the treatment of drug addictions depends on the data given by scientific research, but we have also attended the presentation of works that confer a technical, even handcrafted, dimension to the intervention of therapists. Putting aside the modern dreams of another period in which the scientific dimension of any discipline was vindicated, forgetting its handcrafted and sapiential tradition, it would seem that the moment has come in the treatment of drug addicts to recover both aspects, in other words, that without getting around the precisions of research that is rigorously carried out, we should be aware of the need to deal with the qualitative, affective and handcrafted aspects that are inherent in any job that is based on human relations. In the same way that family doctors are increasingly taking on greater prominence, despite the advances in the various medical specialities, something similar is happening in the field of treating drug addicts. A synthetic vision is being imposed –or at least this is what this author concludes– so as not to scorn any of the contributions that are all valuable and positive that are found in the various chapters of this book, based on the fact that tact should guide the action of therapists who know that their work can always be optimised because, at the end of the day, it depends on them to find the right action for each occasion. Universal formulas serve for the formal sciences, of a logical-mathematical nature and for the theoretical suppositions or physical sciences, but not for disciplines in which the human being is the protagonists or, on occasions, only wants to survive but who, at other times, wishes to give his life a new meaning, which involves a radical change or metanoia. A difficult challenge, but at the end of the day, one that also gives meaning to the therapeutic work of everyone who faces this intricate world of drug addiction; an increasingly more global phenomenon against which we need to fight with high levels of hope and expectation.